Recent Advances in OPHTHALMOLOGY-17

Recent Advances in OPHTHALMOLOGY-17

Editor

Nitin Nema MS DNB
Professor
Department of Ophthalmology
Sri Aurobindo Medical College and
Postgraduate Institute of Medical Sciences
Indore, Madhya Pradesh, India

JAYPEE

JAYPEE BROTHERS MEDICAL PUBLISHERS
The Health Sciences Publisher
New Delhi | London

Jaypee Brothers Medical Publishers (P) Ltd

Headquarters
EMCA House, 23/23-B
Ansari Road, Daryaganj
New Delhi 110 002, India
Landline: +91-11-23272143, +91-11-23272703
+91-11-23282021, +91-11-23245672
e-mail: jaypee@jaypeebrothers.com

Corporate Office
4838/24, Ansari Road, Daryaganj
New Delhi 110 002, India
Phone: +91-11-43574357
Fax: +91-11-43574314
e-mail: jaypee@jaypeebrothers.com

Overseas Office
JP Medical Ltd.
83, Victoria Street, London
SW1H 0HW (UK)
Phone: +44-20 3170 8910
e-mail: info@jpmedpub.com

EU GPSR Authorised Representative
Logos Europe, 9 rue Nicolas Poussin
17000, La Rochelle, France
Phone: +33 (0) 6 67 93 73 78
e-mail: contact@logoseurope.eu

Website: www.jaypeebrothers.com
Website: www.jaypeedigital.com

Inquiries for bulk sales may be solicited at: jaypee@jaypeebrothers.com

Recent Advances in Ophthalmology-17

First Edition: **2025**

ISBN: 978-93-6616-723-7

Printed in India at Sterling Graphics Pvt. Ltd.

Dedication

In loving memory of my parents who still continue to inspire me

Contributors

Aafreen Bari
MD DNB FICO FAICO
Consultant
Department of Cornea, Cataract and Refractive Surgery Services
Dr Rajendra Prasad Centre for Ophthalmic Sciences
All India Institute of Medical Sciences
New Delhi, India

Abdullah S Al-Mujaini
MD FRCSC
Professor
Department of Ophthalmology
Muscat, Sultanate of Oman

Abha Gour
MBBS DO FSCEH
Senior Consultant, Clinician, Scientist
Department of Cornea and Anterior Segment
Eicher Centre of Stem Cell Research
Dr Shroffs Charity Eye Hospital
New Delhi, India

Abhipsa Sharma
MD DNB
Consultant
Department of Strabismus and Neuro-ophthalmology
Nimmagadda Prasad Children's Eye Care Centre
Child Sight Institute
LV Prasad Eye Institute
Visakhapatnam, Andhra Pradesh, India

Abhyuday Saxena
MBBS MS
Resident
Department of Ophthalmology
Regional Institute of Ophthalmology
Sitapur, Uttar Pradesh, India

Abinaya Valliappan
MBBS MS FMRF FICO
Consultant
Department of Pediatric Ophthalmology and Strabismus
Sankara Nethralaya
Chennai, Tamil Nadu, India

Aditya Maitray MS FRMF
Senior Consultant
Department of Vitreoretina
Aravind Eye Hospital
Chennai, Tamil Nadu, India

Akash Belenje
MS FLVPEI
Assistant Consultant (Vitreoretinal Services, Pediatric Retina)
Newborn Eye Health Alliance (NEHA)
Srimati Kanuri Santhamma Center for Vitreo Retinal Diseases
Anant Bajaj Retina Institute
Kallam Anji Reddy Campus
LV Prasad Eye Institute
Hyderabad, Telangana, India

Amol Bansal MBBS MS
Consultant
Department of Strabismus and Neuro-ophthalmology
Jasti V Ramanamma Children's Eye Care Centre, Child Sight Institute
LV Prasad Eye Institute
Hyderabad, Telangana, India

Anand Rajendran DNB FRCS
Head
Department of Vitreoretina
Aravind Eye Hospital
Chennai, Tamil Nadu, India

Anshukita MD FMRF
Consultant
Department of Uvea and Anterior Segment
Sankara Nethralaya
Chennai, Tamil Nadu, India

AR Anand PhD
Associate Professor and Incharge
Department of Microbiology
Sankara Nethralaya
Vision Research Foundation
Chennai, Tamil Nadu, India

Arnav Singh Saroya MS DNB
Fellow
Department of Cornea and
Refractive Surgery
Dr Agarwals Eye Hospital
Chennai, Tamil Nadu, India

Bhavik Panchal DNB FICO
Consultant
Department of Vitreoretina
LV Prasad Eye Institute
Visakhapatnam, Andhra Pradesh, India

Chetan Rao MS
Senior Consultant
Department of Vitreoretina
Bhagwan Mahavir Vitreoretinal Services
Medical Research Foundation
Sankara Nethralaya
Chennai, Tamil Nadu, India

Debolina Deb MBBS MS FVRS
Consultant
Department of Vitreoretina
Aravind Eye Hospital
Chennai, Tamil Nadu, India

Deeksha Thorat MBBS DNB
Clinical Fellow
Department of Cornea and
Anterior Segment
LV Prasad Eye Institute
Hyderabad, Telangana, India

Devendra Maheshwari MS
Consultant
Department of Glaucoma
Aravind Eye Hospital
Tirunelveli, Tamil Nadu, India

Dipankar Das
MBBS MS
Head
Department of Ocular Pathology
and Uvea
Senior Consultant
Ocular Pathology, Uveitis and
Neuro-ophthalmology Services
Sri Sankaradeva Nethralaya
Guwahati, Assam, India

Divyansh K Mishra
DO DNB FVR ICO (London) FAICO FGO PDMRF
Consultant
Vitreoretina and Ocular Oncology
Services
Sankara Eye Hospital
Bengaluru, Karnataka, India

Himanshu Garkoti MS DNB
Fellow
Department of Vitreoretina
and Uvea
Sri Sankaradeva Nethralaya
Guwahati, Assam, India

Inderjeet Kaur PhD
Senior Scientist
Brien Holden Eye Research Centre
LV Prasad Eye Institute
Hyderabad, Telangana, India

Jessica Basumatary MBBS MS
Fellow
Department of Medical Retina
and Uvea
Sri Sankaradeva Nethralaya
Guwahati, Assam, India

Jyotirmay Biswas
MS FMRF FNAMS FIC Path FAICO MNAsc FRCS
(Ed) FACS
Director
Department of Uveitis and
Ocular Pathology
Sankara Nethralaya,
Chennai, Tamil Nadu, India

Kiran Chandra Kedarisetti
MBBS MS
Consultant
Department of Vitreoretina
LV Prasad Eye Institute
Anant Bajaj Retina Institute
Hyderabad, Telangana, India

KS Siddharthan
MS DNB MNAMS FAICO
Medical Director and Senior Consultant
Department of Cornea, Cataract and Refractive Surgery
Eyemed Hospital and Cornea Research Foundation
Coimbatore, Tamil Nadu, India

L Dhanurekha
BSc MSc PhD
Senior Scientist
SNSC Clinical Microbiology Laboratory
Molecular Diagnostics Laboratory
Sankara Nethralaya
Medical Research Foundation
Chennai, Tamil Nadu, India

Lingam Gopal
MS DNBE MSc (Epidemiology)
Distinguished Senior Consultant
Department of Vitreoretina and Neuro-ophthalmology
Bhagwan Mahavir Vitreoretinal Services
Medical Research Foundation
Chennai, Tamil Nadu, India

Madhavi Ramanatha Pillai
DNB MNAMS
Consultant
Department of Glaucoma
Aravind Eye Hospital
Tirunelveli, Tamil Nadu, India

Mahesh P Shanmugam
MBBS DO FRCSEd PhD FAICO
Head
Vitreoretinal and Oncology Services
Sankara Eye Hospitals
Bengaluru, Karnataka, India

Mehak Vohra PhD
Post-doctoral Fellow
Department of Ophthalmology
Swamynathan Laboratory
Morsani College of Medicine
University of South Florida
Tampa, Florida, USA

Muralidhar Ramappa MD
Head
Cornea and Anterior Segment Services
LV Prasad Eye Institute
Hyderabad, Telangana, India

Namrata Sharma
MBBS MD FRCOphth FRCSEd
Professor
Cornea, Cataract and Refractive Surgery Services
Dr Rajendra Prasad Centre for Ophthalmic Sciences
All India Institute of Medical Sciences
New Delhi, India

Neet Mehta DNB
Fellow
Cornea and Anterior Segment Services
Shantilal Shanghvi Cornea Institute
LV Prasad Eye Institute
Hyderabad, Telangana, India

Nitin Nema MS DNB
Professor
Department of Ophthalmology
Sri Aurobindo Medical College and Postgraduate Institute of Medical Sciences
Indore, Madhya Pradesh, India

R Ramakrishnan DO MS
Advisor, Department of Glaucoma
Aravind Eye Hospital
Tirunelveli, Tamil Nadu, India

Raja Narayanan MBBS MS MBA
Network Director (Human Resources)
Consultant
Department of Vitreoretina
Anant Bajaj Retina Institute
LV Prasad Eye Institute
Hyderabad, Telangana, India

Rajendra Prakash Maurya MS PhD
Professor and Head
Department of Ophthalmology
Regional Institute of Ophthalmology
Institute of Medical Sciences
Banaras Hindu University
Varanasi, Uttar Pradesh, India

Raksheeth Nathan Rajagopal
MBBS DNB FICO
Consultant Cornea, Cataract and Refractive Surgeon
Cornea, Cataract and Refractive Services
The Eye Foundation
Coimbatore, Tamil Nadu, India

Ramamurthy Dandapani
MD MNAMS
Chairman and Senior Consultant
Department of Cataract and Refractive Surgery
The Eye Foundation
Coimbatore, Tamil Nadu, India

Ritesh Chainani DNB FVRS
Consultant
Department of Vitreoretina
Aravind Eye Hospital
Chennai, Tamil Nadu, India

Rohit Saxena MD PhD
Professor
Department of Ophthalmology
Dr RP Centre for Ophthalmic Sciences
All India Institute of Medical Sciences
New Delhi, India

Sameera Nayak MSc
Senior Research Fellow
Brien Holden Eye Research Centre
LV Prasad Eye Institute
Hyderabad, Telangana, India

Samya Singh MS FAICO
Senior Resident
Department of Ophthalmology
King George's Medical University
Lucknow, Uttar Pradesh, India

Sandeep Saxena
MS PhD FRCSEd FRCS FRCOphth FACS FAMS FAICO FAcadTM
Professor
Department of Ophthalmology
King George's Medical University
Lucknow, Uttar Pradesh, India

Saurabh Kumar MSc
Senior Research Fellow
Department of Ophthalmology
Brien Holden Eye Research Centre
LV Prasad Eye Institute
Hyderabad, Telangana, India

Shilpi Arya MS DNB
Senior Resident
Department of Ophthalmology
King George's Medical University
Lucknow, Uttar Pradesh, India

Shreesha Kumar Kodavoor
MS DNB MNAMS FAICO
Senior Consultant
Department of Cornea, Cataract and Refractive Surgery
The Eye Foundation
Coimbatore, Tamil Nadu, India

Sneha Gupta MBBS
Junior Resident
Department of Ophthalmology
Regional Institute of Ophthalmology
Institute of Medical Sciences
Banaras Hindu University
Varanasi, Uttar Pradesh, India

Somasheila I Murthy MD DOMS FCPS
Medical Director
Department of Corneal Diseases
Uveitis, Cataract and Refractive Surgery
Shantilal Shangvi Eye Institute
LV Prasad Eye Institute
Hyderabad, Telangana, India

Su Xinyi M Med FRCS PhD
Executive Director
Institute of Molecular and Cell Biology
Agency for Science and Technology
Senior Consultant
National University of Singapore and
Associate Professor
National University of Singapore
Department of Ophthalmology
National University of Singapore
Singapore

Subhadra Jalali MS
Network Director
Newborn Eye Health Alliance (NEHA)
and Quality
Consultant
Department of Retina and Pediatric
Ophthalmology
Srimati Kannuri Santhamma Centre
for Vitreoretinal Diseases
Anant Bajaj Retina Institute
Jasti V Ramanamma Children's
Eye Care Centre
Kallam Anji Reddy Campus
LV Prasad Eye Institute
Hyderabad, Telangana, India

Sumita Agarkar MBBS MS DNB
Director
Department of Pediatric
Ophthalmology and Strabismus
Sankara Nethralaya
Chennai, Tamil Nadu, India

Sunita Chaurasia MD
Director
Ramayamma International Eye Bank
Cornea and Anterior Segment Services
Shantilal Shanghvi Cornea Institute
LV Prasad Eye Institute
Hyderabad, Telangana, India

Tapas Ranjan Padhi
MS DNB FMRF
Visiting Scholar
Pediatric Retina and Visual
Electrodiagnostics
Kellog Eye Center
University of Michigan, USA
Visiting Scholar, ARC, Royal Oak
Michigan, USA
Faculty (Vitreoretinal Services)
Anant Bajaj Retina Institute
Pediatric Retina, Newborn Eye Health
Alliance (NEHA)
Miriam Hyman Children Eye Care Center
LV Prasad Eye Institute
Bhubaneswar, Odisha, India

Tasneem Neemuchwala DO DNB
Fellow
Department of Cornea, Cataract and
Refractive Surgery
The Eye Foundation
Coimbatore, Tamil Nadu, India

Vinay Gupta MSc (Opt) PhD Scholar
Research Associate
Department of Ophthalmology
Dr RP Centre for Ophthalmic Sciences
All India Institute of Medical Sciences
New Delhi, India

Virender Sachdeva MS DNB
Head and Consultant
Department of Neuro-ophthalmology
Nimmagadda Prasad Children's Eye
Care Centre, Child Sight Institute
LV Prasad Eye Institute
Visakhapatnam, Andhra Pradesh, India

Virender Singh Sangwan MBBS MS
Director Innovations, Senior Consultant
Department of Cornea and Anterior
Segment
Eicher-Shroff Centre of Stem Cell Research
Dr Shroffs Charity Eye Hospital
New Delhi, India

Preface

Ophthalmology never stands still. It continues to evolve as new technology, techniques, and knowledge are incorporated in the eye care of patients. Therefore, it is necessary to be aware of the *Recent Advances in Ophthalmology-17* to keep oneself abreast with the newer developments.

Childhood myopia is an extremely common ocular condition seen globally with its prevalence increasing at an alarming rate. Genetic and environmental factors play a key role in the development of myopia in children. Rohit Saxena et al. have described approaches involving prevention, early intervention, and management of childhood myopia.

Bioengineered cornea aims at regenerating and developing a biomimetic cornea that eliminates the need for donor cornea. It is an effective alternative to deal with shortage of human donor corneal tissue. Further, it addresses the biocompatibility challenges seen after corneal transplantation. The regenerative approaches employed in corneal bioengineering are explained by Sangwan et al.

Corneal diseases are the third leading cause of visual disability and blindness in the world after cataract and glaucoma. Pediatric keratoconus, a rapidly progressive ectatic condition of the cornea, may cause corneal blindness if not diagnosed and managed early. A detailed account of advances in diagnosis and treatment of this condition is given by Ramappa et al.

Lamellar keratoplasty retains the healthy recipient cornea while selectively replacing the scarred tissue. Advancement in different techniques of lamellar keratoplasty is elaborately covered by Kodavoor et al. Moreover, the book also gives a lucid description of some of the interesting topics like medical management of glaucoma and noninfectious uveitis, application of polymerase chain reaction in the diagnosis of uveitis, and management of hard cataracts.

Technological advances in ocular imaging help the operating surgeon to capture high-quality images that facilitate the real-time visualization of ocular structures intraoperatively. Integrated intraoperative optical coherence tomography (iOCT) improves surgical accuracy and efficacy as well as enhances decision-making during the surgery. Murthy et al. and Gopal et al. have given a classy description of indications and limitations of iOCT in anterior and posterior segment eye surgeries, respectively.

Posterior segment eye diseases are mostly chronic and identified as the major cause of visual impairment and blindness worldwide. Distinguished authors have done a critical literature review and presented the advancements in management of retinopathy of prematurity, treatment of age-related macular degeneration, diagnosis and management of diabetic macular edema, and pachychoroid disease spectrum.

Optic neuritis is one of the commonly encountered neuro-ophthalmic conditions that may affect both children and adults. Sachdeva et al. have beautifully explained the current concepts in optic neuritis.

Orbital hemangioma is the most prevalent primary tumor of orbit. Update on newer diagnostic methods and recent therapeutic strategies used in the management of oculo-orbital hemangioma has been covered by Maurya et al.

Agarkar et al. have emphasized the use of advance imaging modalities and artificial intelligence in the diagnosis and evaluation of strabismus to improve its treatment outcome. The authors have highlighted the need of meticulous planning and correct decision-making in order to get the best results.

ChatGPT is a large language model that provides text to deliver information. This artificial intelligence platform has potential uses in ophthalmology that is vividly described by Shanmugam et al.

Ophthalmology has advanced by leaps and bounds over the past few decades. *Recent Advances in Ophthalmology-17*, therefore, cannot cover all the advancements. It is believed that postgraduate students and fellows in ophthalmology as well as practicing ophthalmologists will get benefited from this book.

Nitin Nema

Acknowledgments

I am incredibly indebted to all the authors for contributing their exquisite work in *Recent Advances in Ophthalmology-17*. I appreciate the extraordinary dedication, hard work, and time management of all the contributors.

My sincere thanks go to Dr Yashas Goyal, Fellow VST Center for Glaucoma Care, LV Prasad Eye Institute, Hyderabad; Dr Rishabh Rathi, Senior Resident, Department of Ophthalmology, Sri Aurobindo Medical College and PG Institute, Indore; and Dr Aashi Bansal Lunawat, Assistant Professor, Department of Ophthalmology, Sri Aurobindo Medical College and PG Institute, Indore for their invaluable help and cooperation.

I would be failing in my duty if I do not thank my wife and children for their constant support and understanding.

Shri Jitendar P Vij (Group Chairman), and Mr Ankit Vij (Managing Director), Jaypee Brothers Medical Publishers (P) Ltd, New Delhi, India, deserve special appreciation for showing keen interest in the publication of *Recent Advances in Ophthalmology* book. I am thankful to Ms Pragati Singh (Development Editor), and the entire team involved in the publication of the book for their patience, perseverance, and forbearance.

Contents

1 CHAPTER

Prevention and Management of Childhood Myopia

Vinay Gupta, Abhyuday Saxena, Rohit Saxena

ABSTRACT

Childhood myopia is a growing global public health concern with a significant increase in prevalence worldwide, particularly in Asia including India. The condition is influenced by genetic predisposition and environmental factors such as prolonged near work and limited outdoor activities. Advances in the prevention and management of childhood myopia have focused on various strategies to curb its onset and progression. Prominent preventive measures include increasing outdoor activities, which have been shown to reduce myopia onset. Educational interventions to reduce near work and promote eye-friendly habits, alongside public health campaigns, play crucial roles in awareness and behavioral changes. Management strategies have seen significant developments, especially in pharmacological and optical interventions. Pharmacological approaches, particularly low-dose atropine eye drops, have proven effective in slowing myopia progression with minimal side effects. The optical interventions include extra-depth-of-focus contact lenses, orthokeratology (Ortho-K), and myopia-control spectacles designed to create peripheral defocus and slow eye elongation. Technological innovations, including advanced diagnostic tools and artificial intelligence, have enhanced early detection, monitoring, and personalized treatment plans. Public health initiatives, such as school-based screening programs and awareness campaigns, are critical in early detection and intervention. Future directions include advancements in genetic research, the development of new pharmacological agents, and long-term studies to evaluate the efficacy and safety of myopia control interventions. A multidisciplinary approach integrating ophthalmology, optometry, education, and public health is essential for addressing the myopia epidemic, ultimately improving outcomes for children worldwide.

Keywords: Myopia, childhood myopia, myopia control, myopia management, myopia interventions

INTRODUCTION

Myopia, also known as *near-sightedness*, is a refractive error where distant objects appear blurry while close ones can be seen clearly. Myopia has emerged as a global public health issue and is recognized by the World Health

Organization's global initiative for the elimination of avoidable blindness as an immediate priority ocular condition.[1] The global prevalence of myopia is on the rise, particularly in East Asia, where up to 80–90% of school-aged children are affected.[2] Although lower rates of myopia among children have been reported in South Asia, North America, and Europe, the situation is expected to become alarming as nearly half of the world's population is predicted to be myopic by 2050.[3,4] The earliest survey conducted in India in the 1970s showed a myopia prevalence of 4.79% among school children in Chandigarh.[5] Recent meta-analyses report an overall myopia prevalence of approximately 7.5% among 5–15-year-old in India, documenting a rising trend over the last four decades.[6] In rural areas, the prevalence has increased from 4.6% during 1980–2008 to 6.8% from 2009 to 2019. While the prevalence does not seem to be alarming percentage-wise, considering our large population, particularly children and young adults, it amounts to a staggering count of approximately 20 million children.

The increased prevalence of myopia over the past few decades has raised concerns due to its association with severe eye complications later in life, such as retinal detachment, glaucoma, and myopic maculopathy.[7,8] The etiology of myopia involves a combination of genetic predisposition and environmental factors. Myopia develops due to an elongation of the eyeball (axial elongation), which causes light to focus in front of the retina instead of directly on it. This process is influenced by several factors, including multiple genes that have been linked to myopia, affecting eye growth and refractive development; excessive near work and limited exposure to natural light that are critical environmental factors; and dysregulation of eye growth signaling pathways, including dopamine and retinal defocus mechanisms.[9] Children with myopic parents are at a higher risk, indicating a strong genetic component. Additionally, environmental influences such as prolonged near work (e.g., reading and screen time), lack of outdoor activities, and urbanization have been identified as significant contributors.[10]

At an individual level, myopia is associated with low self-esteem and a poor quality of life. The estimated global productivity loss due to uncorrected myopia and myopic macular degeneration is approximately 244 billion USD per year,[11] with Asia being the most affected region. In India, based on the prevalence of uncorrected refractive error and the cost of spectacle provision, it would cost approximately 6.3 billion INR (US$131.6 million) to 24.6 billion INR (US$513.7 million) to provide the entire affected population with readymade or custom spectacles, respectively.[12] The clinical and socioeconomic impact of myopia is expected to increase with its rising prevalence. Therefore, the focus has shifted to preventing the incidence and progression of myopia.[13] Conventional myopia-correction spectacles/contact lens do not help in preventing myopia progression. Interventions specifically aim to prevent the progression of myopia currently being studied and preferred by practitioners.

As such, understanding and advancing strategies for the prevention and management of myopia in children have become a critical focus for researchers, clinicians, and public health policymakers.

ADVANCES IN PREVENTION STRATEGIES

Outdoor Activity

Increasing outdoor activity (up to 120 min/day) has been consistently shown to reduce the onset of myopia.[14] Natural light exposure is believed to play a crucial role, potentially through mechanisms involving dopamine release in the retina, which inhibits eye elongation. Public health initiatives encouraging children to spend more time outdoors have been implemented in various countries, demonstrating significant success in myopia prevention.[14,15]

Educational Interventions

Educational programs aimed at reducing near work and promoting eye-friendly habits have also been effective. These include:

- Regular breaks during near work [20-20-20 rule given by American Academy of Ophthalmology-American Association for Pediatric Ophthalmology and Strabismus (AAO-AAPOS):[16] every 20 minutes, look at something 20 feet away for at least 20 seconds]
- Parental education on limiting screen time and encouraging outdoor play.

Other Lifestyle Interventions

Other lifestyle interventions, including ensuring adequate ambient indoor lighting, maximizing natural lighting, and maintaining adequate posture (preferably sitting), are also recommended for myopia prevention.[13]

Identify Premyopia

A refractive state of the eye of ≤+0.75 D and >–0.50 D (spherical equivalent refractive error <+0.75 D but >–0.50 D) in children, where a combination of baseline refraction, age, and other quantifiable risk factors indicates a high likelihood of developing myopia, is referred to as *premyopia*.[17] These children merit preventative interventions.

The management of premyopia is not yet well defined. It is important to compare their refractive error to age-normal values. Specific binocular vision disorders, such as increased accommodative lag and a higher accommodative convergence/accommodation (AC/A) ratio, may be present in premyopes and require evaluation. Preventative measures for premyopic children include lifestyle and environmental modifications.[13]

ADVANCES IN MANAGEMENT STRATEGIES

Effective myopia management begins with a comprehensive approach that involves analyzing the patient's risk profile and selecting individuals who meet the specific inclusion criteria for the chosen treatment method. Educating both the patient and the parents about the benefits and potential risks associated with myopia control treatments is essential for informed decision-making. Following this, conducting a basic ocular examination, including cycloplegic refraction and other relevant treatment-related assessments, helps guide treatment planning **(Flowchart 1.1)**.

It is crucial to maintain regular follow-up appointments at scheduled intervals to monitor progress and record relevant parameters accurately. The essential investigation at the time of enrollment includes slit-lamp examination, fundus examination, distance and near visual acuity evaluation, cycloplegic refraction, and measurement of axial length.[13] The intraocular pressure, pupillometry, amplitude of accommodation, and measurement of other ocular biometry parameters, such as keratometry, anterior chamber depth, and lens thickness, could be recorded. The first follow-up visit (1 month after starting myopia prevention intervention) is to monitor any side effects (if any) and assess compliance (can be done telephonically). Afterward, 6-monthly follow-ups are to be done, and all essential investigations should be performed at 1 year, 2 years, and so on to assess the treatment efficacy.

Additionally, ongoing observation of the child's ocular health and prompt examination as needed ensure timely intervention if any issues arise. Analyzing changes in refractive error/axial length over time allows for adjustments to the clinical management plan as necessary, ensuring personalized and effective myopia management for each patient. The recent guidelines for the management of childhood myopia are summarized in **Flowchart 1.2.**[13]

Various methods have been described in the literature to control myopia by either slowing its progression or preventing its onset. Several strategies, such as undercorrection of myopia, alignment-fit gas-permeable contact

Flowchart 1.1: Overview of management strategies.

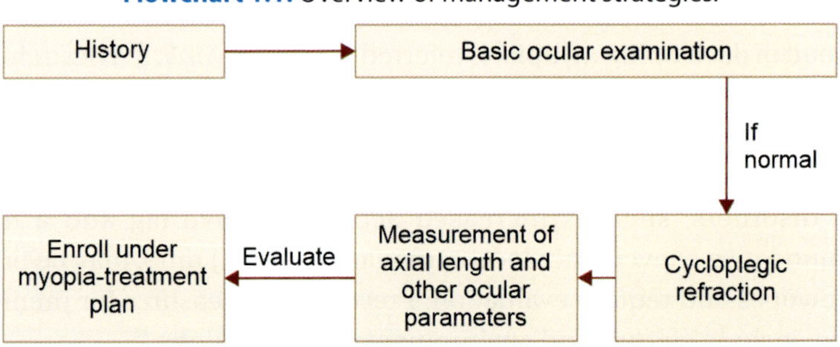

Flowchart 1.2: Guidelines for the management of childhood myopia.

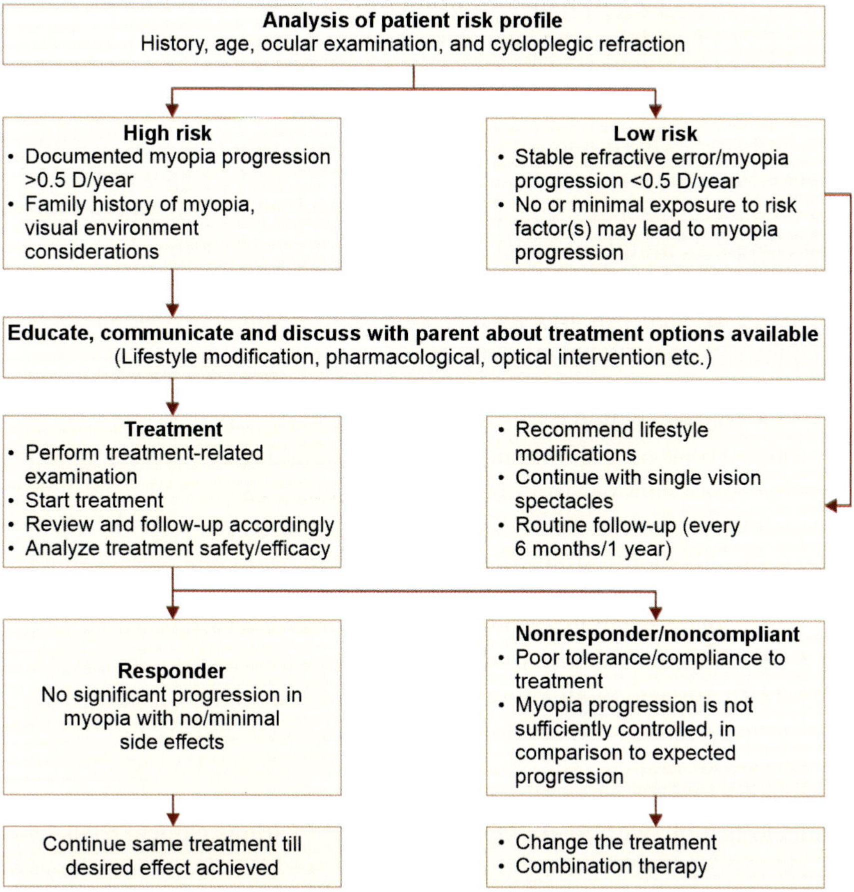

Source: Saxena R, Dhiman R, Gupta V, et al. Prevention and management of childhood progressive myopia: National consensus guidelines. Indian J Ophthalmol. 2023;71(7):2873-81.

lenses, and bifocal or multifocal spectacles, have been shown to be ineffective for myopia control.[18] More effective methods include atropine eye drops, orthokeratology (Ortho-K), bifocal contact lenses, especially segmented spectacles, etc. On average, each of these myopia control methods provides around 50% reduction in the progression of myopia.[18]

Pharmacological Intervention(s)

Low-dose Atropine

Low-dose atropine eye drops have emerged as a promising pharmacological intervention to slow myopia progression. Atropine is an anticholinergic agent that blocks parasympathetic acetylcholine muscarinic receptors on the sphincter pupillae muscle, leading to mydriasis and cycloplegia.[19] The debate about atropine's antimyopia effect centers around whether it is due to accommodative mechanisms or unclear biochemical reactions. Earlier accommodative theories, which suggested that increased accommodative demand led to myopia progression, were dismissed when atropine's protective effect was observed even in animals without an accommodative mechanism.[18] The nonaccommodative theory proposes that atropine's effect is based on local retinal actions and biochemical changes affecting the scleral matrix, slowing scleral growth.[20] Another less-popular theory posits that atropine's protective effect results from enhanced ultraviolet exposure due to pupillary dilation, which downregulates inflammatory processes and decreases axial growth, though this lacks strong evidence. Despite the lack of consensus on the exact mechanism, the most accepted theory currently is that atropine's direct and indirect effects on the retina reduce scleral stretch and halt axial elongation.[20,21]

Clinical trials have shown inconclusive findings regarding the correlation between the effect of atropine on myopia progression and axial length elongation.[22] However, it is suggested that changes in crystalline lens power may contribute to the antimyopia effect observed with low-dose atropine.[23] Also, the involvement of muscarinic receptors in the posterior segment of the eye is considered a possible mode of action for low-dose atropine treatment.[24] These insights underscore the complex interplay between atropine and ocular structures in modulating myopia progression, highlighting the need for further research to elucidate the underlying mechanisms and optimize treatment strategies. Numerous studies have demonstrated the dose-dependent effectiveness of atropine in slowing myopia progression and axial elongation, with tolerable side effects.[25-30] Various clinical trials [e.g., ATOM (Atropine in the Treatment of Myopia),[26] LAMP (Low-concentration Atropine for Myopia Progression),[27] CHAMP,[28] and I-ATOM[29]] conducted worldwide have reported that low concentration(s) of atropine (0.0–0.05%) are effective in reducing myopia progression with minimal side effects. Higher concentrations of atropine (1%) are associated with significant side effects such as photophobia, glare, and difficulty with near vision due to strong cycloplegia. Lower concentrations (0.01–0.05%) have been found to be effective with minimal side effects, making them more suitable for long-term use in children.

The ATOM 1 study[30] conducted in Singapore, involved 400 children aged 6–12 years. The study found that 1% atropine significantly slowed myopia progression by 77% over 2 years compared to placebo (mean progression of –0.28 D/year in the atropine group vs. –1.20 D/year in the placebo group). The ATOM 2 study[26] tested lower concentrations of atropine (0.5, 0.1, and 0.01%) and demonstrated that all concentrations were effective in slowing myopia progression, with 0.01% atropine showing the best balance between efficacy and minimal side effects. The LAMP study[27] compared 0.05,

0.025, and 0.01% atropine in Chinese children aged 4–12 years. The 0.05% concentration showed the highest efficacy in slowing myopia progression and axial elongation, with a mean progression of –0.27 D/year compared to –0.81 D/year in the placebo group. Lower concentrations also showed effectiveness but with fewer side effects. I-ATOM study[29] was a multicentric randomized controlled trial conducted in India, showing a 56% reduction in myopia progression after 1 year of topical atropine (0.01%) treatment among children with mild-to-moderate myopia. Topical low-dose atropine (0.01%) is commercially available in many countries, including India.

Other Topical Agents

The role of several other antimuscarinic agents in myopia management has also been explored. Pirenzepine, a relatively selective M1/M4 receptor antagonist, showed promise with fewer side effects, such as less mydriasis and cycloplegia compared to atropine.[31] However, recent trials for pirenzepine were halted due to its lower efficacy and the inconvenience of twice-daily dosing.

Tropicamide and scopolamine are other anticholinergic agents that have been less thoroughly explored and have not gained much traction due to similar side effects and insufficient follow-up research.[32]

7-Methylxanthine (7MX), an adenosine antagonist found in caffeine, has shown potential in slowing myopia progression by stabilizing the collagen in the posterior sclera.[33] This drug is currently approved for myopia management in Denmark.

Timolol, a beta-adrenergic receptor blocker, was also tested for myopia control but failed to show significant benefits in reducing myopia progression.[34]

Optical Interventions

It is well known that uncorrected myopia causes light rays to focus in front of the retina, with some rays partially focusing on the periphery "behind" the retina **(Fig. 1.1A)**. Traditional single-vision glasses correct central vision by focusing light on the retina, but this causes most peripheral light rays to focus behind the retina, creating hyperopic defocus **(Fig. 1.1B)**. The eye is thought to respond to this hyperopic defocus by increasing axial length.[35] The current theory suggests that creating myopic defocus, where peripheral light rays focus slightly in front of the retina **(Fig. 1.1C)**, can slow down myopia progression and is, therefore, the preferred method of correction.[18]

Defocus Incorporated Multiple Segments

Defocus Incorporated Multiple Segments (DIMS) spectacle is a novel optical intervention designed to control myopia progression in children.[36]

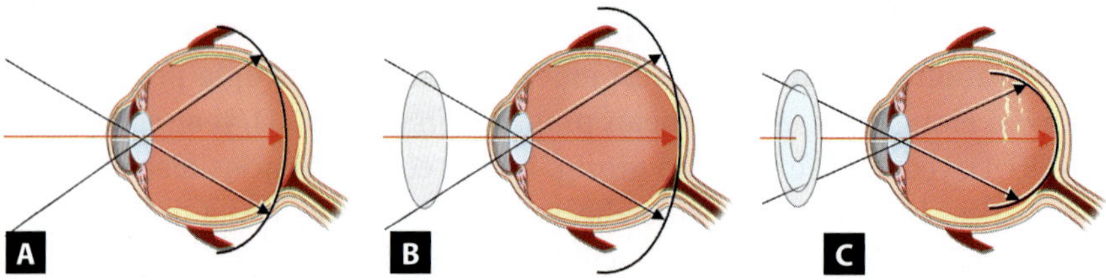

Figs. 1.1A to C: Overview of difference between traditional and specialized myopia correction spectacles: (A) Uncorrected myopia; (B) Traditional single-vision correction; (C) Preferred correction.

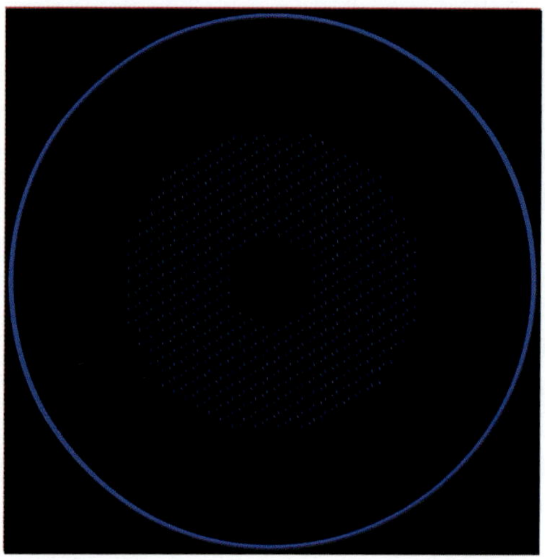

Fig. 1.2: DIMS spectacle design with a center clear zone with a segment of positive power in the periphery. (DIMS: defocus incorporated multiple segments)

These spectacles use a unique lens design to create a dual-focus optical system that aims to slow down the elongation of the eyeball associated with myopia. The design is based on the principle of myopic defocus imposed on both the central and the peripheral retina. The DIMS lens comprises a central optical zone for clear distance vision and multiple defocus segments arranged in a honeycomb pattern around this central zone **(Fig. 1.2)**. These defocus segments create myopic defocus, meaning that they focus light in front of the retina. The dual-focus system works as follows:

- *Central zone:* This part of the lens provides clear, sharp vision for the wearer by focusing light directly on the retina, ensuring normal visual acuity.
- *Defocus segments:* Surrounding the central zone are numerous tiny segments that introduce myopic defocus. These segments ensure that peripheral light rays focus in front of the retina rather than behind it, as is typical with traditional single-vision lenses.

It is postulated that the myopic defocus signals the eye to slow down axial elongation, counteracting the typical growth pattern associated with myopia progression.[37]

A randomized controlled trial conducted in Hong Kong included 160 Chinese children aged 8–13 years.[38] The children were divided into two groups: One group wore DIMS spectacles and the other wore traditional single-vision lenses. After 2 years, the DIMS group showed a 52% reduction in myopia progression compared to the control group (mean myopia progression of –0.41 D/year in the DIMS group vs. –0.85 D/year in the control group). Axial elongation was also significantly slower in the DIMS group, with an average elongation of 0.21 mm/year compared to 0.55 mm/year in the control group. The results from another study supported that DIMS lenses provided sustained myopia control without adverse effects over the 6-year study period.[39]

Spectacles with Highly Aspheric Lenslets

Spectacles with highly aspherical lenslets (HAL) represent an advanced approach to myopia control. Spectacles incorporating aspheric lenslets operate on the principle of generating a three-dimensional volume of myopic defocus in front of the retina **(Fig. 1.3)**.[40] HAL spectacles incorporate a multitude of HAL distributed across the lens surface, surrounding a central clear zone. Each lenslet, typically ranging from 0.6 to 1.1 mm in diameter,

Illustration of the study device providing a volume of myopic defocus (VoMD) (white shell) in front of the retina through 11 concentric rings of contiguous lenslets (A = depth of VoMD and B = distance from the retina).

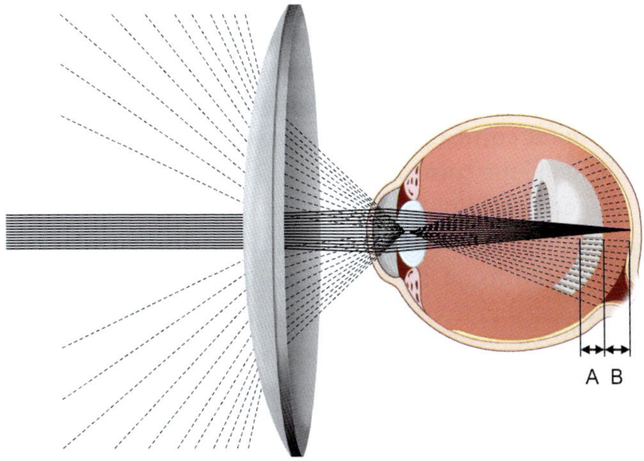

Fig. 1.3: Illustration of HAL spectacle providing a volume of myopia defocus. (HAL: highly aspherical lenslets)

Source: Bao J, Yang A, Huang Y, Li X, Pan Y, Ding C, et al. One-year myopia control efficacy of spectacle lenses with aspherical lenslets. Br J Ophthalmol. 2020;106(8):1171-6.

contributes to this effect. Within the lens, 11 concentric rings are formed by contiguous aspherical lenslets. This design strategy ensures that the optical properties of the lens create a specific distribution of light in front of the retina, promoting myopic defocus across a range of viewing distances.[40]

A randomized controlled trial involving 170 children aged 8–13 years compared HAL lenses with traditional single-vision lenses.[40] After 1 year, the HAL group showed a 67% reduction in myopia progression (mean progression of –0.28 D/year) compared to the control group (mean progression of –0.81 D/year). Axial elongation was also significantly reduced in the HAL group, with an average increase of 0.13 mm/year versus 0.36 mm/year in the control group. This study reported high levels of comfort and adaptability among children wearing HAL spectacles. The aspherical lenslets did not interfere with central vision, and no significant adverse effects were noted. The compliance rate was high, indicating that the lenses were well accepted by the children and their parents.

Notably, DIMS and HAL spectacles represent one of the least invasive methods for managing myopia progression and are straightforward to use, making them an attractive option for both patients and clinicians alike. Other recently introduced spectacle designs like cylindrical annular refractive element[41] and diffusion optics technology[42] are also being used to prevent myopia progression. By utilizing these special designs, these spectacles offer a targeted approach to managing myopia progression, potentially providing benefits beyond traditional corrective glasses.

Orthokeratology

Orthokeratology involves the use of especially designed rigid gas-permeable contact lenses worn overnight to temporarily reshape the cornea, providing clear vision during the day without the need for glasses or contact lenses.[43] The primary action of Ortho-K lenses is to flatten the central cornea and steepen the mid-peripheral cornea. This reshaping process temporarily corrects myopia by changing the cornea's curvature, allowing light to focus correctly on the retina, and providing clear vision. As the Ortho-K lenses flatten the central cornea, they also create a peripheral myopic defocus. This means that while the central vision is corrected, light rays entering the eye from the periphery are focused in front of the retina. This myopic defocus is believed to send a signal to the eye to slow down its axial elongation, which is a key factor in myopia progression. Studies suggest that this altered visual input prevents the eye from elongating further, thereby slowing the progression of myopia.[44]

The Retardation of Myopia in Orthokeratology (ROMIO) study[45] was a randomized controlled trial that included 78 children aged 6–10 years, with one group using Ortho-K lenses and the other group wearing single-vision spectacles. Over 2 years, the Ortho-K group showed a 43% reduction in myopia progression compared to the spectacle group. The mean axial elongation in the Ortho-K group was 0.27 mm, compared to 0.46 mm in the control group. The Study of Myopia Control with Orthokeratology (SMART) study[46] included 102 children aged 7–12 years. The participants were divided into an Ortho-K group and a control group wearing single-vision glasses. After 2 years, the mean axial elongation in the Ortho-K group was significantly less (0.31 mm) compared to the control group (0.64 mm), demonstrating a 51% reduction in myopia progression. The Longitudinal Orthokeratology Research in Children (LORIC) study[47] had 35 children aged 7–12 years wearing Ortho-K lenses for 2 years. The results showed a 32% reduction in axial elongation compared to a historical control group not using Ortho-K lenses. The mean axial elongation in the Ortho-K group was 0.29 mm, compared to 0.43 mm in the control group.

The greatest benefit of this therapy is typically observed within the first 2 years of use, although its effectiveness may diminish over time. One of the primary advantages of these lenses is that they eliminate the need for daytime correction, providing convenience for the wearer. However, despite their potential benefits, these lenses face challenges with low acceptance rates in many countries, including India. Additionally, there is a risk of microbial keratitis associated with their use,[48] highlighting the importance of careful monitoring and adherence to proper hygiene protocols. Common side effects include mild discomfort during the initial adaptation period and a slight risk of eye infections, which can be minimized with proper lens hygiene and regular follow-up visits with an eye care professional.

Specialized Contact Lens

The management of myopia may involve the off-label use of presbyopic-correction methods, such as multifocal contact lenses.[49] The daily disposable lenses are specifically designed and approved for myopia control in certain countries.[50] Another type of soft contact lens, (Extended Depth of Focus or EDOF CL) offers a unique solution, functioning as a center-distance lens with peripheral add to extend the depth of focus.[51] EDOF contact lenses function through a unique optical design that manipulates how light focuses on the retina. EDOF lenses create multiple focal points by utilizing advanced optics, such as aspheric lens designs and higher-order aberrations. This results in a continuous range of clear vision from near to distance, reducing the demand for accommodation and minimizing accommodative lag, which is often associated with myopia progression. Similar to other myopia-control lenses, EDOF lenses are designed to shift peripheral light rays to focus in front of the retina (myopic defocus), thereby reducing the stimulus for the eye to elongate.

A randomized controlled trial involved 72 children aged 9–14 years, divided into an EDOF lens group and a control group wearing single-vision contact lenses.[52] After 1 year, the EDOF group showed a 36% reduction in myopia progression compared to the control group. The mean myopia progression in the EDOF group was –0.70 D/year, compared to –0.88 D/year in the control group. Another study involved 508 children aged 8–13 years, comparing the effects of EDOF contact lenses to single-vision contact lenses over a 2-year period.[51] Results indicated that the EDOF group experienced a significant reduction in both myopia progression (24–32%) and axial elongation (22–32%).

Regular follow-up visits with an eye care professional are essential to monitor lens fit and ocular health and ensure compliance with proper lens hygiene to minimize the risk of complications such as eye infections. Notably, these lenses are readily available in India, providing access to advanced myopia-management technologies. Furthermore, for individuals with myopia and astigmatism, toric multifocals have been successfully utilized, highlighting the versatility and efficacy of modern contact lens options in addressing myopia prevention.

Combination Therapy

Combination therapy for myopia management involves strategic patient selection and careful consideration of interventions to combine.[53] Patients who exhibit rapid progression of myopia and/or demonstrate poor compliance with a single intervention may benefit from combination therapy. Choosing the appropriate interventions to combine is crucial for optimizing treatment outcomes. Options may include combining atropine with spectacles, Ortho-K, or multifocal contact lenses. Alternatively, spectacles can be paired with environmental modifications to enhance efficacy. Other combinations, such as atropine with spectacles and environmental modifications, may also be considered.

Light Therapy

Light therapy for myopia presents a complex picture, with research findings sometimes appearing contradictory. While red light, a form of long-wavelength light, would theoretically induce hyperopic defocus and potentially exacerbate myopia, studies have shown unexpected results.[54] For instance, experiments on rhesus monkeys raised in quasi-monochromatic red light revealed little difference in refractive error performance.[55] Similarly, another study reported that rhesus monkeys wearing long-wavelength-pass (red) filters exhibited apparent hyperopia. Despite these initial observations, light therapy has emerged as a new treatment modality for myopia management. Although limited data exists to support its use, recent studies have shown promising results.[56] Both repeated low red-light (RLRL) therapy and blue-light therapy have proven effective in inhibiting axial length elongation, offering potential avenues for further investigation and clinical application.

Technological Innovations

Digital Devices and Applications

The advent of digital technology has introduced several innovative tools to manage myopia. Applications and devices that monitor and control screen time, provide reminders for breaks, and encourage outdoor activity are becoming increasingly popular among parents and educators.[57] Additionally, digital eye strain management applications help to ensure that children use electronic devices in an eye-friendly manner.

Advanced Diagnostic Tools

Improved diagnostic tools, such as optical coherence tomography (OCT) and axial length measurement devices, allow for early detection and precise monitoring of myopia progression.[58,59] These technologies enable personalized treatment plans and more accurate assessments of intervention efficacy.

Artificial Intelligence

Artificial intelligence (AI) and machine-learning algorithms are being developed to predict myopia progression and customize treatment plans based on individual risk factors.[60-62] These tools analyze large datasets to identify patterns and recommend optimal prevention and management strategies for each child.

Public Health Initiatives

Awareness Campaigns

Governments and health organizations worldwide have launched campaigns to raise awareness about myopia.[63] These campaigns focus on educating parents, teachers, and healthcare providers about the importance of early detection and intervention.[64,65] Initiatives such as World Myopia Day highlight the global impact of myopia and promote preventive measures.

School-based Programs

School-based screening programs for myopia are essential for early detection and intervention.[66] These programs often include vision screenings, educational workshops, and collaboration with parents to ensure that children receive appropriate eye care. Some programs also incorporate outdoor activity breaks and classroom modifications to reduce near-work strain.

Policy Development

Policymakers are increasingly recognizing the need for regulations and guidelines to address the myopia epidemic. Policies promoting outdoor activities, regulating screen time, and ensuring access to affordable eye care are critical components of a comprehensive strategy to combat myopia.

Future Directions

Genetic Research

Advancements in genetic research hold promise for understanding the underlying mechanisms of myopia and developing targeted therapies.[67] Identifying genetic markers associated with myopia can lead to personalized prevention and treatment strategies, potentially reducing the risk for those with a strong genetic predisposition.

New Pharmacological Agents

Research is ongoing to identify new pharmacological agents that can effectively control myopia progression with fewer side effects. These may include novel compounds targeting specific biochemical pathways involved in eye growth and refractive development.

Longitudinal Studies

Long-term studies are essential to evaluate the efficacy and safety of various myopia-control interventions. These studies will provide valuable data on the sustainability of treatment effects and potential long-term complications, guiding clinical practice and informing future research directions.

Integration of Multidisciplinary Approaches

A multidisciplinary approach combining ophthalmology, optometry, education, and public health is crucial for addressing the myopia epidemic. Collaborative efforts can lead to more comprehensive and effective prevention and management strategies, ultimately improving outcomes for children worldwide.

CONCLUSION

The rise in childhood myopia is a significant public health concern with far-reaching implications. However, advances in prevention and management strategies offer hope for mitigating this growing problem. By promoting outdoor activities, implementing educational interventions, utilizing pharmacological and optical treatments, and leveraging technological innovations, we can effectively reduce the prevalence and progression of myopia in children. Continued research and public health initiatives will be essential in ensuring that future generations enjoy better eye health and quality of life.

REFERENCES

1. Parajasegram R. VISION 2020 the right to sight: from strategies to action. Am J Ophthalmol. 1999;128:359-60.
2. Lin LL, Shih YF, Hsiao CK, Chen CJ. Prevalence of myopic in Taiwanese school children: 1983 to 2000. Ann Acad Med Singapore. 2004;33:27-33.
3. Morgan IG, Ohno-Matsui K, Saw SM. Myopia. Lancet. 2012;379:1739-48.
4. Pan CW, Ramamurthy D, Saw SM. Worldwide prevalence and risk factors for myopia. Ophthalmic Physiol Opt. 2012;32(1):3-16.
5. Jain IS, Jain S, Mohan K. The epidemiology of high myopia: changing trends. Indian J Ophthalmol. 1983;31(6):723-8.
6. Agarwal D, Saxena R, Gupta V, Mani K, Dhiman R, Bhardawaj A, et al. Prevalence of myopia in Indian school children: meta-analysis of last four decades. PLoS One. 2020;15(10):e0240750.
7. Marcus MW, de Vries MM, Junnoy Montolio FG, Jansonius NM. Myopia as a risk factor for open-angle glaucoma: a systematic review and meta-analysis. Ophthalmology. 2011;118(10):1989-94.
8. Hayashi K, Ohno-Matsui K, Shimada N, Moriyama M, Kojima A, Hayashi W, et al. Long-term pattern of progression of myopic maculopathy: a natural history study. Ophthalmology. 2010;117(8):1595-611.
9. Flitcrot DI. The complex interactions of retinal, optical and environmental factors in myopia Aetiology. Prog Retin Eye Res. 2012;31(6):622-60.
10. Saxena R, Gupta V, Prasad P, Bhardwaj A, Vashist P. Prevalence of myopia and its risk factors in rural school children in North India: the North India myopia rural study (NIM-R Study). Eye (Lond). 2022;36(10):2000-5.
11. Fricke TR, Holden BA, Wilson DA, Schlenther G, Naidoo KS, Resnikoff S, et al. Global cost of correcting vision impairment from uncorrected refractive error. Bull World Health Organ. 2012;90:728-38.
12. Angell B, Ali F, Gandhi M, Mathur U, Friedman DS, Jan S, et al. Ready-made and custom-made eyeglasses in India: a cost-effectiveness analysis of a randomised controlled trial. BMJ Open Ophthalmol. 2018;3:e000123.
13. Saxena R, Dhiman R, Gupta V, Phuljhele S, Mahajan A, Rakheja V, et al. Prevention and management of childhood progressive myopia: national consensus guidelines. Indian J Ophthalmol. 2023;71(7):2873-81.
14. He X, Sankaridurg P, Wang J, Chen J, Naduvilath T, He M, et al. Time outdoors in reducing myopia: a school-based cluster randomized trial with objective monitoring of outdoor time and light intensity. Ophthalmology. 2022;129(11):1245-54.
15. Wu PC, Chen CT, Chang LC, Niu YZ, Chen ML, Liao LL, et al. Increased time outdoors is followed by reversal of the long-term trend to reduced visual acuity in Taiwan primary school students. Ophthalmology. 2020;127(11):1462-9.
16. Screen time and e-learning. Children eye foundation of AAPOS. American Association for Pediatric Ophthalmology and Strabismus (AAPOS). [online]

Available from https://aapos.org/glossary/screen-time-and-online-learning. [Last accessed September, 2024].
17. Flitcroft DI, He M, Jonas JB, Jong M, Naidoo K, Ohno-Matsui K, et al. IMI-defining and classifying myopia: a proposed set of standards for clinical and epidemiologic studies. Invest Ophthalmol Vis Sci. 2019;60(3):20-30.
18. Dhiman R, Rakheja V, Gupta V, Saxena R. Current concepts in the management of childhood myopia. Indian J Ophthalmol. 2022;70(8):2800-15.
19. Upadhyay A, Beuerman RW. Biological mechanisms of atropine control of myopia. Eye Contact Lens. 2020;46(3):129-35.
20. McBrien NA, Stell WK, Carr B. How does atropine exert its anti-myopia effects? Ophthalmic Physiol Opt J Br Coll Ophthalmic Opt Optom. 2013;33(3):373-8.
21. Chia A, Chua W-H, Wen L, Fong A, Goon YY, Tan D. Atropine for the treatment of childhood myopia: changes after stopping atropine 0.01%, 0.1% and 0.5%. Am J Ophthalmol. 2014;157(2):451-7.
22. Zhao C, Cai C, Ding Q, Dai H. Efficacy and safety of atropine to control myopia progression: a systematic review and meta-analysis. BMC Ophthalmol. 2020;20(1):478.
23. Saxena R, Gupta V, Dhiman R, Phuljhele S, Kumar P, Sharma N, et al. Effect of low-dose atropine (0.01%) on crystalline lens power among school-aged children with progressive myopia. Ophthalmic Physiol Opt. 2023;43(6):1406-11.
24. Kumar P, Saxena R, Dhiman Phuljhele S, Kumar V, Chawla R, et al. Evaluation of the levels of low-dose topical atropine (0.01%) in aqueous and vitreous humor in human eyes. Optom Vis Sci. 2023;100(8):530-6.
25. Saxena R, Gupta V, Dhiman R, Joseph E, Agarkar S, Neena R, et al. Low-dose atropine 0.01% for the treatment of childhood myopia: a Pan-India multicentric retrospective study. Br J Ophthalmol. 2024;108(4):588-92.
26. Chia A, Chua WH, Cheung YB, Wong WL, Lingham A, Fong A, et al. Atropine for the treatment of childhood myopia: safety and efficacy of 0.5%, 0.1%, and 0.01% doses (Atropine for the Treatment of Myopia 2). Ophthalmology. 2012;119(2):347-54.
27. Yam JC, Jiang Y, Tang SM, Law AKP, Chan JJ, Wong E, et al. Low-concentration Atropine for Myopia Progression (LAMP) Study: a randomized, double-blinded, placebo-controlled trial of 0.05%, 0.025% and 0.01% atropine eye drops in myopia control. Ophthalmology. 2019;126(1):113-24.
28. Zadnik K, Schulman E, Flitcroft I, Fogt JS, Blumenfeld LC, Fong TM, et al. Efficacy and safety of 0.01% and 0.02% atropine for the treatment of pediatric myopia progression over 3 years: a randomized clinical trial. JAMA Ophthalmol. 2023;141(10):990-9.
29. Saxena R, Dhiman R, Gupta V, Kumar P, Matalia J, Roy L, et al. Atropine for the treatment of childhood myopia in India: multicentric randomized trial. Ophthalmology. 2021;128(9):1367-9.
30. Chua WH, Balakrishnan V, Chan YH, Tong L, Ling Y, Quah BL, et al. Atropine for the treatment of childhood myopia. Ophthalmology. 2006;113(12):2285-91.
31. Bartlett JD, Niemann K, Houde B, Allred T, Edmondson MJ, Crockett RS. A tolerability study of pirenzepine ophthalmic gel in myopic children. J Ocul Pharmacol Ther Off J Assoc Ocul Pharmacol Ther. 2003;19(3):271-9.
32. Abraham S. Control of myopia with tropicamide. A progress report. J Pediatr Ophthalmol. 1966;3:10-22.

33. Trier K, Munk Ribel-Madsen S, Cui D, Brøgger Christensen S. Systemic 7-methylxanthine in retarding axial eye growth and myopia progression: a 36-month pilot study. J Ocul Biol Dis Infor. 2008;1(2-4):85-93.
34. Jensen H. Myopia progression in young school children. A prospective study of myopia progression and the effect of a trial with bifocal lenses and beta blocker eye drops. Acta Ophthalmol Suppl. 1991;200:1-79.
35. Russo A, Boldini A, Romano D, Mazza G, Bignotti S, Morescalchi F, et al. Myopia: mechanisms and strategies to slow down its progression. J Ophthalmol. 2022;20:1004977.
36. Carlà MM, Boselli F, Giannuzzi F, Gambini G, Caporossi T, De Vico U, et al. Overview on defocus incorporated multiple segments lenses: a novel perspective in myopia progression management. Vision (Basel). 2022;6(2):20.
37. Zhang HY, Lam CSY, Tang WC, Leung M, To CH. Defocus incorporated multiple segments spectacle lenses changed the relative peripheral refraction: a 2-year randomized clinical trial. Invest Ophthalmol Vis Sci. 2020;61(5):53.
38. Lam CSY, Tang WC, Tse DY, Lee RPK, Chun RKM, Hasegawa K, et al. Defocus incorporated multiple segments (DIMS) spectacle lenses slow myopia progression: a 2-year randomised clinical trial. Br J Ophthalmol. 2020;104(3): 363-8.
39. Lam CS, Tang WC, Lee PH, Zhang HY, Qi H, Hasegawa K, et al. Myopia control effect of defocus incorporated multiple segments (DIMS) spectacle lens in Chinese children: results of a 3-year follow-up study. Br J Ophthalmol. 2022;106(8):1110-4.
40. Bao J, Yang A, Huang Y, Li X, Pan Y, Ding C, et al. One-year myopia control efficacy of spectacle lenses with aspherical lenslets. Br J Ophthalmol. 2022;106(8):1171-6.
41. Liu X, Wang P, Xie Z, Sun M, Chen M, Wang J, et al. One-year myopia control efficacy of cylindrical annular refractive element spectacle lenses. Acta Ophthalmol. 2023;101(6):651-7.
42. Rappon J, Chung C, Young G, Hunt C, Neitz J, Neitz M, et al. Control of myopia using diffusion optics spectacle lenses: 12-month results of a randomised controlled, efficacy and safety study (CYPRESS). Br J Ophthalmol. 2023;107(11):1709-15.
43. Bullimore MA, Johnson LA. Overnight orthokeratology. Cont Lens Anterior Eye. 2020;43(4):322-32.
44. Cho P, Tan Q. Myopia and orthokeratology for myopia control. Clin Exp Optom. 2019;102(4):364-77.
45. Cho P, Cheung SW. Retardation of myopia in orthokeratology (ROMIO) study: a 2-year randomized clinical trial. Invest Ophthalmol Vis Sci. 2012;53(11): 7077-85.
46. Pauné J, Morales H, Armengol J, Quevedo L, Faria-Ribeiro M, González-Méijome JM. Myopia control with a novel peripheral gradient soft lens and orthokeratology: a 2-year clinical trial. Biomed Res Int. 2015;2015:507572.
47. Cho P, Cheung SW, Edwards M. The longitudinal orthokeratology research in children (LORIC) in Hong Kong: a pilot study on refractive changes and myopic control. Curr Eye Res. 2005;30(1):71-80.
48. Watt K, Swarbrick HA. Microbial keratitis in overnight orthokeratology: review of the first 50 cases. Eye Contact Lens. 2005;31(5):201-8.
49. Remón L, Pérez-Merino P, Macedo-de-Araújo RJ, Amorim-de-Sousa AI, González-Méijome JM. Bifocal and multifocal contact lenses for presbyopia and myopia control. J Ophthalmol. 2020;1:8067657.

50. Ruiz-Pomeda A, Villa-Collar C. Slowing the progression of myopia in children with the MiSight contact lens: a narrative review of the evidence. Ophthalmol Ther. 2020;9(4):783-95.
51. Sankaridurg P, Bakaraju RC, Naduvilath T, Hen X, Weng R, Tilia D, et al. Myopia control with novel central and peripheral plus contact lenses and extended depth of focus contact lenses: 2-year results from a randomised clinical trial. Ophthalmic Physiol Opt. 2019;39(4):294-307.
52. Shen EP, Chu HS, Cheng HC, Tsai TH. Center-for-near extended-depth-of-focus soft contact lens for myopia control in children: 1-year results of a randomized controlled trial. Ophthalmol Ther. 2022;11(4):1577-88.
53. Wolffsohn JS, Whayeb Y, Logan NS, Weng R; International Myopia Institute Ambassador Group. IMI-global trends in myopia management attitudes and strategies in clinical practice-2022 update. Invest Ophthalmol Vis Sci. 2023;64(6):6.
54. Tang J, Liao Y, Yan N, Dereje SB, Wang J, Luo Y, et al. Efficacy of repeated low-level red-light therapy for slowing the progression of childhood myopia: a systematic review and meta-analysis. Am J Ophthalmol. 2023;252:153-63.
55. Zhang P, Zhu H. Light signaling and myopia development: a review. Ophthalmol Ther. 2022;11(3):939-57.
56. Jiang Y, Zhu Z, Tan X, Kong X, Zhong H, Zhang J, et al. Effect of repeated low-level red-light therapy for myopia control in children: a multicenter randomized controlled trial. Ophthalmology. 2022;129(5):509-19.
57. Li Y, Yip MYT, Ting DSW, Ang M. Artificial intelligence and digital solutions for myopia. Taiwan J Ophthalmol. 2023;13(2):142-50.
58. Li Y, Zheng F, Foo LL, Wong QY, Ting D, Hoang QV, et al. Advances in OCT imaging in myopia and pathologic myopia. Diagnostics (Basel). 2022;12(6):1418.
59. López-Muñoz A, Gargallo-Martínez B, Sánchez-González MC, Capote-Puente R, De-Hita-Cantalejo C, Romero-Luna M, et al. Key factors in early diagnosis of myopia progression within ocular biometric parameters by Scheimpflug technology. Life (Basel). 2023;13(2):447.
60. Zhang J, Zou H. Insights into artificial intelligence in myopia management: from a data perspective. Graefes Arch Clin Exp Ophthalmol. 2024;262(1):3-17.
61. Zhang C, Zhao J, Zhu Z, Li Y, Li K, Wang Y, et al. Applications of artificial intelligence in myopia: current and future directions. Front Med (Lausanne). 2022;9:840498.
62. Foo LL, Ng WY, Lim GYS, Tan TE, Ang M, Ting DSW. Artificial intelligence in myopia: current and future trends. Curr Opin Ophthalmol. 2021;32(5):413-24.
63. Ang M, Flanagan JL, Wong CW, Müller A, Davis A, Keys D, et al. Review: myopia control strategies recommendations from the 2018 WHO/IAPB/BHVI meeting on myopia. Br J Ophthalmol. 2020;104(11):1482-7.
64. Ortiz-Peregrina S, Solano-Molina S, Martino F, Castro-Torres JJ, Jiménez JR. Parental awareness of the implications of myopia and strategies to control its progression: a survey-based study. Ophthalmic Physiol Opt. 2023;43(5):1145-59.
65. Li Q, Guo L, Zhang J, Zhao F, Hu Y, Guo Y, et al. Effect of school-based family health education via social media on children's myopia and parents' awareness: a randomized clinical trial. JAMA Ophthalmol. 2021;139(11):1165-72.
66. Huang LM, Fan XM, Xie YH, Meng ZY, Chen T, Dai BF, et al. Improving myopia awareness via school-based myopia prevention health education among Chinese students. Int J Ophthalmol. 2023;16(5):794-9.
67. Wang YM, Lu SY, Zhang XJ, Chen LJ, Pang CP, Yam JC. Myopia genetics and heredity. Children (Basel). 2022;9(3):382.

2 CHAPTER

Bioengineered Cornea

Abha Gour, Mehak Vohra, Virender Singh Sangwan

ABSTRACT

Corneal bioengineering has emerged as a beacon of hope in conquering vision loss due to corneal diseases. This chapter delves into the innovative techniques and breakthroughs in bioengineering that are reshaping our approach to corneal repair and regeneration. From utilizing advanced biomaterials to integrating stem cell therapy and 3D bioprinting, we explore cutting-edge methods that promise to restore vision and significantly enhance the quality of life for patients worldwide.

Keywords: Corneal blindness, corneal transplants, bioengineering, scaffolds, corneal implants, collagen scaffolds, 3D bioprinting, animal models

INTRODUCTION

Corneal blindness affects nearly 11.5 million people globally due to factors such as poor nutrition, infections from agricultural work, or workplace injuries. This condition is mainly found in developing countries, where limited resources and infrastructure complicate treatment efforts.[1] Annually, only 1 in 70 needy patients receives a corneal transplant.[2] In India, corneal opacities represent 8.2% of all blindness, ranking second to cataracts, contributing to 3.2% of the worldwide blindness burden.[3] Unlike cataract surgery, treating corneal blindness involves complex and varied approaches, including transplants.

Corneal transplantation is also the most successful organ transplant; it can restore vision adequately but faces challenges like high failure rates over time and a shortage of donor corneas. With 12.7 million people globally awaiting transplants and diminishing donor availability due to aging populations,[4] stem cell therapy and corneal bioengineering emerge as promising alternatives to address these issues.

CONCEPT OF BIOENGINEERING

Using autologous tissue has been the gold standard for reconstructing tissue defects, but it still faces significant limitations and complications. The success of keratoplasty depends on multiple factors, including donor and patient characteristics, tissue retrieval and storage conditions, and the availability of skilled surgeons.

An ideal solution for corneal blindness would be a graft that does not require a donor, can be mass-produced, is easily distributed, involves simple surgical techniques, and minimizes or eliminates the need for sutures. Despite the high patient load, India has significantly enhanced its infrastructure to boost keratoplasty rates over the years, creating a conducive environment for such innovations to bridge the gap between demand and supply.

Keratoprosthesis was intended to fulfill this role; however, its use is currently limited to high-risk cases as a last resort. It still requires a corneal graft, such as the Boston KPro types 1 and 2, thus not eliminating the need for donor corneas **(Fig. 2.1)**.

To understand the concept of bioengineering, it is vital to understand the structure and function of the normal cornea. The cornea, an intricate avascular structure, consists of three primary layers: Epithelium, stroma, and endothelium, and contains three main types of cells: Epithelial, fibroblasts/keratocytes, and endothelial cells. The stroma constitutes about 90% of the corneal thickness and is maintained by proteoglycans and type I collagen secreted by keratocytes. A healthy cornea transmits approximately 75% of light to the lens, providing a sharp vision that relies on transparency, maintained by the arrangement of collagen fibers and water content within its structure. Additionally, the corneal epithelial layer's self-renewal properties help maintain its clarity. Damage or disease in the cornea can lead to reduced visual acuity and, in severe cases, result in corneal blindness.

Tissue engineering is a technique aimed at regenerating organs and tissues, specifically to develop a biomimetic replacement that can serve as a partial or complete substitute for diseased corneas. This approach seeks to address the shortage of optical-grade donor corneas by creating transplants that eliminate the need for donor screening and can be mass-produced, distributed widely, and customized to meet individual patient needs.

An ideal graft for corneal replacement should meet the following criteria:

- *Functional:* It must be optically transparent with an adequate refractive index to ensure images are correctly focused on the retina.
- *Mechanically strong:* The graft should protect internal eye structures while being permeable to nutrients and oxygen, essential for the survival of corneal cells.
- *Biomimetic:* The ability to support host stromal cell colonization is critical for the graft to integrate successfully with adjacent structures.
- *Nonantigenic and noninflammatory:* The implant should not trigger a strong immune response, preventing vascularization and opacification that could lead to its biodegradation or calcification.

TECHNIQUES USED IN CORNEAL BIOENGINEERING

Multiple techniques have been successfully used in corneal bioengineering, which are described below.

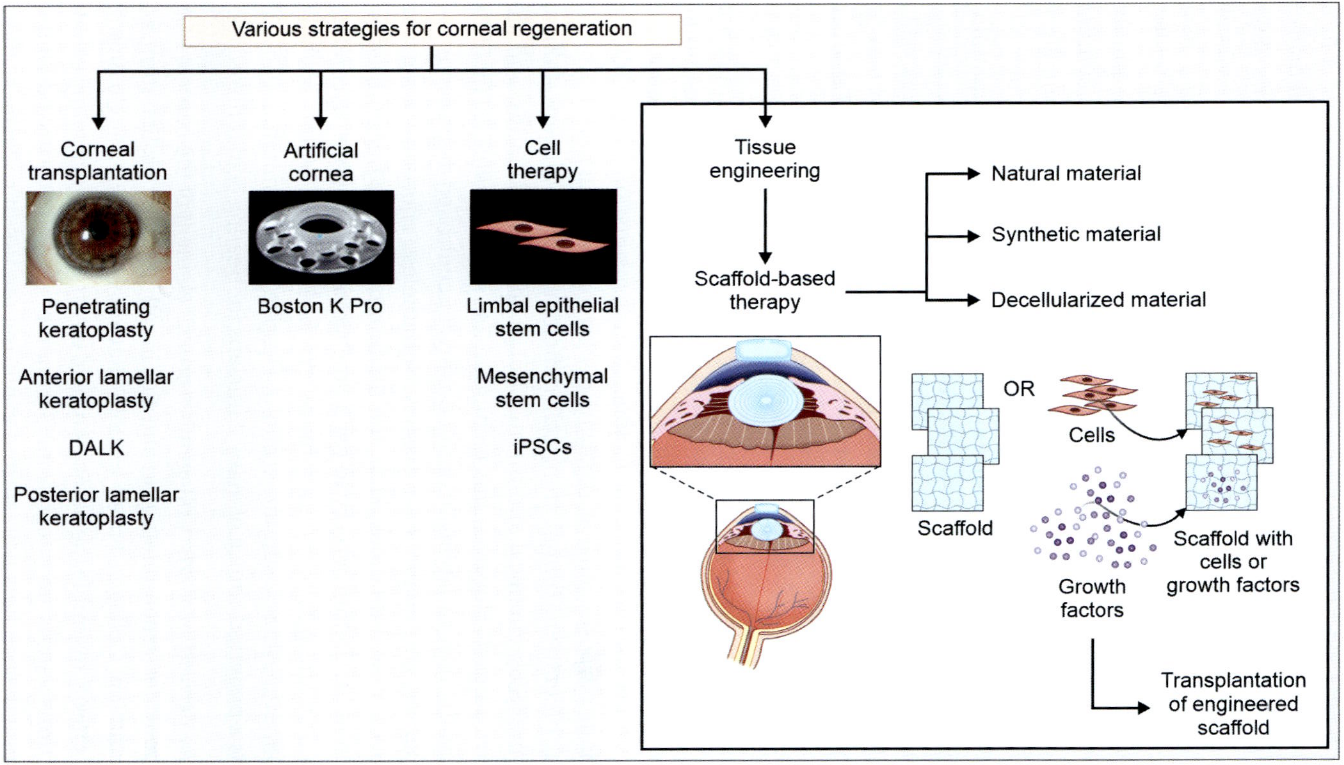

Fig. 2.1: Various strategies for corneal regeneration. (DALK: deep anterior lamellar keratoplasty)

Scaffolds, Biomaterials, and 3D Printing

Scaffold-based Approaches

Scaffold-based therapy is a technique used to address corneal damage by providing a structure that mimics the natural extracellular matrix (ECM) of the cornea. This scaffold is a supportive framework for corneal cells' attachment, proliferation, and differentiation, thus, facilitating tissue regeneration. Various types of scaffolds have been studied for corneal regeneration, including natural materials such as collagen, fibrin, amniotic membrane (AM), and decellularized corneal tissue, as well as synthetic polymers like poly (lactic-co-glycolic acid) (PLGA), poly (ethylene glycol) (PEG), and polycaprolactone (PCL). These materials can be engineered to possess properties such as stiffness, proper topography, biocompatibility, and biodegradability, which are vital for successful tissue regeneration. In addition, the scaffold should withstand suturing without tearing, as well as physiological forces like intraocular pressure, eyelid motion, and tear film motion. Some of the salient properties of the scaffold are listed in **Table 2.1**.

Material Selection

Amniotic membrane: AM is a thick basement membrane in the human body that helps heal epithelial cells while preventing fibroblast proliferation and myofibroblast differentiation. It also contains several antiangiogenic, anti-inflammatory, and neurotrophic factors. AM transplantation is currently used for various purposes, such as repairing persistent epithelial defects, treating corneal ulceration, limbal stem cell deficiency, acute Stevens-Johnson syndrome (SJS), chemical and thermal burns, infectious keratitis, and after refractive surgery. However, this technique has some drawbacks, including tissue availability, variability in donor quality, uncontrolled degradation, and improper storage and processing issues. Nonetheless, efforts are being made to address these limitations. First, the membranes can be freeze-dried and rehydrated just before surgery to overcome storage limitations. Second, the mechanical strength of the membrane can be improved by incorporating a nanofiber mesh as a support scaffold. Despite all the limitations, the AM remains a preferred choice of many clinicians for treating ocular disorders.

Collagen-derived scaffolds: Collagen is a crucial element of the corneal ECM, which provides structural support and aids in cell adhesion, proliferation, and differentiation. Collagen-based scaffolds have become increasingly popular as they closely resemble the natural corneal environment, facilitating cellular interactions and tissue integration. Germain et al.[9] and Orwin and Hubel[10] were some researchers who started exploring the use of collagen scaffolds in the initial days. However, they faced some challenges regarding its poor mechanical properties. To modify these properties of collagen scaffold, many

TABLE 2.1: Desired properties of scaffold for corneal regeneration.

Property of the scaffold	*Rationale/description*
Shape	Radius of approximately 7.8 mm is needed to avoid refractive error
Size	Depends on the type of injury and medical condition to treat. But for full thickness, 500–600 μm is appropriate
Transparency	Transmittance and refractive index close to human cornea. Acceptable transmittance value should be ≥87% and refractive index around 1.373[5]
Compressive modulus and tensile strength	Native cornea has a modulus of 300 kPA and a tensile strength of 3.8 MPa. Therefore, tuning the stiffness of the scaffold by either polymer/crosslinker concentration or crosslinking time is important
Swelling	Minimizing swelling is essential to ensure the scaffold's structural integrity, optical clarity, and compatibility with the surrounding tissues. Excessive swelling can lead to mechanical instability, distortion of the scaffold structure, and impaired integration with the host tissue
Porosity	The scaffold should have a porous structure to allow for nutrient and waste exchange, as well as cell infiltration, proliferation, and migration. An average porosity of 85% and pore diameter of 62 μm have been shown to support a population of corneal keratocytes in the scaffold[6]
Sterility	To minimize the risk of infection and adverse immune responses, scaffolds must be manufactured and handled under sterile conditions
Cytocompatibility	The scaffold should support the viability, growth, proliferation, migration, and differentiation of the corneal cells. Epithelial cells should demonstrate positive expression for markers such as CK3/12, connexin 43, and p63α, whereas stromal keratocytes should stain positively for markers including CD34, ALDH3, and ABCB5[7]
Other biological and clinical features	Low immune rejection rate, re-epithelization with proper barrier functions of the epithelial cells to reduce the risk of infection, should not aid blood vessel formation, promote corneal nerve innervation and biodegrade and promote stromal regeneration[8]

physical treatments or chemical agents were used to achieve intermolecular cross-linking of collagen. Among the physical treatments, ultraviolet (UV) irradiation, gamma radiation, and dehydro-thermal treatment (DHT)[11] are the most commonly used, while using crosslinkers like glutaraldehyde, 1-ethyl-3-(3-dimethyl aminopropyl)-carbodiimide hydrochloride (EDC) chemical modifications can be accomplished mainly by utilizing covalent linkages of amine/imine groups.[12] Though cross-linking strategies of the pure collagen scaffold enhanced the mechanical and structural properties, it was observed that it also introduced negative effects on cellular response in vivo. Hence, a mixture of natural or synthetic polymers is used to overcome the limitations of the mono-component system. Natural polymers [such as chitosan, silk fibroin, hyaluronic acid [HA], and alginate] are widely used in tissue engineering due to their similar features to native ECM. Synthetic polymers, such as poly (ε-caprolactone) (PCL), polylactic acid (PLA), PEG, polyglycolide (PGA), PLGA, and polyvinyl alcohol (PVA), are widely used for tissue engineering.

Decellularized corneal scaffolds: These are a promising option for corneal replacement when severe ocular surface damage or a high risk of rejection from allotransplantation is present. Decellularization involves removing cells and their debris to obtain an acellular scaffold composed of just the ECM. Sodium dodecyl sulfate (SDS) or hypertonic salt like NaCl with nucleases or nonionic detergents like Triton X-100 are the most effective methods for removing cells from human corneal tissue. The main advantage of using decellularized corneas is that the obtained scaffold is biochemically identical to the original tissue.[13] Additionally, the exquisite collagen arrangement in the corneal stroma can be maintained, which is difficult to replicate using other biomaterials. Although human corneas are mainly used for this purpose, studies have reported using porcine corneas due to their anatomical similarities to human corneas and broader availability. A recent study found that the porcine cornea had the highest similarity score to the humans compared to 13 other animals that could be used for decellularization. These animals included dogs, cats, sheep, goats, cows, horses, and rabbits. As far as its application is concerned, its efficacy has been defined both in vitro and in vivo setups, along with its success story in humans, where thin sections of human corneas were decellularized and implanted into patients with keratoconus to increase their stromal thickness and delay the need for transplantation.[14] Furthermore, AiNear Corneal Engineering Co. Ltd., a Chinese company, has developed a product that utilizes dehydrated decellularized porcine corneas. This product has successfully treated patients with fungal keratitis and herpes simplex keratitis, conditions with a high risk of graft rejection.[15] Hence, overall reports on the use of this product have been overwhelmingly positive.

3D Bioprinting

3D bioprinting is a multidisciplinary field that allows scientists to fabricate objects into a desired shape using a suitable bio-ink. This gives high-resolution and diversified patterns. The success of 3D bioprinting depends on the precise deposition of bio-inks in a desired pattern, corresponding to organotypic anatomic cues. This offers the advantages of personalizing refractive power, complex multilayer structure, and spatial heterogeneities.[16] 3D bioprinting has started to gain popularity as a corneal substitute, with its proven feasibility in many fields of tissue engineering, such as skin, cardiac muscle, and oral and maxillofacial tissue. For corneal 3D bioprinting, the bio-ink comprises biomaterial encapsulating the cells. This is then printed on biocompatible substrates layer by layer, forming a biomimetic 3D scaffold with uniform cell distribution.[17] Over the years, different bio-fabrication strategies have been employed to engineer corneal structures. Different types of 3D bioprinting strategies have been explored, such as pressure-assisted or extrusion-based, inkjet-based, acoustic and magnetic-based, laser-assisted, and stereolithography (SLA)-based techniques.

Numerous attempts have been made to create bio-printed corneas, with one of the earliest being in 2016. In that study, alginate-gelatin-collagen-based bio-ink and human corneal epithelial cells were used, but the transparency of the resulting corneas was poor.[18] Since then, various bio-inks have been tested, including alginate with methacrylate collagen, agarose blended with collagen, and corneal ECM, in combination with corneal stromal keratocytes.[19] For bioprinting to be successful, bio-ink must possess certain essential properties such as sufficient biomechanical strength, withstand pressure (equivalent or higher liquid pressure than the intraocular pressure), transparency, porosity, biocompatibility, and high cell viability. It should also encourage proper cell morphology and proper expression of specific proteins. The bio-ink must biodegrade to enable the cells to form their ECM and support themselves. In addition, the bio-ink must be permeable to oxygen and nutrients to ensure cell survival, even in the deeper layers of the construct. To meet these requirements, it is common to chemically modify the material. In summary, bioprinting corneas is a complex process that requires the perfect combination of bio-ink properties to achieve successful results. However, further research and development could lead to a revolutionary breakthrough in the field of ophthalmology.

Diverse Bioprinting Technologies

A variety of technologies are employed to regenerate corneal tissue by bioprinting **(Fig. 2.2)** which are described below.

Extrusion: This is a widely used and affordable technology for corneal bioprinting. The basic principle involves applying pressure to a cartridge to continuously dispense material through a nozzle.[20] This pressure can be generated through pneumatic or mechanical force to increase throughput. Using the appropriate nozzle size, up to 5 million cells per milliliter can be printed while maintaining cellular viability.[19] However, if the bio-ink is too viscous or if the nozzle size is inappropriate, the print head may become clogged, which is the only disadvantage of this technique.[21]

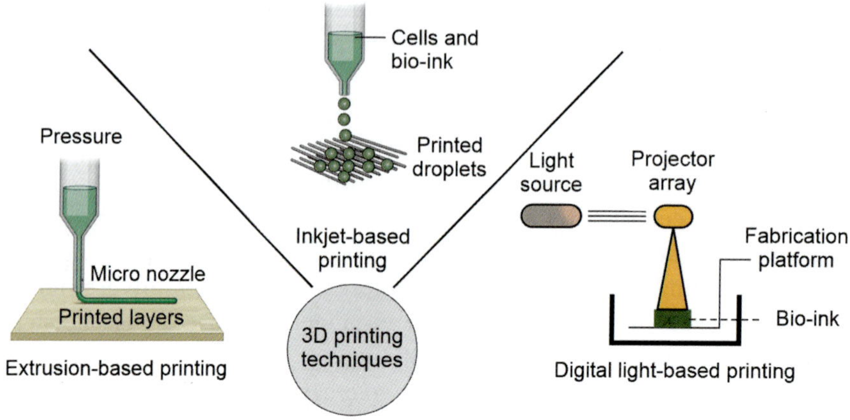

Fig. 2.2: Graphical representation of 3D printing techniques.

Inkjet assisted: A drop-on-demand bioprinting technique compatible with cells was investigated for creating 3D corneal tissues. In this technique, cells and bio-ink can be dispensed as a drop regulated using custom-made software. The software can control the interval between the drops and the distance between each deposited spot. The bioprinter uses a pressurized air supply mounted onto the print head with an electromagnetic microvalve. The pressurized air supply allows for the printing of dome-shaped 3D constructs with high printability and structural integrity. In 2019, Campos et al.[22] used a drop-on-demand inkjet-based bioprinting strategy based on an electromagnetic microvalve to construct 3D models that mimic the human cornea. They embedded primary human corneal keratocytes (hCKs) in an agarose/Col I bio-ink and dispensed the drops of bio-ink in a regulated manner, which resulted in a bio-printed cornea with reasonable optical transparency. In addition, they also showed that the viability and morphology of the hCKs were well maintained in the bio-printed construct even after 7 days in culture in vitro. However, there were few disadvantages to using the technique: First, the gel formed was on the softer side with a mechanical strength of around 15–20 kPa, and second, there was a long production time to make a single 3D printed cornea (more than 1 hour).

Light-based bioprinting: Light-based 3D bioprinting involves digital light processing (DLP) printing, SLA-based printing, and laser-assisted printing (LAP). SLA was the first type of light-assisted 3D printing, followed by DLP and LAP. These methods use a precise light projection to polymerize materials with high printing resolution, accuracy, and speed. Due to its gentle printing conditions, it is also suitable for printing live cells with high cell viability.[17] Gelatin methacrylate (GelMA) and HA are common bio-inks explored in these techniques along with corneal limbal epithelial or corneal stromal cells.

Of the three techniques, DLP is the fastest as all layer dots are processed at once. However, resolution is still a problem while creating curvature despite its resolution being as low as 10 μm.[23]

Challenges in 3D Bioprinting

Bioprinting has several advantages, such as automation, reproducibility, and the ability to print specific shapes. However, creating corneas using bioprinting has some limitations. One of the main limitations is that bioprinted corneas have poor optical properties compared to real corneal tissue. Although the bio-ink material used in printing is typically transparent, the final printed construct's surface is often rough, causing uneven light refraction. This is due to the printing process, which requires each printed layer to be slightly offset to generate a curved shape by printing flat layers. Another potential limitation of bioprinting is the difficulty replicating the collagen fibril organization found in the stroma. Hence, each bioprinting technique possesses specific strengths and weaknesses. In addition to all the mentioned limitations, another aspect that needs to be considered while translating the research from the laboratory to the benchside is its commercial value. The high cost of the printed cornea can be a significant limiting factor in the near future. However, despite these limitations, researchers are making great progress in improving and developing 3D-printed corneas using better bio-inks, which holds great potential.

Use of Bioengineered Cornea in Human Trials

In a study by Islam et al.,[5] a biomaterials-enabled proregeneration strategy using cell-free corneal implants made of recombinant human collagen and phosphorylcholine was tested in an open-label study of six unilaterally blind patients at high risk for donor allograft rejection. These patients underwent anterior lamellar keratoplasty and were followed for an average of 24 months. Early results showed that patients with acute ulceration experienced relief from pain within 1–2 weeks post operation and those with severe infection-induced scarring or ulceration saw notable vision improvement. However, patients with immune or degenerative conditions saw no vision improvement, though the procedure did enhance nerve regeneration and touch sensitivity in all participants. Three patients achieved significant vision improvements, and the rest stabilized enough for potential follow-up surgeries. While outcomes were better in mini-pigs, suggesting limitations in predictive accuracy for severely pathological human corneas, the study confirmed cell-free implants' safety and potential efficacy for high-risk patients.

In another 4-year study by Fagerholm et al.,[24] 10 patients with conditions like keratoconus or central scarring received biosynthetic corneal implants made from recombinant human collagen extracted from yeast. These implants were compared to traditional donor corneas used in penetrating keratoplasty. The biosynthetic implants, which were less rigid and required suturing, showed superior optical transparency with transmission rates over 87% and integrated well into patient corneas, maintaining consistent shape and thickness. Assessments included techniques like slit-lamp microscopy and in vivo confocal microscopy, revealing that the regenerated epithelium mirrored healthy corneal structure and the implants attracted stromal cells over time, though some areas remained cell-free. Notably, the biosynthetic implants supported more organized nerve structures than the donor corneas and did not provoke significant immune responses, avoiding the need for immunosuppressive therapy. Overall, the implants improved visual acuity significantly, demonstrating their potential as a viable alternative to donor corneas in transplant surgeries.

Buznyk et al.[25] developed corneal implants using a composite of cross-linked recombinant human collagen type III (RHCIII) and 2-methacryloyloxyethyl phosphorylcholine (MPC), a synthetic phospholipid known for its antifouling properties which got Food and Drug Administration (FDA) approval for vascular stent coatings. The combination is designed to prevent neovascularization. The study involved three high-risk patients who underwent the removal of diseased corneal tissue and implantation of the biosynthetic material. Follow-up assessments for 12 months included visual acuity, slit-lamp bio-microscopy, and confocal microscopy. The implants matched the optical properties of healthy corneas but had lower mechanical strength, though sufficient for surgical use. Epithelialization was complete within 6 weeks, and the implants showed no neovascularization or significant complications over 9–12 months. Early postoperative issues like mild edema and haze responded to topical steroids, stabilizing without long-term immunosuppression. Initial results indicate that these implants can effectively replace diseased corneas in high-risk patients and support further treatments to enhance visual outcomes.

In the latest study involving two clinical cohorts, a bioengineered porcine collagen implant (BPCDX), which underwent double crosslinking, was used for minimally invasive vision restoration in advanced keratoconus.[26] Inserted into an intrastromal pocket within the recipient's cornea, the BPCDX implant is made from medical-grade type I porcine collagen, adhering to good manufacturing practices (GMP) to ensure high safety and quality. Combining chemical and photochemical treatments, the double crosslinking process enhances the implant's structural integrity, increasing its strength and resistance to enzymatic degradation. Comparative studies using a collagenase solution showed that BPCDX degrades slower than its single-crosslinked counterpart, indicating greater durability. Clinical data from Iran and India demonstrated that the implant improved corneal thickness and curvature and maintained transparency without adverse events, scars, or further surgeries. Over 24 months, these improvements were sustained, significantly enhancing visual acuity and showing the potential of BPCDX as a durable treatment for advanced keratoconus. These results support the adoption of this suture-free technique as a standard treatment for keratoconus.

FUTURE DIRECTIONS

Advances in biomaterials have led to a revolutionary method for managing corneal issues like fibrosis and inflammation. Developing a biomaterial-based sacrificial matrix incorporating bioactive molecules offers significant potential as a cutting-edge treatment for these complex eye conditions. This innovative therapeutic strategy is based on the natural principles of tissue regeneration, where the biomaterials support initial healing and create a favorable environment for ongoing regeneration. In keeping with this strategy, the authors have achieved successful results in animal studies by excising the partial-thickness scar and replacing it with a biomimetic hydrogel scaffold designed to promote corneal regeneration. We have developed a biodegradable hydrogel,[27] Kuragel, in the functionalized gelatin and HA form photo-cross-linkable hydrogel with transparency and compressive modulus similar to healthy human cornea. Kuragel composition is also tuned to achieve sufficient adhesive strength for sutureless integration to host tissue, with minimal swelling post administration. Studies in the New Zealand rabbit mechanical injury model affecting corneal epithelium and stroma demonstrate that Kuragel efficiently promotes re-epithelialization within 1 month of administration, while stroma and sub-basal nerve plexus regenerate within 3 months **(Figs. 2.3A to S)**. This promising method requires that the endothelium remains unaffected and, hence, does not address all corneal pathologies that necessitate a transplant.

In collaboration with the Defence Research and Development Organization, the authors are also undertaking an ambitious translational project that seeks to offer a groundbreaking solution to developing the entire cornea. This cutting-edge initiative aims to eliminate reliance on human tissue by ingeniously crafting a suturable material that possesses the necessary structural characteristics to mimic the cornea and also maintains exceptional corneal clarity.

Meanwhile, the bioactive molecules critically drive this regenerative process; each element has its limitations when used alone. A holistic approach that combines multiple components and integrates concepts from tissue engineering and regenerative medicine is more effective in achieving positive outcomes.

CONCLUSION

The significance of these innovative breakthroughs cannot be overstated. By obviating the need for human tissue, these projects hold the potential to

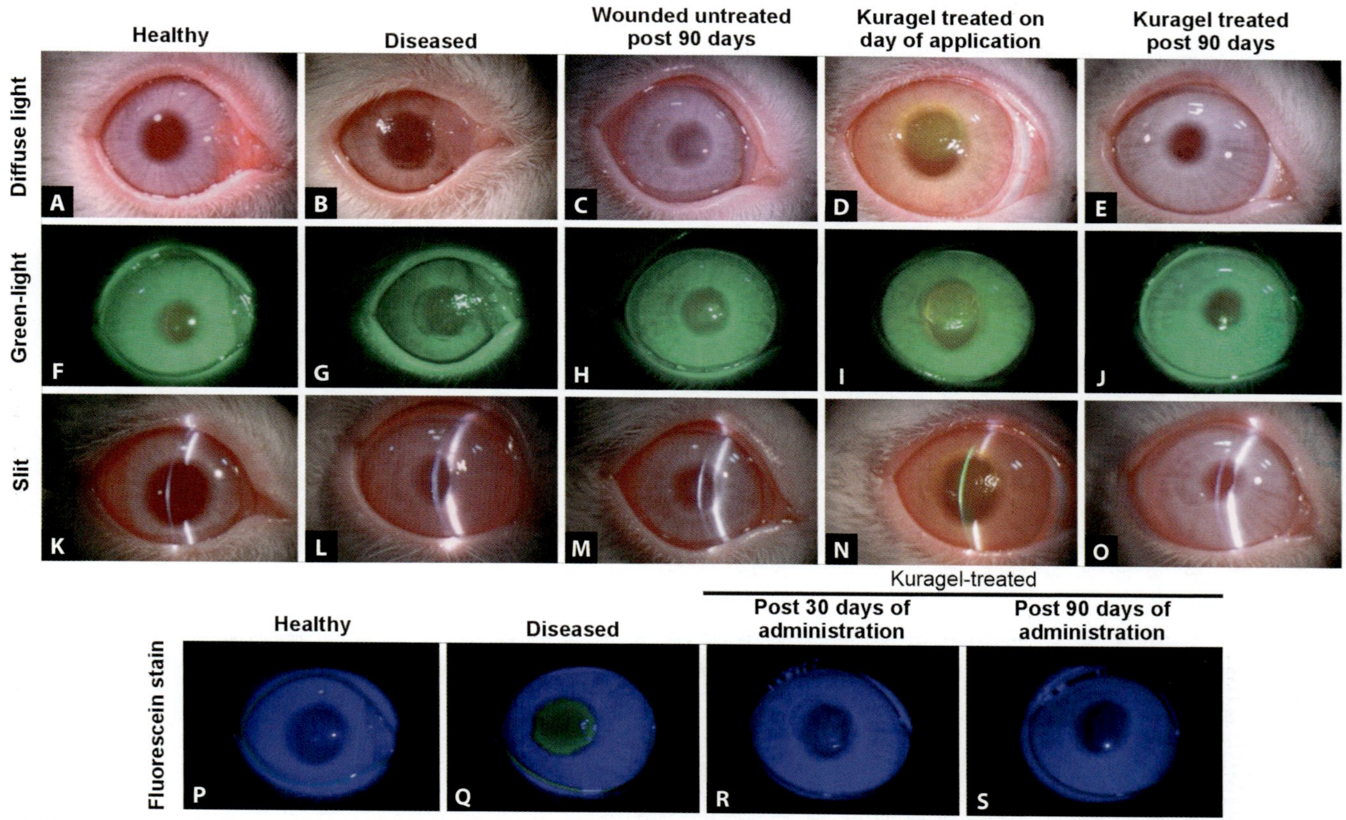

Figs. 2.3A to S: Slit-lamp examination of healthy, diseased, wounded untreated and Kuragel-treated rabbit cornea at the time of administration and post 90 days of treatment: (A to E) Diffuse light indicates cornea clarity; (F to J) Green light indicates neovascularization; (K to O) Slit-beam indicates complete corneal curvature; (P to S) Fluorescein stain indicates an epithelial defect in the cobalt blue filter.

address the persistently challenging issue of corneal transplantation, which is hindered by limited availability and compatibility constraints. Moreover, developing a suturable material specifically designed for corneal applications presents a versatile and scalable approach that can benefit a wider population of patients needing corneal restoration.

With the current pace of development, we can confidently achieve tangible advancements that will profoundly impact the field of ophthalmology and improve the lives of countless individuals needing corneal restoration.

REFERENCES

1. Wang M, Li Y, Wang H, Li M, Wang X, Liu R, et al. Corneal regeneration strategies: from stem cell therapy to tissue engineered stem cell scaffolds. Biomed Pharmacother. 2023;165:115206.
2. Oliva MS, Schottman T, Gulati M. Turning the tide of corneal blindness. Indian J Ophthalmol. 2012;60(5):423-7.
3. Vashist P, Senjam SS, Gupta V, Gupta N, Shamanna BR, Wadhwani M, et al. Blindness and visual impairment and their causes in India: results of a nationally representative survey. PLoS One. 2022;17(7):0271736.
4. Gain P, Jullienne R, He Z, Aldossary M, Acquart S, Cognasse F, et al. Global survey of corneal transplantation and eye banking. JAMA Ophthalmol. 2016;134(2):167-73.
5. Islam MM, Buznyk O, Reddy JC, Pasyechnikova N, Alarcon EI, Hayes S, et al. Biomaterials-enabled cornea regeneration in patients at high risk for rejection of donor tissue transplantation. NPJ Regen Med. 2018;3:2.
6. Vrana NE, Builles N, Justin V, Bednarz J, Pellegrini G, Ferrari B, et al. Development of a reconstructed cornea from collagen-chondroitin sulfate foams and human cell cultures. Invest Ophthalmol Vis Sci. 2008;49(12):5325-31.
7. Miyashita H, Shimmura S, Kobayashi H, Taguchi T, Asano-Kato N, Uchino Y, et al. Collagen-immobilized poly(vinyl alcohol) as an artificial cornea scaffold that supports a stratified corneal epithelium. J Biomed Mater Res B Appl Biomater. 2006;76(1):56-63.
8. Roshandel D, Eslani M, Baradaran-Rafii A, Cheung AY, Kurji K, Jabbehdari S, et al. Current and emerging therapies for corneal neovascularization. Ocul Surf. 2018;16(4):398-414.
9. Germain L, Auger FA, Grandbois E, Guignard R, Giasson M, Boisjoly H, et al. Reconstructed human cornea produced in vitro by tissue engineering. Pathobiology. 1999;67(3):140-7.
10. Orwin EJ, Hubel A. In vitro culture characteristics of corneal epithelial, endothelial, and keratocyte cells in a native collagen matrix. Tissue Eng. 2000; 6(4):307-19.
11. Wang W, Zhang Y, Ye R, Ni Y. Physical crosslinkings of edible collagen casing. Int J Biol Macromol. 2015;81:920-5.
12. Suchy T, Supova M, Sauerova P, Verdanova M, Sucharda Z, Ryglova S, et al. The effects of different cross-linking conditions on collagen-based nanocomposite scaffolds-an in vitro evaluation using mesenchymal stem cells. Biomed Mater. 2015;10(6):065008.

13. Wilson SL, Sidney LE, Dunphy SE, Dua HS, Hopkinson A. Corneal decellularization: a method of recycling unsuitable donor tissue for clinical translation? Curr Eye Res. 2016;41(6):769-82.
14. Alio Del Barrio JL, Alio JL. Cellular therapy of the corneal stroma: a new type of corneal surgery for keratoconus and corneal dystrophies. Eye Vis (Lond). 2018; 5:28.
15. Cengiz N, Wareham CS. Ethical considerations in xenotransplantation: a review. Curr Opin Organ Transplant. 2020;25(5):483-8.
16. Zema L, Melocchi A, Maroni A, Gazzaniga A. Three-dimensional printing of medicinal products and the challenge of personalized therapy. J Pharm Sci. 2017;106(7):1697-705.
17. Zhang J, Hu Q, Wang S, Tao J, Gou M. Digital light processing based three-dimensional printing for medical applications. Int J Bioprint. 2020;6(1):242.
18. Wu Z, Su X, Xu Y, Kong B, Sun W, Mi S. Bioprinting three-dimensional cell-laden tissue constructs with controllable degradation. Sci Rep. 2016;6:24474.
19. Kim H, Jang J, Park J, Lee KP, Lee S, Lee DM, et al. Shear-induced alignment of collagen fibrils using 3D cell printing for corneal stroma tissue engineering. Biofabrication. 2019;11(3):035017.
20. Yilmaz B, Tahmasebifar A, Baran ET. Bioprinting technologies in tissue engineering. Adv Biochem Eng Biotechnol. 2020;171:279-319.
21. Adhikari J, Roy A, Das A, Ghosh M, Thomas S, Sinha A, et al. Effects of processing parameters of 3D bioprinting on the cellular activity of bioinks. Macromol Biosci. 2021;21(1):e2000179.
22. Campos DDF, Rohde M, Ross M, Anvari P, Blaeser A, Vogt M, et al. Corneal bioprinting utilizing collagen-based bioinks and primary human keratocytes. J Biomed Mater Res A. 2019;107(9):1945-53.
23. Wu Y, Su H, Li M, Xing H. Digital light processing-based multi-material bioprinting: processes, applications, and perspectives. J Biomed Mater Res A. 2023;111(4):527-42.
24. Fagerholm P, Lagali NS, Ong JA, Merrett K, Jackson WB, Polarek JW, et al. Stable corneal regeneration four years after implantation of a cell-free recombinant human collagen scaffold. Biomaterials. 2014;35(8):2420-7.
25. Buznyk O, Pasyechnikova N, Islam MM, Iakymenko S, Fagerholm P, Griffith M. Bioengineered corneas grafted as alternatives to human donor corneas in three high-risk patients. Clin Transl Sci. 2015;8(5):558-62.
26. Rafat M, Jabbarvand M, Sharma N, Xeroudaki M, Tabe S, Omrani R, et al. Bioengineered corneal tissue for minimally invasive vision restoration in advanced keratoconus in two clinical cohorts. Nat Biotechnol. 2023;41(1):70-81.
27. Agrawal P, Tiwari A, Chowdhury SK, Vohra M, Gour A, Waghmare N, et al. Kuragel: a biomimetic hydrogel scaffold designed to promote corneal regeneration. iScience. 2024;27(5):109641.

3 CHAPTER

Diagnosis and Management of Pediatric Keratoconus

Neet Mehta, Sunita Chaurasia, Muralidhar Ramappa

ABSTRACT

Keratoconus is a noninflammatory, progressive ectatic condition of the cornea. Pediatric keratoconus (PKC) differs significantly from the adult-onset form, primarily due to delays in initial diagnosis and the rapidity of progression of the disease. This rapid progression is attributed to the pliable and elastic nature of the cornea in children, which is not biologically cross-linked, and plausible risk factors such as incessant eye rubbing due to uncorrected refractive errors, unrecognized allergies, or blepharokeratoconjunctivitis. As a result, the condition is often presented at an advanced stage, making management in young children particularly challenging and prone to complications like hydrops and their consequences like scarring, vascularization, or apical scarring. Therefore, early diagnosis, prompt guidance against eye rubbing, proper management of allergic or blepharitic eye conditions, and timely preventive interventions are crucial for effective management. This discussion focuses on recent advances in PKC diagnosis and treatment modalities.

Keywords: Pediatric keratoconus, corneal ectasia, collagen cross-linking, contact lenses

INTRODUCTION

Pediatric keratoconus (PKC) is a corneal ectasia that affects children and adolescents below 18 years of age. The prevalence of PKC is approximately 0.16%.[1] This condition tends to follow a very aggressive course compared to adult keratoconus, with rapid progression and an advanced stage of disease at the time of diagnosis.[2] Nearly 40% of PKC cases are associated with some form of systemic allergy, with vernal keratoconjunctivitis (VKC) being the most common ocular association.[3,4] These cases pose a significant burden on society as they impact the social, economic, and educational development of the affected individuals and their families. Early detection and timely, appropriate intervention lead to better outcomes in children.

DIAGNOSIS

Pediatric keratoconus typically manifests as bilateral, asymmetrical corneal ectasia. Its clinical features resemble those seen in adults, including frequent changes in spectacles, the presence of scissors reflex on retinoscopy, the oil droplet sign (Charleux sign) observed through a distant direct ophthalmoscope or retro-illumination, and Munson's and Rizzuti's signs on torchlight examination in advanced keratoconus. Slit-lamp examination often reveals a central or inferior-paracentral cone, with the base of the cone clearly defined by an epithelial iron line known as Fleischer's ring, visible through a cobalt blue filter. Other findings may include Vogt striae, prominent corneal nerves, apical scarring, and, occasionally, the presence of hydrops. Many cases also exhibit signs of ocular allergies, such as papillary reaction, limbal thickening, and perilimbal conjunctival pigment stippling, suggesting an association with VKC. Unlike adults, PKC may present with a positive family history, associated systemic syndromes, and some degree of amblyopia due to its asymmetric nature.[5]

Diagnostic Dilemma

Diagnosing keratoconus in pediatric patients can be challenging. While slit-lamp evaluation is the gold standard for diagnosis, the characteristic changes are typically observed in moderate-to-severe stages of the disease. As a result, these changes may not be very obvious in the early stages of keratoconus, leading to cases going undiagnosed in children. Early screening, along with prompt treatment, is, therefore, recommended in this age group to prevent poor outcomes associated with unmanaged keratoconus.[6] Mass screening for keratoconus is particularly recommended in children with high-risk features,[7] which are mentioned below:

- Allergic eye disease
- Children living in high altitude/high ultraviolet (UV) exposure
- Geographic areas with a high incidence of PKC
- Children with Down's syndrome
- Family history of PKC
- School children with myopia and myopic astigmatism

Apart from these, certain clinical features predispose them to higher rates of progression and more aggressive course. These include:

- Thinner corneal thickness
- Higher average central corneal keratometry
- Increased posterior corneal elevation
- History of severe eye rubbing
- History of allergic eye disease

Review of Literature

Studies have shown that certain factors, such as smoking[8] and glycosylated end products,[9] induce collagen cross-linking (CXL), which increases corneal stiffening and may offer a protective mechanism against the progression of corneal ectasia. Conversely, eye rubbing, genetic susceptibility, female gender, and hypothyroidism are associated with an increased risk of progressive keratoconus.

Several classifications have been proposed and utilized in clinical settings to achieve a more consistent grading of keratoconus severity. Among the most commonly used are the Amsler-Krumeich classification[10,11] which is based on the mean corneal power, astigmatism, transparency, and thinnest corneal thickness **(Table 3.1)** and the newer Belin ABCD grading system,[12] which takes into consideration the anterior and posterior curvatures around the area of maximum thinning apart from pachymetry and distance best-corrected visual acuity (BCVA) **(Table 3.2)**.

TABLE 3.1: Amsler–Krumeich classification of keratoconus.

Grades	*Characteristics*
Stage 1	• Eccentric steeping • Myopia and astigmatism <5 D • Mean central K readings <48 D
Stage 2	• Myopia and astigmatism from 5 to 8 D • Mean central K readings <53 D • Absence of scarring • Minimum corneal thickness >400 μm
Stage 3	• Myopia and astigmatism from 8 to 10 D • Mean central K readings >53 D • Absence of scarring • Minimum corneal thickness from 300 to 400 μm
Stage 4	• Refraction not measurable • Mean central K readings >55 D • Central corneal scarring • Minimum corneal thickness 200 μm

TABLE 3.2: New ABCD system for classification of keratoconus.

ABCD criteria	*A ARC (3 mm Zone)*	*B PRC (3 mm Zone)*	*C Thinnest pach (μm)*	*D BDVA*	*Scarring*
Stage 0	>7.25 mm (<46.5 D)	>5.90 mm (<57.25 D)	>490	=20/20 (=1.0)	–
Stage I	>7.05 mm (<48.0 D)	>5.70 mm (<59.25 D)	>450	<20/20 (<1.0)	–, +, ++
Stage II	>6.35 mm (<53.0 D)	>5.15 mm (<65.5 D)	>400	<20/40 (<0.5)	–, +, ++
Stage III	>6.15 mm (<55.0 D)	>4.95 mm (<68.5 D)	>300	<20/100 (<0.2)	–, +, ++
Stage IV	<6.15 mm (>55.0 D)	<4.95 mm (>68.5 D)	= 300	<20/400 (<0.05)	–, +, ++

(ARC: anterior radius of curvature; BDVA: best distance visual acuity; PRC: posterior radius of curvature)

While keratoconus is a clinical diagnosis typically made via slit-lamp examination, early recognition often relies on other diagnostic imaging modalities, including corneal topography, tomography, anterior segment optical coherence tomography (AS-OCT), aberrometry, and ocular response analyzers (ORA).

Corneal topography: Placido disk-based corneal topography, which measures the anterior curvature, was once the gold standard for early diagnosis and detection of astigmatism progression and keratometry values. These, however, have the limitation of measuring only the anterior curvature and not taking into account the changes in the posterior curvature.

Corneal tomography: Tomographers, such as Scheimpflug imaging, optical coherence tomography (OCT), and slit-scan tomography, are particularly effective and measure both anterior and posterior curvatures and have now taken precedence in the early recognition of this condition **(Figs. 3.1A and B)**. There are various parameters that are predictors of an ectatic cornea which includes inferior–superior dioptric asymmetry, central corneal power, Sim-K astigmatism, skewed radial axis, etc. Based on these parameters, numerous indices have been established like Rabinowitz criteria,[13] KISA% Index,[14] Belin/Ambrósio Enhanced Ectasia Display, Maeda and Klyce, etc. For instance, the Pentacam (Oculus, Germany), using Scheimpflug technology,

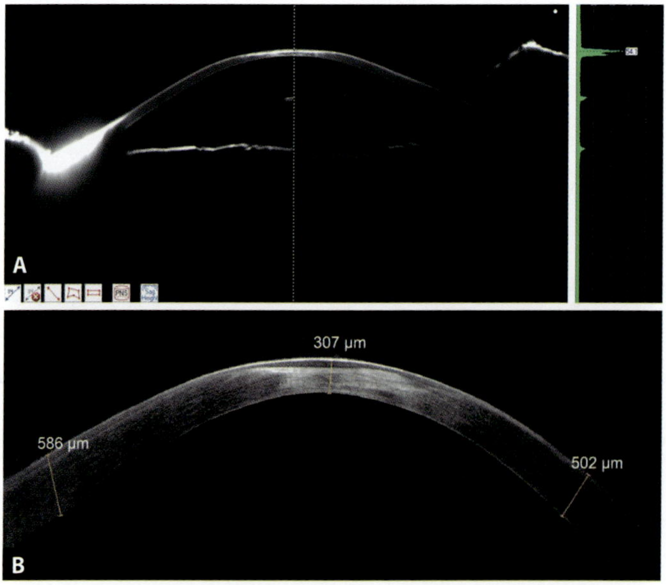

Figs. 3.1A and B: (A) Scheimpflug image of keratoconus along with corresponding densitometry scan; (B) Anterior segment optical coherence tomography in keratoconus showing ectasia along with central compensatory epithelial thickening.

employs the Belin/Ambrósio Enhanced Ectasia Display (BAD) program[15] to assess the likelihood of corneal ectasia by combining pachymetry maps with anterior and posterior elevation maps **(Figs. 3.2 and 3.3)**. These methods are superior in detecting early keratoconus, as posterior curvature changes can be observed even in mild cases. Ultrasound pachymetry remains an effective method to determine and monitor the progression of corneal thickness.

Epithelial mapping: The epithelial thickness map **(Fig. 3.4)** serves as a supplementary tool for diagnosing keratoconus in cases where topography and tomography are suggestive, but not definitive of keratoconus. The two most commonly used techniques for obtaining epithelial maps are OCT and high-frequency digital ultrasound. It is seen that in keratoconus, the epithelium tends to compensate for the underlying stromal ectasia by thinning at the apex of the cone and thickening around it. This creates a pattern resembling a "donut."[16,17] In case of advanced ectasia due to Bowman's layer fragmentation, the overlying epithelium thickness increases, while the stroma may actually have significant thinning which can cause a discrepancy while planning for CXL for these patients.

Corneal hysteresis: The Ocular Response Analyzer is a noncontact tonometer that measures the cornea's deformation response to an air puff **(Fig. 3.5)**. Corneal biomechanics seeks to understand and forecast changes in corneal structure over time and their potential impact on vision. *Corneal hysteresis* is defined as the difference between the pressure at which the cornea bends inward during air-puff applanation and the pressure at which it bends outward. This difference, measured in millimeters of mercury, assesses the elasticity of the cornea. This value is usually lower in patients with keratoconus than in healthy controls; however, much overlap exists with the normal population and may diminish the diagnostic potential of this measurement.[18]

Progressive Keratoconus

Progressive keratoconus is defined as an increase in one or more diopters of K-max over 12 months.[19] In the pediatric age group, the disease progresses very rapidly, necessitating more frequent follow-ups compared to adult keratoconus, which can be monitored for progression every 6 months.

MANAGEMENT

Pediatric keratoconus tends to have a higher rate of progression and usually presents in a more advanced stage. Early cases may benefit from a simple spectacle prescription; however, as irregular astigmatism progresses, children often become uncomfortable with glasses and present with a history of frequent changes and dissatisfaction with spectacles. It is crucial to emphasize that eye rubbing should be strictly avoided, as it is associated with increased

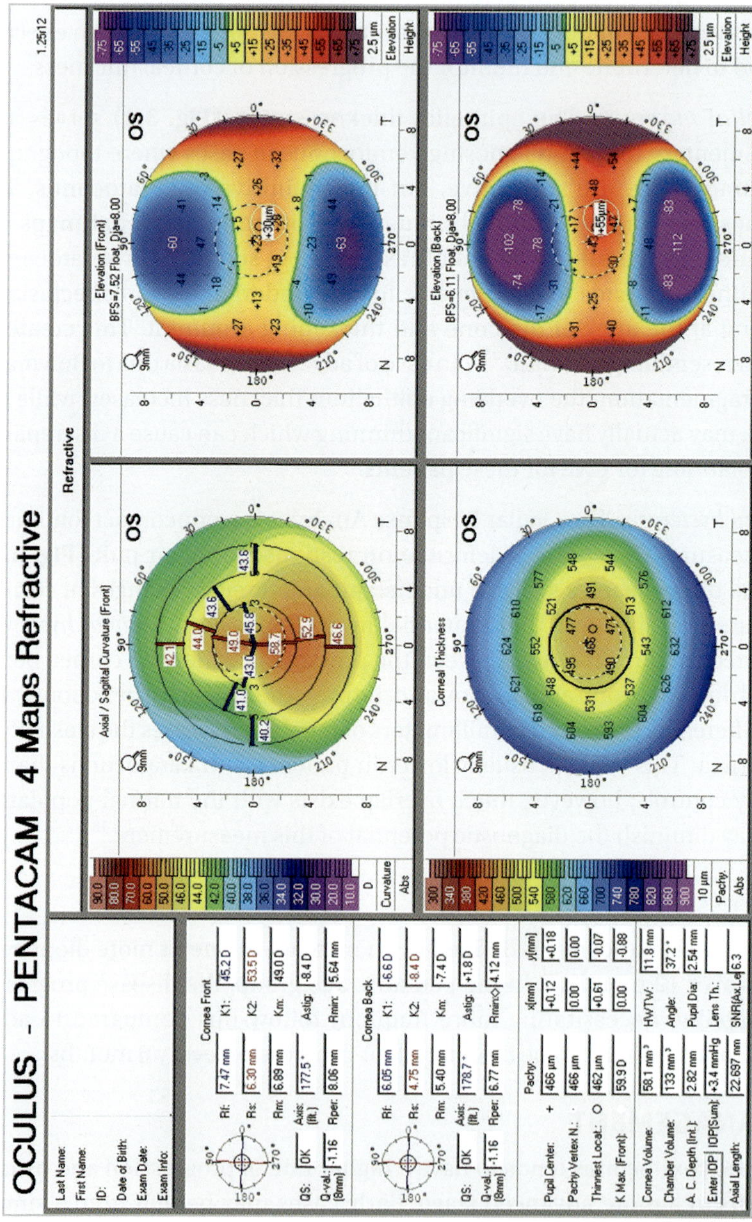

Fig. 3.2: Tomography of keratoconus showing the curvature, thickness, and elevation maps.

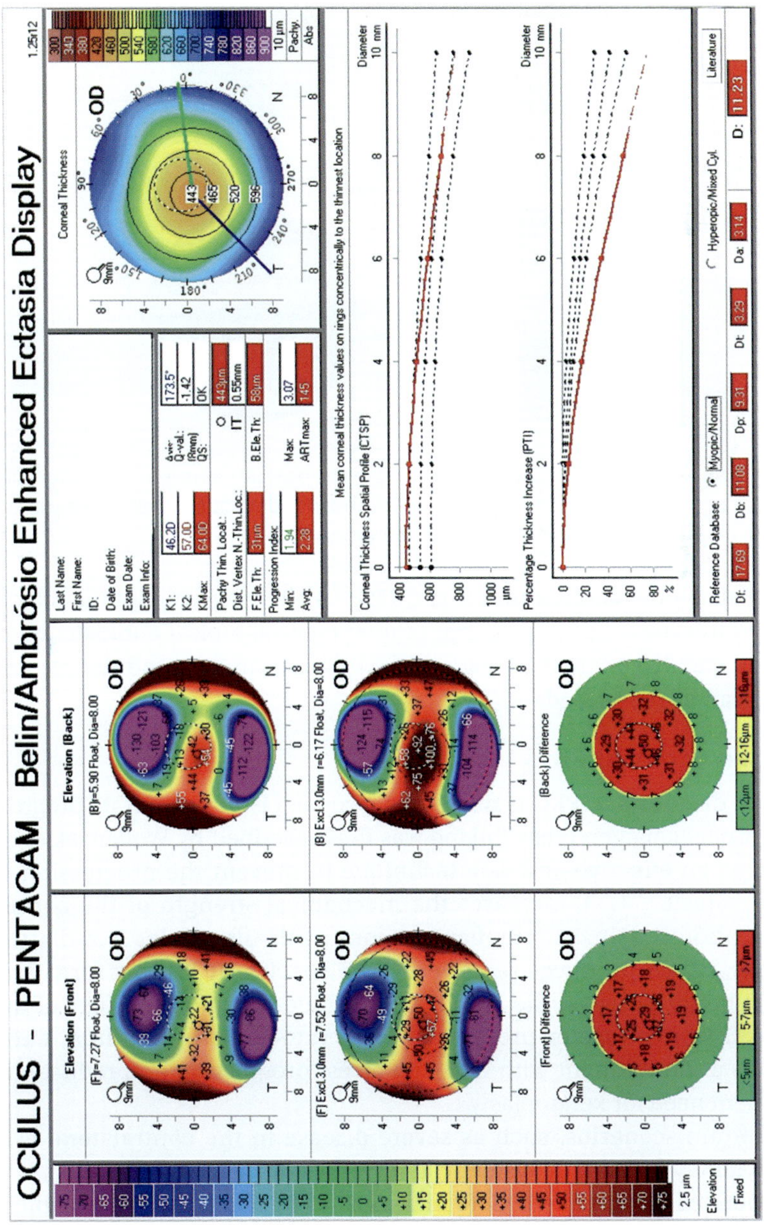

Fig. 3.3: Belin/Ambrósio-enhanced ectasia display in keratoconus.

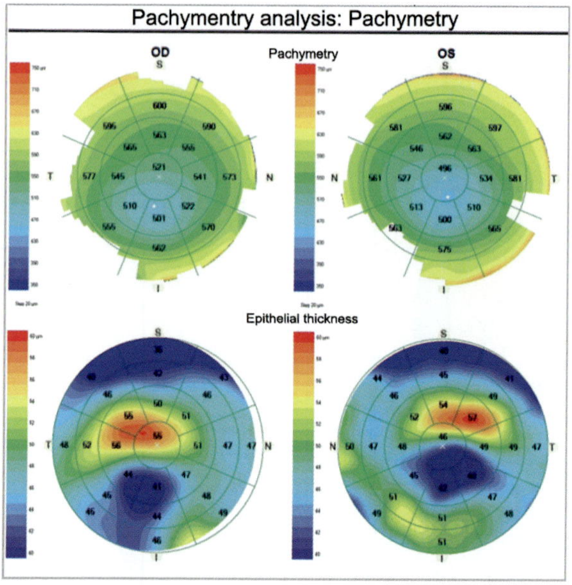

Fig. 3.4: Epithelial mapping on anterior segment optical coherence tomography showing the focal area of epithelial thickening corresponding to the area of ectasia as a surrogate marker for the diagnosis of keratoconus.

levels of matrix metalloproteinase-13 (MMP-13), leading to apoptotic activity of the keratocytes.[20] To keep allergies under control, topical antihistamines, mast cell stabilizers, dual-acting agents, topical immunomodulators, and steroids can be prescribed.

Collagen Cross-linking

Once the diagnosis of PKC is made, the next step is to prevent its progression. Corneal collagen cross-linking was first described by Wollensak et al. in 2003 as an effective and safe technique to prevent the progression of corneal ectasia.[21] CXL increases the mechanical strength of the cornea using a photosensitizer (riboflavin) along with ultraviolet A radiation (370 nm), which produces reactive oxygen species (ROS) that form new covalent bonds between the amino acid residues in collagen fibers of the cornea. Given the faster progression of keratoconus in children, early diagnosis and treatment with CXL can arrest progression and reduce the subsequent need for keratoplasty.

In certain scenarios, such as severe disease in the contralateral eye, positive family history, or systemic associations like Down syndrome, it is recommended to expedite CXL to maximize its benefits. The contraindications for CXL are the same as those in adults, including a corneal thickness of <400 μm, severe allergic conjunctivitis, severe dry eyes, corneal opacities, or infection. Various protocols have been proposed for CXL to optimize outcomes.

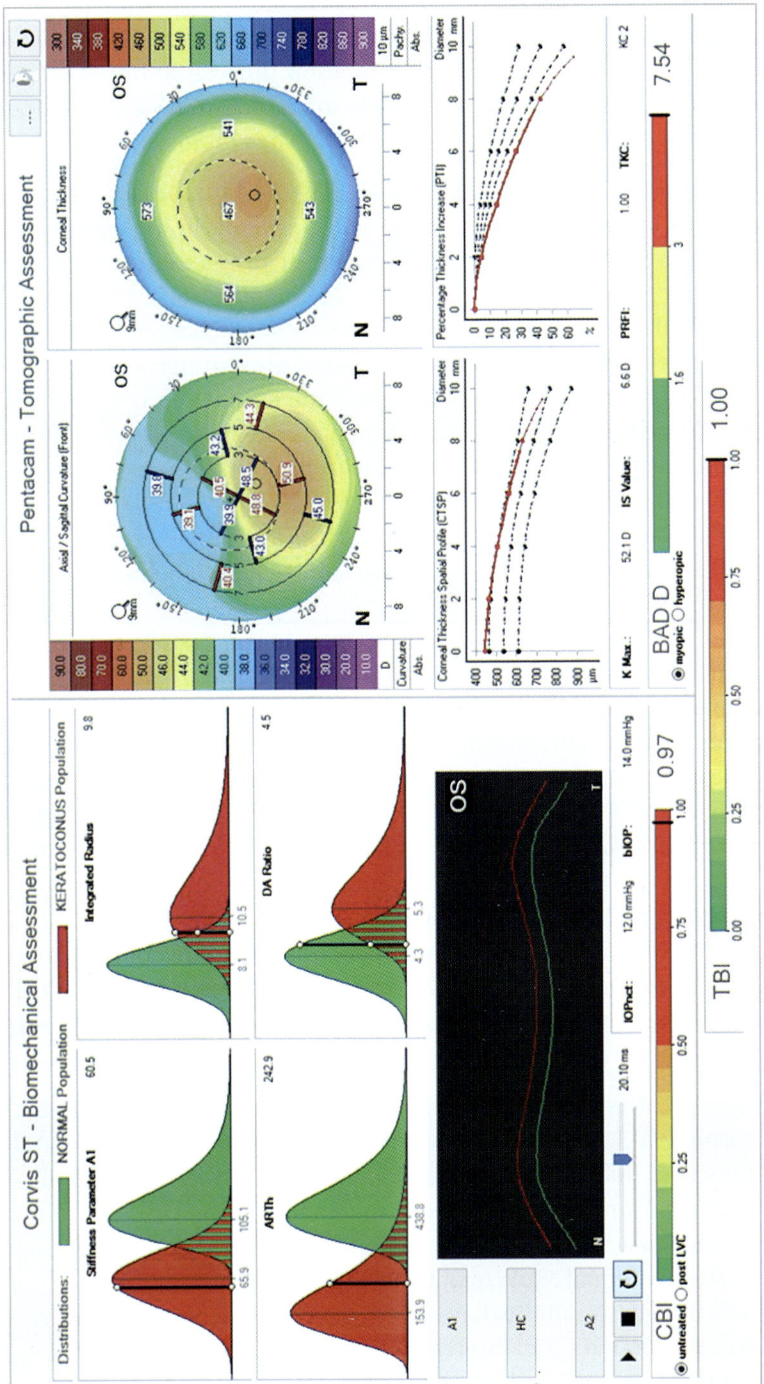

Fig. 3.5: Ocular response analyzer.

Standard Dresden protocol for CXL: The original cross-linking protocol involves the removal of the central corneal epithelium up to 9 mm. Riboflavin 0.1% is then applied as a photosensitizer, one drop every 2 minutes for 30 minutes. This is followed by an irradiation time of 30 minutes using 370 nm ultraviolet-A (UVA) light with an irradiance of 3 mW/cm^2. This protocol is commonly referred to as the *Dresden protocol.*[21]

Transepithelial CXL: Transepithelial CXL (TE CXL) presents a significant advancement in the field of corneal CXL, particularly for cases where epithelial debridement can be challenging or problematic, such as in children under topical anesthesia. The conventional epi-off CXL procedure has its drawbacks, including postoperative pain, corneal haze, infection risks, and other potential complications like reactivation of herpes and sterile infiltrations. In contrast, epi-on CXL, where the epithelium remains intact during the procedure, offers several advantages like reduced postoperative pain, lower infection rates, and the ability to perform the procedure in an outpatient setting.

One of the key challenges with epi-on CXL is the limited permeability of intact epithelium to molecules with a high molar mass, such as riboflavin, which is crucial for the cross-linking process. To address this limitation, modifications to the technique have been introduced. These modifications include the use of agents like benzalkonium (BAK), benzoate application, and iontophoresis, which help promote the penetration of riboflavin through the intact epithelium. One specific modification is the use of 0.1% riboflavin in a 15% dextran solution supplemented with trometamol and EDTA, known as Ricrolin-TE.[22,23] These additives facilitate the penetration of riboflavin into the corneal stroma, allowing for effective cross-linking even with the epithelium intact. Despite these advancements, studies still generally consider conventional epi-off CXL as superior to epi-on CXL. This is likely due to factors such as better riboflavin penetration and overall efficacy in halting keratoconus progression. However, ongoing research and refinements in techniques may continue to improve the outcomes of epi-on CXL, making it a viable option for certain patient populations and clinical scenarios.

Accelerated CXL: It is an innovative approach aimed at reducing the duration of the corneal CXL procedure while maintaining its effectiveness. The concept involves delivering a higher irradiance of UVA light, which allows for a shorter exposure time compared to the standard protocol. For example, protocols might use 9 mW/cm^2 for 10 minutes or 30 mW/cm^2 for 4 minutes instead of the traditional 3 mW/cm^2 for 30 minutes.[24-26]

Several comparative studies have investigated the outcomes of accelerated versus nonaccelerated CXL. Interestingly, nonaccelerated CXL has shown significant flattening of Kmax (maximum keratometry) and improvements in BCVA and Kmax compared to accelerated CXL. While the exact reasons for this disparity are not fully understood, animal studies suggest that nonaccelerated CXL may lead to superior anterior stromal stiffening compared to the accelerated approach.

In addition to accelerated CXL, other modifications in the CXL technique are being explored to enhance its efficacy and safety. These include the following:

- *Cross-hatched grid pattern for epithelial debridement:* This technique involves creating a cross-hatched pattern during epithelial removal, which may improve the distribution of riboflavin and UVA absorption in the cornea, potentially enhancing the cross-linking effect.
- *Contact lens-assisted cross-linking:* Using a contact lens during the CXL procedure can help maintain a consistent and controlled environment, improve riboflavin penetration, and enhance UVA delivery to the cornea, leading to more predictable outcomes.

These modifications represent ongoing efforts to optimize the CXL procedure, tailor it to individual patient needs, and improve outcomes in conditions like keratoconus and corneal ectasia. Further research and clinical studies are needed to fully understand the benefits and limitations of these modified techniques and their long-term effects on corneal biomechanics and visual outcomes.

Pulsed CXL: It is a promising variation of the corneal CXL procedure that aims to optimize the availability of oxygen during the treatment process, potentially enhancing its depth and efficacy. Oxygen plays a crucial role in the cross-linking process as it contributes to the formation of ROS that facilitate CXL.[27]

In accelerated CXL protocols, where higher irradiance and shorter exposure times are used, there is concern that there may not be sufficient time for oxygen replenishment in the corneal stroma. This could potentially limit the effectiveness of the treatment. Pulsed CXL addresses this issue by utilizing pulsing of the UVA irradiation. By pulsing the UVA light, intervals of darkness are introduced, allowing more oxygen to diffuse into the corneal stroma during these periods of rest. This increased oxygen availability is theorized to enhance the depth and efficacy of the cross-linking process.

However, it is essential to note that there is currently limited data available on pulsed CXL compared to traditional continuous UVA irradiation methods. Research and clinical studies are ongoing to evaluate the safety, efficacy, and long-term outcomes of pulsed CXL. As more data becomes available, this technique may offer a valuable alternative or adjunct to standard CXL protocols, particularly in cases where optimizing oxygen availability is critical for treatment success.

Topography-guided CXL: It is an advanced technique that customizes the corneal CXL procedure based on the specific topographic features of an individual's cornea. This approach allows for the treatment to be tailored according to the unique cone shape and distribution of corneal thinning, providing a more personalized intervention. In topography-guided CXL, UV intensity is modulated based on the corneal topography data, targeting the areas with the most significant irregularities and steepening. This method aims to enhance the efficacy of the CXL procedure by focusing the treatment more precisely where it is needed. A randomized controlled trial has demonstrated that topography-guided CXL can yield superior results in terms of spherical equivalent and visual acuity at 12 months post-treatment compared to standard CXL. This suggests that by customizing the UV irradiation pattern according to corneal topography, better refractive and visual outcomes can be achieved for patients with keratoconus or other corneal ectatic disorders. As with other advanced CXL techniques, ongoing research and long-term studies are needed to further validate the benefits of topography-guided CXL and establish standardized protocols for its implementation in clinical practice.[28]

Safety Margin of CXL

While CXL is safe in long-term follow-ups of adults,[29] in the pediatric age group, the longest follow-up available in a study is 7.5 years.[30] Complications include epithelial defects, ulceration, infection, sterile infiltration, endothelial damage, and rarely limbal cell loss.

Contact Lens

Contact lenses provide superior quality of vision to these patients as compared to glasses and a variety of options are available, including soft toric contact lenses, conventional rigid gas permeable (RGP) lenses, Rose K lenses, miniscleral lenses, and scleral lenses. Soft lenses **(Fig. 3.6A)** can be tried in the initial stage of the disease, while the mild-to-moderate disease can be fitted with monocurve gas permeable lenses and more advanced keratoconus benefits from a bicurve GP lens.[31,32]

Intracorneal Ring Segment

Around 20% of keratoconus cases are managed using intracorneal ring segment (ICRS).[33] Cases that can benefit from ICRS include those intolerant to contact lens wear, with a minimum corneal thickness of 400 μm at the corneal midperiphery, no central corneal scarring, and no history of corneal transplantation. ICRSs **(Fig. 3.6B)** are short PMMA arc/ring segments that cause central flattening. While these are safe and reversible in adults, it is not the preferred treatment in PKC due to rapid progression advanced presentation in this age group, eye rubbing tendencies, risk of extrusion, and noncompliance. There is also a high chance of implant extrusion in

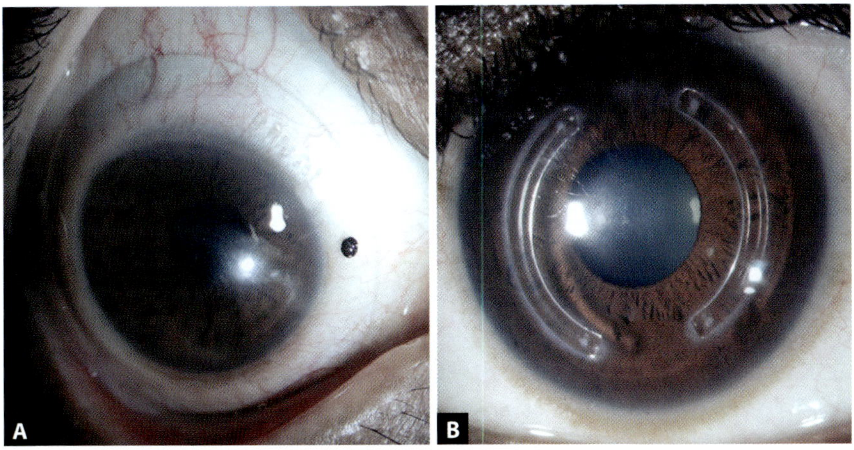

Figs. 3.6A and B: (A) Scleral contact lens in a patient with keratoconus; (B) Intracorneal ring segment used as a surgical modality in cases of keratoconus.

cases of keratoconus with VKC. One study combining CXL with ICRS shows promising results. Thus, these can be considered a less-invasive alternative to keratoplasty in selected cases.[34]

MANAGEMENT OF COMPLICATIONS

Hydrops

Several methods have been described for managing acute hydrops. Since hydrops is a self-limiting condition, conservative management with medical therapy such as hypertonic saline, steroids, and intraocular pressure-lowering medications is preferred for mild hydrops <5 mm. However, resolution can often take several months and may not always result in a favorable outcome, especially in eyes with a large area of involvement. Moreover, extensive hydrops affecting the peripheral cornea can also lead to corneal neovascularization, increasing the risk of graft rejection and failure in subsequent keratoplasty. Surgical management of hydrops includes intracameral gas injection[35] such as perfluoro propane (C_3F_8)/sulfur hexafluoride (SF_6), performing venting incisions, full-thickness compression suturing, penetrating keratoplasty, mini-Descemet stripping endothelial keratoplasty, and intracameral injection of platelet-rich plasma. Surgical management also includes a modified technique of compression sutures that includes partial thickness compression sutures of 50–60% depth **(Figs. 3.7A and B)**, which has shown the quickest resolution of corneal edema as compared to all other surgical methods.[36,37] Also, the risk of having hydrops in the contralateral eye is as high as 87% within a year after first; hence, expedited CXL would help minimize this risk.

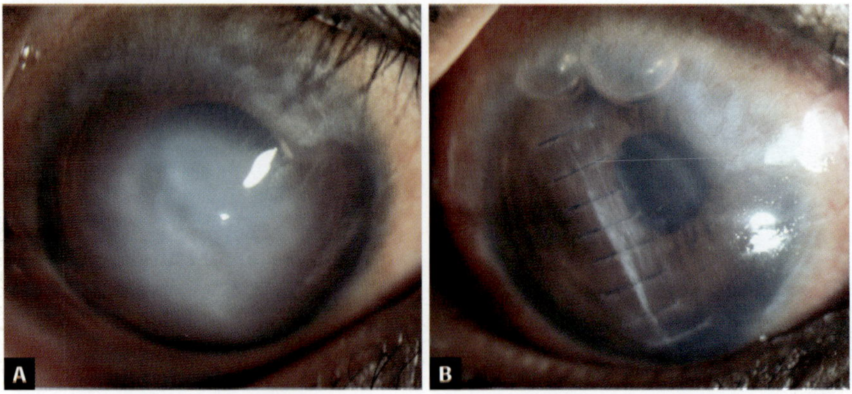

Figs. 3.7A and B: (A) Clinical photograph of hydrops; (B) Postoperative day 1 image of the same patient postmodified technique of compression suture showing significant resolution of corneal edema in 24 hours.

PENETRATING KERATOPLASTY

Penetrating keratoplasty (PK) is usually reserved for advanced cases of keratoconus, with visual axis scarring and irregular astigmatism not suitable for contact lens fitting. Keratoconus is the most common acquired nontraumatic indication for corneal transplantation in children.[38] In the Indian scenario, keratoconus precedes postinfection adherent leukoma as the second most common indication of nontraumatic keratoplasty.[39] It is of utmost importance to medically treat any underlying allergic conjunctivitis before taking up these cases for surgical intervention. Preoperatively, it is important to assess patient compliance with medication and regular follow-up. Among all indications of keratoplasty in the pediatric age group, keratoconus has the best long-term survival outcomes. Despite this, keratoplasty in the pediatric age group has its challenges. These can be overcome by taking appropriate precautions during surgery. Same-sized grafts are usually taken in cases of keratoconus. Over the last decade, the need for keratoplasty has come down significantly owing to early recognition and timely application of CXL promptly, thus retarding the progress.

DEEP ANTERIOR LAMELLAR KERATOPLASTY

Deep anterior lamellar keratoplasty (DALK) has now become the procedure of choice because of its better structural stability and lower incidence of graft rejection. There are various modifications of DALK. DALK can be performed with manual trephination or as a femtosecond laser-assisted procedure.[40,41] Furthermore, stromal bed dissection in DALK can be done by a manual method till the pre-Descemet's layer known as predescemetic DALK (pd-DALK) or by baring Descemet's membrane (d-DALK) by air either (Anwar's big-bubble technique), hydro, or viscoelastic dissection.[42,43] The success rates of getting a big bubble to achieve a plane between Dua's layer and the Descemet membrane are higher in keratoconus, considering the weaker ectatic stromal lamella. The visual outcomes of PK for keratoconus in pediatric patients are good, with one study reporting logMAR ≥ 0.3 at the last visit, mean age of 10.6 ± 4.3 years.[44] In the DALK group, Ashar et al. noted that more than 75% of their patients had a BCVA of better than 20/80 at their last visit. Comparing the outcomes of big-bubble DALK versus predescemetic DALK, Karimian and Feizi[43] found that the former had better outcomes but no significant difference in the subgroup analysis. Femtosecond laser-assisted DALK showed comparable BCVA and manifest astigmatism, but the spherical equivalent was on the lower side compared to mechanical trephination.[45]

STROMAL AUGMENTATION/TISSUE ADDITION SURGERIES

Bowman's Membrane Transplantation

Bowman's layer transplantation (BLT) is a technique of isolated transplantation of Bowman's layer harvested from a donor cornea that provides additional strength to the ectatic cornea, flattens the anterior curvature, thus improving visual acuity, and also arrests the disease progression. While it was earlier used for treating post-PRK subepithelial scaring,[46] it was in 2014 that Van Dijk et al.[47] described this technique in the treatment of keratoconus with contact lens intolerance.[47] In this technique, a BL graft is prepared from the donor tissue via either the manual method or using a femtosecond laser.[48] The tissue is then rinsed in a 70% alcohol solution for 30 seconds to remove any epithelial cells and stored in appropriate preservation media. This is then inserted in a lamellar dissection plane created in the host cornea. This procedure has shown a decrease in corneal curvature, increased pachymetry, better spectacle-corrected visual acuity, and improved contact lens tolerance. Apart from these, BLT is a sutureless technique and has a much lesser risk of allograft rejection as BL is essentially an acellular tissue. Disadvantages include a tedious procedure, a steeper learning curve for graft preparation, and mild interface haze.[49]

Bowman's Layer Onlay Grafting

This is a new technique that has come up that does not involve corneal dissection and the clinical outcomes are comparable to the BLT (inlay technique).[50]

Stromal Lenticule Addition Keratoplasty

The stromal lenticule addition keratoplasty (SLAK) procedure involves insertion of a negative meniscus-shaped lenticule that is thinner in the center and thicker in the periphery, into a stromal pocket in the host cornea. As the stromal pocket is made under the guidance of a femtosecond laser, it is relatively an easy procedure. It causes a central flattening effect along with stromal augmentation, with good postoperative results.[51,52]

Intralamellar Keratoplasty

An intralamellar keratoplasty (ILK) technique involves creating a stromal pocket in the host cornea and a stromal lenticule from the donor cornea using a femtosecond laser and subsequently inserting the latter into the host cornea.[53]

Corneal Allogenic Intrastromal Ring Segments

Corneal allogenic intrastromal ring segments (CAIRS) is a new procedure developed by Jacob et al.,[54] which involves insertion of allogenic semicircular corneal ring segments that are pretreated with 0.1% riboflavin in 20% dextran, into the host cornea similar to the ICRS. Following implantation, the cornea is subjected to accelerated CXL to strengthen the bonds between the segment and the host collagen fibers.

Femtosecond Intrastromal Lenticular Implantation

The femtosecond intrastromal lenticular implantation (FILI) technique involves a donut-shaped stromal lenticule insertion into the host cornea followed by an accelerated CXL. This lenticule was inserted at a depth of 100 µm from the epithelial surface, unlike the ICRSs which are usually implanted at 80% depth.[55]

CELL-BASED EVOLVING THERAPIES FOR STROMAL REGENERATION

Over the past decade, cellular therapy involving corneal cell expansion and tissue engineering has gained interest as a potential alternative to conventional keratoplasty. Stem cells have found a role in stromal keratocyte regeneration. Autologous ocular stem cells have limitations of difficulties in isolation and availability in high density; extraocular stem cells have been studied and have successfully been differentiated into human keratocytes in vivo. These cells can be harvested from various tissues like adipose tissue, hematopoietic stem cells, dental pulp, and umbilical cord blood.

Adipose-derived Mesenchymal Stem Cell Transplantation

Adipose-derived adult (mesenchymal) stem cell (ADASC) transplantation, a novel technique, involves the use of mesenchymal stem cells derived from adipose cells. Autologous ADASCs were obtained by liposuction. These were injected into the corneal stroma through a femtosecond-assisted lamellar pocket into the host cornea. The authors reported production of new collagen at the stromal level and subsequently increase in the BCVA and decrease in anterior Km and Kmax values.[56]

CONCLUSION

Pediatric keratoconus poses a challenging condition due to its advanced stage of presentation, rapid progression, and poor visual outcomes in case of late intervention.[57] The treatment needs to be customized based on the presentation, age, and severity of involvement. These include the use of various types of CXL for preventing progression and the use of contact lenses, ICRS, or keratoplasty for visual rehabilitation. Although keratoplasty has significantly improved in safety, resulting in excellent anatomical and functional outcomes for pediatric eyes, there are still concerns that need attention to further improve prognosis. DALK is favored over penetrating keratoplasty due to its superior structural stability, preservation of the host endothelium, and lower rejection rates. Literature has evidenced that over the last decade, the need for lamellar or full-thickness keratoplasty has come down significantly owing to the application of CXL promptly, thus retarding the progress. Apart from these, newer cell-based therapies for stromal augmentation and mechanical-surgical-based stromal augmentation techniques may be the future for keratoconus management in view of their less-invasive nature and arresting disease progression.

REFERENCES

1. Moshirfar M, Heiland MB, Rosen DB, Ronquillo YC, Hoopes PC. Keratoconus screening in elementary school children. Ophthalmol Ther. 2019;8:367-71.
2. Gokhale NS. Epidemiology of keratoconus. Indian J Ophthalmol. 2013;61(8):382-3.
3. Abelson MB, Granet D. Ocular allergy in pediatric practice. Curr Allergy Asthma Rep. 2006;6:306-11.
4. Gordon-Shaag A, Millodot M, Shneor E, Liu Y. The genetic and environmental factors for keratoconus. Biomed Res Int. 2015;2015:795738.
5. Sahebjada S, Fenwick EK, Xie J, Snibson GR, Daniell MD, Baird PN. Impact of keratoconus in the better eye and the worse eye on vision-related quality of life. Invest Ophthalmol Vis Sci. 2014;55:412-6.
6. Omar IAN. Keratoconus screening among myopic children. Clin Ophthalmol. 2019;13:1909-12.
7. Anitha V, Vanathi M, Raghavan A, Rajaraman R, Ravindran M, Tandon R. Pediatric keratoconus – current perspectives and clinical challenges. Indian J Ophthalmol. 2021;69(2):214.
8. Spoerl E, Raiskup-Wolf F, Kuhlisch E, Pillunat LE. Cigarette smoking is negatively associated with keratoconus. J Refract Surg. 2008;24(7):737-40.
9. Kuo IC, Broman A, Pirouzmanesh A, Melia M. Is there an association between diabetes and keratoconus? Ophthalmology. 2006;113(2):184-90.

10. Amsler M. Classic keratocene and rough keratocene; Unitary arguments. Ann Ocul. 1947;180:112.
11. Amsler M. Keratocone classique et keratocone fruste; arguments unitaires. Ophtalmologica. 1946;111:96-101.
12. Belin MW, Duncan JK. Keratoconus: the ABCD grading system. Klin Monbl Augenheilkd. 2016;233(6):701-7.
13. Rabinowitz YS. Videokeratographic indices to aid in screening for keratoconus. J Refract Surg. 1995;11(5):371-9.
14. Rabinowitz YS, Rasheed K. KISA% index: a quantitative videokeratography algorithm embodying minimal topographic criteria for diagnosing keratoconus. J Cataract Refract Surg. 1999;25(10):1327-35.
15. Belin MW, Ambrosio R. Scheimpflug imaging for keratoconus and ectatic disease. Indian J Ophthalmol. 2013;61(8):401-6.
16. de Toledo MC, Gonçalves BV. Keratoconus. In: Almodin E, Nassaralla BA, Sandes J (Eds). Corneal Epithelial Thickness Mapping in Keratoconus. Singapore: Springer; 2022.
17. Yang Y, Pavlatos E, Chamberlain W, Huang D, Li Y. Keratoconus detection using OCT corneal and epithelial thickness map parameters and patterns. J Cataract Refract Surg. 2021;47(6):759-66.
18. Yuhas PT, Fortman MM, Mahmoud AM, Robert CJ. Keratoconus cone location influences ocular biomechanical parameters measured by the Ocular Response Analyzer. Eye and Vis (Lond). 2024;11(1):2.
19. Raiskup-Wolf F, Hoyer A, Spoerl E, Pillunat LE. Collagen crosslinking with riboflavin and ultraviolet-A light in keratoconus: long-term results. J Cataract Refract Surg. 2008;34:796-801.
20. McMonnies CW. Mechanisms of rubbing-related corneal trauma in keratoconus. Cornea. 2009;28:607-15.
21. Wollensak G, Spoerl E, Seiler T. Riboflavin/ultraviolet-A-induced collagen cross-linking for the treatment of keratoconus. Am J Ophthalmol. 2003;135(5):620-7.
22. Salman AG. Transepithelial corneal collagen crosslinking for progressive keratoconus in a pediatric age group. J Cataract Refract Surg. 2013;39(8):1164-70.
23. Buzzonetti L, Petrocelli G. Transepithelial corneal cross-linking in pediatric patients: early results. J Refract Surg. 2012;28(11):763-7.
24. Soeters N, van der Valk R, Tahzib NG. Corneal cross-linking for treatment of progressive keratoconus in various age groups. J Refract Surg. 2014;30(7):454-60.
25. Amer I, Elaskary A, Mostafa A, Hazem HA, Omar A, Abdou A. Long-term visual, refractive and topographic outcomes of "epi-off" corneal collagen cross-linking in pediatric keratoconus: standard versus accelerated protocol. Clin Ophthalmol. 2020;14:3747-54.
26. Dias J, Diakonis VF, Lorenzo M, Gonzalez F, Porras K, Douglas S, et al. Corneal stromal elasticity and viscoelasticity assessed by atomic force microscopy after different cross-linking protocols. Exp Eye Res. 2015;138:1-5.
27. Zhu Y, Reinach PS, Zhu H, Li L, Yang F, Qu J, et al. Continuous-light versus pulsed-light accelerated corneal crosslinking with ultraviolet-A and riboflavin. J Cataract Refract Surg. 2018;44(3):382-89.
28. Nordstrom M, Schiller M, Fredriksson A, Behndig A. Refractive improvements and safety with topography-guided corneal crosslinking for keratoconus: 1-year results. Br J Ophthalmol. 2017;101(7):920-5.

29. El Rami H, Chelala E, Dirani A, Fadlallah A, Fakhoury H, Cherfan C, et al. An update on the safety and efficacy of corneal collagen cross-linking in pediatric keratoconus. BioMed Res Int; 2015. pp.1-7.
30. Bakshi E, Barkana Y, Goldich Y, Avni I, Zadok D. Corneal cross-linking for progressive keratoconus in children: our experience. Int J Kerat Ect Cor Dis. 2012;1(1):53-6.
31. Sultan P, Dogan C, Iskeleli G. A retrospective analysis of vision correction and safety in keratoconus patients wearing Toris K soft contact lenses. Int Ophthalmol. 2016;36(6):799-805.
32. Lunardi LH, Arroyo D, Andrade Sobrinho MV, Lipener C, Rosa JM. Descriptive analysis of the type and design of contact lenses fitted according to keratoconus severity and morphology. Arq Bras Oftalmol. 2016;79(2):82-4.
33. Kankariya VP, Kymionis GD, Diaknois VF, Yoo SH. Management of pediatric keratoconus—evolving role of corneal collagen cross-linking: an update. Ind J Ophthalmol. 2013;61(8):435-40.
34. Saleem MIH, Ibrahim Elzembely HA, AboZaid MA, Elagouz M, Saeed AM, Ali Mohammed O, et al. Three-year outcomes of cross-linking PLUS (combined cross-linking with femtosecond laser intracorneal ring segments implantation) for management of keratoconus. J Ophthalmol. 2018;6907573.
35. Basu S, Vaddavalli PK, Ramappa M, Shah S, Murthy SI, Sangwan VS. Intracameral perfluoropropane gas in the treatment of acute corneal hydrops. Ophthalmology. 2011;118(5):934-9.
36. Daza J, Ramappa M, Murthy S, Chaurasia S. Strategies and application of compression sutures with a modified technique for rapid resolution of large (Grade III) hydrops: a prospective interventional study. Cornea. 2024;20.
37. Chaurasia S, Ramappa M, Murthy S. Rapid resolution of large and non-resolving corneal hydrops using a modified technique of compression sutures. Semin Ophthalmol. 2022;37(5):637-42.
38. Mukhtar S, Ambati BK. Pediatric keratoconus: a review of the literature. Int Ophthalmol. 2018;38(5):2257-66.
39. Ganekal S, Gangangouda C, Dorairaj S, Jhanji V. Early outcomes of primary pediatric keratoplasty in patients with acquired, atraumatic corneal pathology. J AAPOS. 2011;15:353-55.
40. Vanathi M, Panda A, Vengayil S, Chaudhuri Z, Dada T. Pediatric keratoplasty. Surv Ophthalmol. 2009;54:245-71.
41. Ashar JN, Pahuja S, Ramappa M, Vaddavalli PK, Chaurasia S, Garg P. Deep anterior lamellar keratoplasty in children. Am J Ophthalmol. 2013;155:570-74.
42. Tan DT, Por YM. Current treatment options for corneal ectasia. Curr Opin Ophthalmol. 2007;18:279-83.
43. Karimian F, Feizi S. Deep anterior lamellar keratoplasty: indications, surgical techniques and complications. Middle East Afr J Ophthalmol. 2010;17:28-37.
44. Patel HY, Ormonde S, Brookes NH, Moffatt LS, McGhee CN. The indications and outcome of paediatric corneal transplantation in New Zealand: 1991-2003. Br J Ophthalmol. 2005;89(4):404-8.
45. Buzzonetti L, Petrocelli G, Valente P, Petroni S, Parrilla R, Iarossi G. Refractive outcome of keratoconus treated by big-bubble deep anterior lamellar keratoplasty in pediatric patients: two-year follow-up comparison between mechanical trephine and femtosecond laser assisted techniques. Eye Vis (Lond). 2019;6:1.

46. Lie J, Droutsas K, Ham L, Dapena I, Ververs B, Otten H, et al. Isolated Bowman layer transplantation to manage persistent subepithelial haze after excimer laser surface ablation. J Cataract Refract Surg. 2010;36(6):1036-41.
47. van Dijk K, Parker J, Tong CM, Ham L, Lie JT, Groeneveld-van Beek EA, et al. Midstromal isolated Bowman layer graft for reduction of advanced keratoconus: a technique to postpone penetrating or deep anterior lamellar keratoplasty. JAMA Ophthalmol. 2014;132(4):495-501.
48. Parker JS, Huls F, Cooper E, Graves P, Groeneveld-van Beek EA, Lie J, et al. Technical feasibility of isolated Bowman layer graft preparation by femtosecond laser: a pilot study. Eur J Ophthalmol. 2017;27(6):675-7.
49. Zygoura V, Birbal RS, van Dijk K, Parker JS, Baydoun L, Dapena I, et al. Validity of Bowman layer transplantation for keratoconus: visual performance at 5–7 years. Acta Ophthalmol. 2018;96(7):901-2.
50. Dapena I, van der Star L, Groeneveld-van Beek EA, Quilendrino R, van Dijk K, Parker JS, et al. Bowman layer onlay grafting: proof-of-concept of a new technique to flatten corneal curvature and reduce progression in keratoconus. Cornea. 2021;40(12):1561-66.
51. Mastropasqua L, Nubile M, Salgari N, Mastropasqua R. Femtosecond laser-assisted stromal lenticule addition keratoplasty for the treatment of advanced keratoconus: a preliminary study. J Refract Surg. 2018;34(1):36-44.
52. Fasolo A, Galzignato A, Pedrotti E, Chierego C, Cozzini T, Bonacci E, et al. Femtosecond laser-assisted implantation of corneal stroma lenticule for keratoconus. Int Ophthalmol 2021;41(5):1949-57.
53. Tan BU, Purcell TL, Torres LF, Schanzlin DJ. New surgical approaches to the management of keratoconus and post-LASIK ectasia. Trans Am Ophthalmol Soc. 2006;104:212-20.
54. Jacob S, Patel SR, Agarwal A, Ramalingam A, Saijimol AI, Raj JM. Corneal allogenic intrastromal ring segments (CAIRS) combined with corneal cross-linking for keratoconus. J Refract Surg. 2018;34(5):296-303.
55. Ganesh S, Brar S. Femtosecond intrastromal lenticular implantation combined with accelerated collagen cross-linking for the treatment of keratoconus – initial clinical result in 6 eyes. Cornea. 2015;34(10):1331-9.
56. Alió Del Barrio JL, El Zarif M, de Miguel MP, Azaar A, Makdissy N, Harb W, et al. Cellular therapy with human autologous adipose-derived adult stem cells for advanced keratoconus. Cornea. 2017;36(8):952-60.
57. Ramappa M. Commentary: a perspective on pediatric keratoconus: one size does not fit all. Indian J Ophthalmol. 2021;69(2):225-6.

4 CHAPTER

Lamellar Keratoplasty

Shreesha Kumar Kodavoor, Tasneem Neemuchwala,
KS Siddharthan, Arnav Singh Saroya,
Ramamurthy Dandapani

ABSTRACT

Lamellar keratoplasty (LK) has undergone significant advancements in recent years, revolutionizing the field of corneal transplantation. This chapter highlights the latest developments and techniques in LK, focusing on both anterior and posterior lamellar procedures. Anterior lamellar keratoplasty (ALK) techniques, such as deep anterior lamellar keratoplasty (DALK), have gained popularity due to their ability to preserve the healthy endothelial layer. Improved instrumentation and surgical expertise have led to enhanced outcomes, including faster visual recovery, reduced risk of graft rejection, and improved graft survival rates. Moreover, the advent of femtosecond laser-assisted techniques has enabled precise dissection, facilitating smoother graft–host interface and minimizing intraoperative complications. Posterior lamellar keratoplasty (PLK), particularly Descemet's stripping endothelial keratoplasty (DSEK) and Descemet membrane endothelial keratoplasty (DMEK), has witnessed remarkable advancements in donor tissue preparation, surgical instrumentation, and surgical techniques. Novel approaches, such as preloaded donor tissue insertion systems and intraoperative optical coherence tomography (OCT) guidance, have contributed to improved surgical efficiency and enhanced outcomes. Furthermore, innovations in tissue storage and transportation have extended the viability of donor tissue, widening the donor pool and reducing waiting times for patients. The advent of tissue engineering and regenerative medicine holds promise for developing bioengineered corneal substitutes, offering a potential solution to the global shortage of donor corneas.

Keywords: Lamellar keratoplasty, Bowman's layer transplant, deep anterior lamellar keratoplasty, sutureless femtosecond laser-assisted anterior lamellar keratoplasty, Descemet membrane endothelial keratoplasty, ultrathin Descemet's stripping endothelial keratoplasty, descemetorhexis without endothelial keratoplasty

INTRODUCTION

The landscape of corneal transplantation has been profoundly reshaped by the emergence of lamellar keratoplasty (LK). Recent years have witnessed significant strides in LK, ushering in a new era of enhanced outcomes and broader treatment options for individuals with corneal diseases. This transformative progress is dedicated to the preservation of healthy corneal tissue, mitigating complications, and optimizing visual results. Within this chapter, we delve into the cutting-edge advancements that characterize the latest breakthroughs in lamellar keratoplasty techniques.

Lamellar keratoplasty can be broadly categorized into two distinct approaches: Replacement of epithelium and stroma, known as *anterior lamellar keratoplasty (ALK)*, and replacement of Descemet's membrane (DM), termed *posterior lamellar keratoplasty (PLK)*.

Anterior lamellar keratoplasty comprises various procedures which include:

- Bowman's layer transplantation (BLT)
- Deep anterior lamellar keratoplasty (DALK)

There are various techniques of DALK which are as follows:

- Sutureless femtosecond laser-assisted anterior lamellar keratoplasty (FALK)
- Tuck in femtosecond laser-assisted anterior lamellar keratoplasty (T-FALK)
- Double docking procedure for DALK (DD-DALK)

Posterior lamellar keratoplasty includes:

- Descemet's stripping endothelial keratoplasty (DSEK)/Descemet's stripping automated endothelial keratoplasty (DSAEK)
- Pre-Descemet's endothelial keratoplasty (PDEK)
- Descemet membrane endothelial keratoplasty (DMEK)

ADVANCEMENTS IN ANTERIOR LAMELLAR KERATOPLASTY

Isolated Bowman's Layer Transplantation

This is an emerging and evolving method, although not routinely practiced. Its primary applications include serving as an inlay graft into the mid-stroma of the cornea for managing keratoconus **(Figs. 4.1A to C)** and as an onlay graft to address persistent subepithelial haze observed in some cases following excimer laser surface ablation.[1]

One study shows the potential use of femtosecond laser (FSL) technology for harvesting the donor Bowman's layer. Initial feasibility analysis has indicated compelling outcomes, showcasing the creation of a thick and relatively smooth posterior cut edge in the FSL group. In contrast, the manually dissected group exhibited a virtually isolated Bowman's layer, with irregular remnants of dispersed stroma.[2]

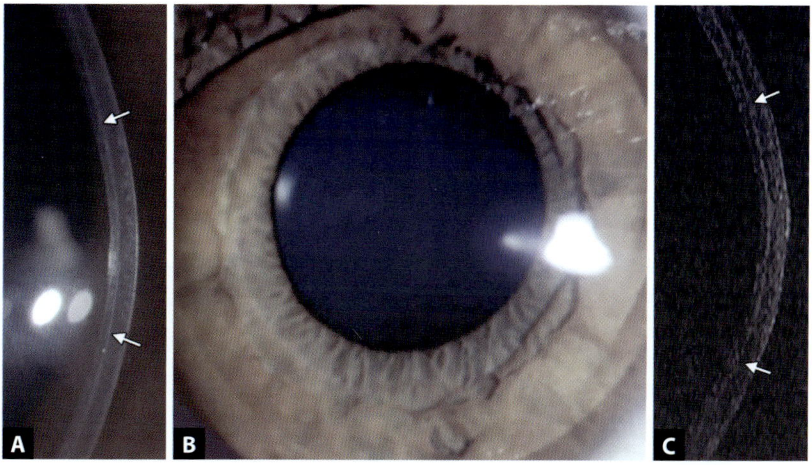

Figs. 4.1A to C: Slit-lamp images and optical coherence tomography (OCT) image after Bowman layer transplantation. The (A, B) slit-lamp images and (C) OCT images were obtained 6 months after Bowman layer transplantation. The Bowman layer transplant (white arrows) is visible as a thin, white line within the recipient stroma (A and C), whereas the cornea is clear and without any interface haze or stromal reaction (B).

Sutureless Femtosecond Laser-assisted Anterior Lamellar Keratoplasty

The depth of the pathology is measured by anterior segment OCT (ASOCT). The procedure employs a FSL to create a lamellar cut in the recipient's cornea, precisely matched with donor corneal tissue. The thickness of the donor cut is adjusted based on the depth of the lesions, with an additional 10–20% thickness allowance to compensate for potential donor tissue swelling. Subsequently, the scarred corneal tissue in the recipient is carefully removed and replaced by the corneal donor lenticule **(Figs. 4.2 and 4.3)**. After the replacement, the incision is dried, and the adhesion of the flap is checked to ensure proper alignment and attachment. A bandage soft contact lens is finally placed over the cornea.[3]

A variation of the FALK method was documented by Bonfadini et al., employing the Ziemer FSL from Ziemer Ophthalmic Systems AG, Port, Switzerland. This modification introduces two distinct dissection depths: Midstromal (exceeding 250 µm of posterior residual corneal bed thickness) and pre-Descemet (approximately 50 µm of posterior residual corneal bed thickness). The foundational principles of this modified approach align with those previously described for the conventional FALK method.[4]

Tuck in Femtosecond Laser-assisted Anterior Lamellar Keratoplasty

It is a sutureless and glueless technique, offering a novel and effective alternative for managing superficial anterior corneal scars. The depth of the anterior corneal scar is assessed using ASOCT. The procedure involves the precise preparation of both donor and recipient lenticules through the application of FSL technology. Following the removal of the recipient's anterior scarred lenticule, the donor lenticule is positioned onto the recipient's bed. The margins of the donor lenticule are tucked in beneath the recipient cornea **(Figs. 4.4A to C)**, creating a secure fit.[5]

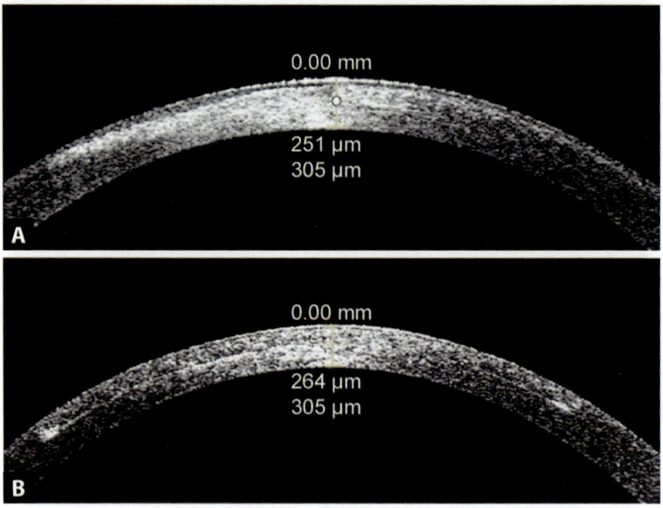

Figs. 4.2A and B: Anterior segment noncontact optical coherence tomography for corneal scarring depth evaluation reveals the depth of the lesion-scarring (A) preoperatively and (B) after femtosecond laser-assisted sutureless anterior lamellar keratoplasty.

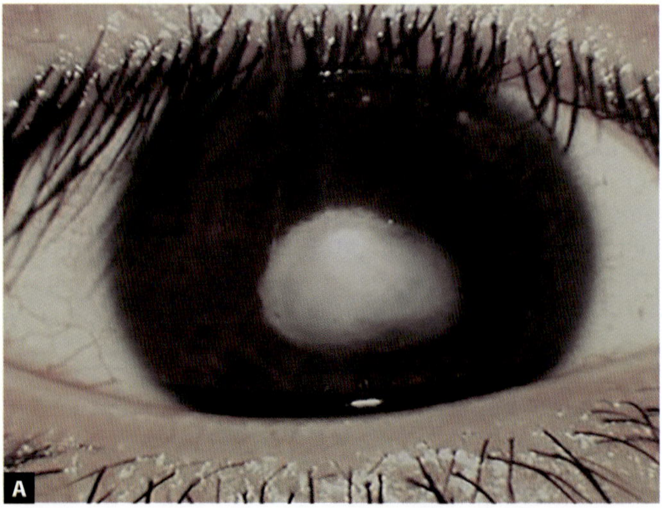

Fig. 4.3A

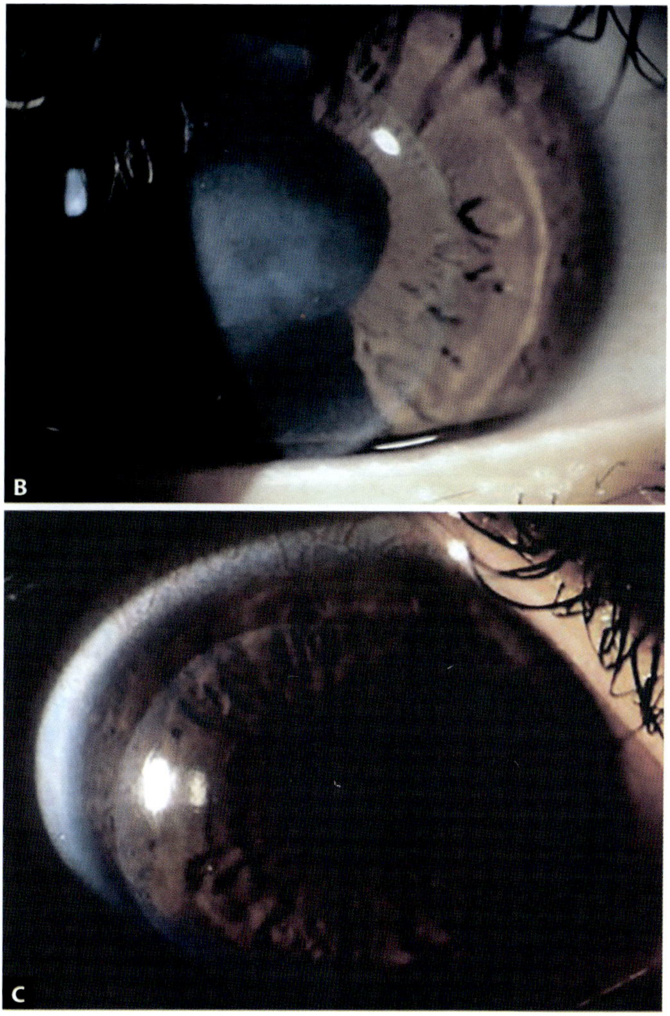

Figs. 4.3B and C

Figs. 4.3A to C: (A) Corneal slit-lamp photograph of a 19-year-old male with a paracentral scar and best-corrected visual acuity (BCVA) of 20/60. (B) 10 months after femtosecond laser-assisted sutureless anterior lamellar keratoplasty, there was residual corneal scarring. (C) Phototherapeutic keratectomy was performed after lifting the anterior lamellar graft, with a complete restoration of corneal clarity and improvement in BCVA to 20/25.

Double Docking Procedure for Deep Anterior Lamellar Keratoplasty

It represents a secure surgical technique utilizing the precision of FSL technology and intraoperative optical coherence tomography (iOCT). In this procedure, the FSL and iOCT work in tandem to provide direct visual control during the first lamellar resection, often referred to as the *first docking*. This initial step is crucial for minimizing the risk of corneal perforation,

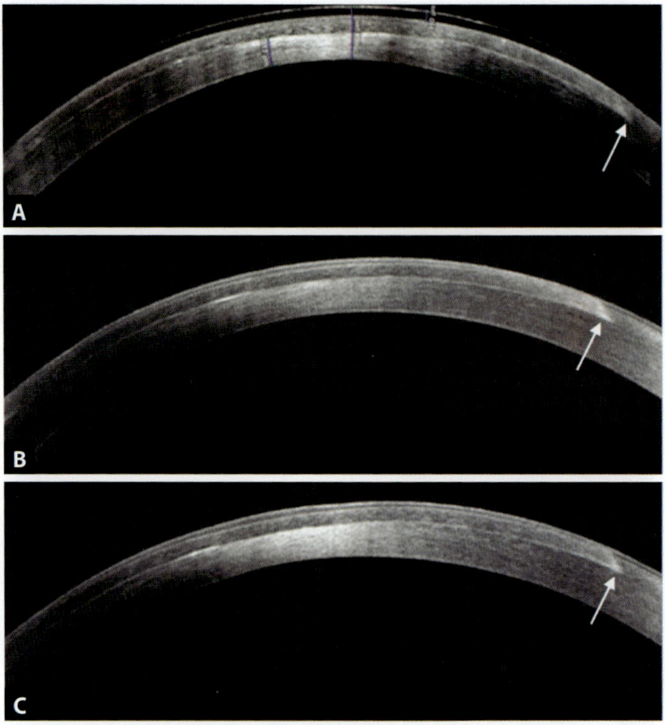

Figs. 4.4A to C: ASOCT images of a patient who underwent T-FALK showing good healing at the graft–host junction at (A) 1 day, (B) 1 month, and (C) 3 months. Also note the angle of 45° that allows good apposition of the graft–host junction after the T-FALK procedure. (ASOCT: anterior segment optical coherence tomography; T-FALK: tuck in femtosecond laser-assisted anterior lamellar keratoplasty)

particularly in comparison to the use of a manual trephine. The lamellar resection performed during the first docking is instrumental in positioning the needle or cannula close to the Descemet membrane, a prerequisite for the successful formation of a big bubble (BB). Following the BB formation, a second docking is done to cut the residual irregular posterior stroma using the FSL. Subsequently, the residual stroma is removed using forceps **(Figs. 4.5A to L)**. This second docking to eliminate the residual stroma minimizes the need for extensive surgical dissection, thereby enhancing the learning curve associated with this intricate and challenging technique. The DD-DALK method ensures a safe and controlled approach to deep anterior lamellar keratoplasty.[6]

Algorithm for Performing DALK Using Preoperative OCT in Keratoconus Eyes

Through the application of ASOCT, a noncontact method rooted in low-coherence interferometry principles, Sandali and colleagues introduced a novel classification system delineating structural corneal alterations observed

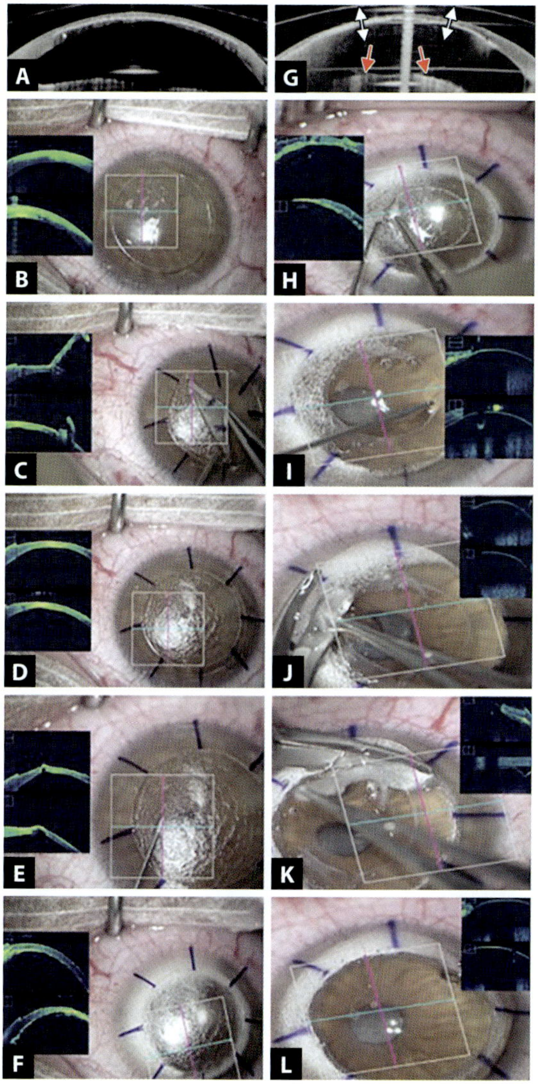

Figs. 4.5A to L: FSL-assisted DALK with the double-docking technique. After the first docking, an FSL-assisted anterior lamellar cut is performed (A). Under an operative microscope with integrated OCT, the lamellar cut is checked (B) and then the anterior stromal lamella is removed using the spatula and forceps (C, D). A 30-G needle is inserted in the residual stroma under OCT guidance (E) and then air is injected to create the BB (F). After the second docking, DM is visible with the FSL integrated OCT (G, red arrows). The cylindrical vertical cut is set and performed on the residual stroma (G), the white arrows indicating the vertical cut setting. Then, the residual stroma is peeled off with forceps (H), and the viscoelastic substance is used to push back DM (I). The residual peripheral stroma is removed using scissors (J, K). The stroma has been fully removed and bare DM was preserved before grafting the donor's anterior stroma (L). (BB: big bubble; DALK: deep anterior lamellar keratoplasty; DM: Descemet membrane; FSL: femtosecond laser; OCT: optical coherence tomography)

during the progression of keratoconus. This classification system, informed by the corneal microarchitecture changes characteristic of keratoconus eyes, facilitates the assessment and grading of disease severity.[7]

The classification is as follows:

- *Stage 1:* Thinning of epithelial and stromal layers at the conus; corneal layers with normal aspect
- *Stage 2A:* Hyper-reflective anomalies at the Bowman's layer level with epithelial thickening
- *Stage 2B:* Stage 2A + stromal opacities
- *Stage 3A:* Posterior displacement of the hyper-reflective structures at the Bowman's layer level with increased epithelial thickening + stromal thinning
- *Stage 3B:* Stage 3A + stromal opacities
- *Stage 4:* Pan stromal scar
- *Stage 5A:* Acute onset with Descemet membrane rupture with dilacerations of collagen lamellae, large fluid-filled intrastromal cysts, and epithelial edema formation
- *Stage 5B:* Healing stage of 5A with pan stromal scarring with the remaining aspect of Descemet membrane rupture

Based on this classification, an algorithm for performing DALK using preoperative OCT of the recipient cornea has been made **(Flowchart 4.1)**:[8]

Flowchart 4.1: Algorithm for performing DALK using preoperative OCT of the recipient cornea.

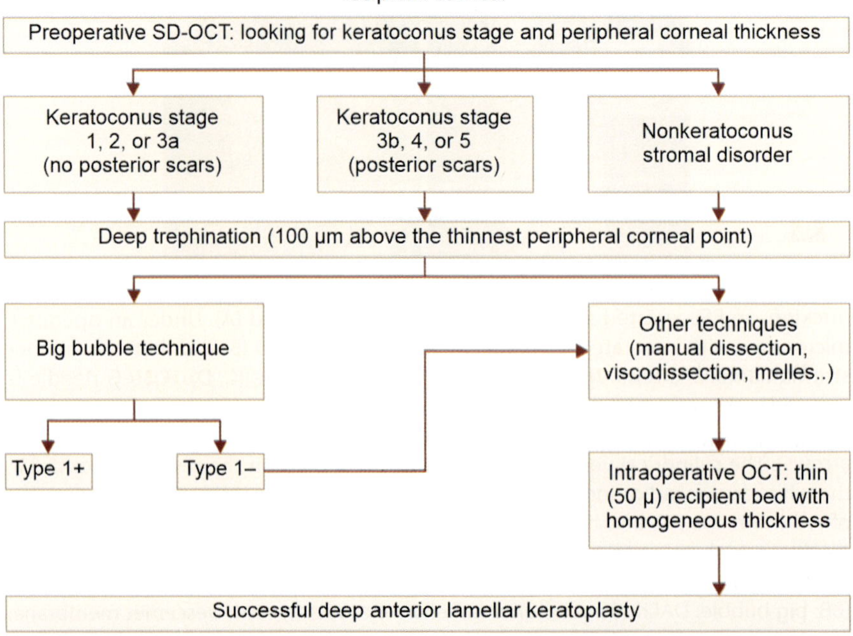

(DALK: deep anterior lamellar keratoplasty; OCT: optical coherence tomography)

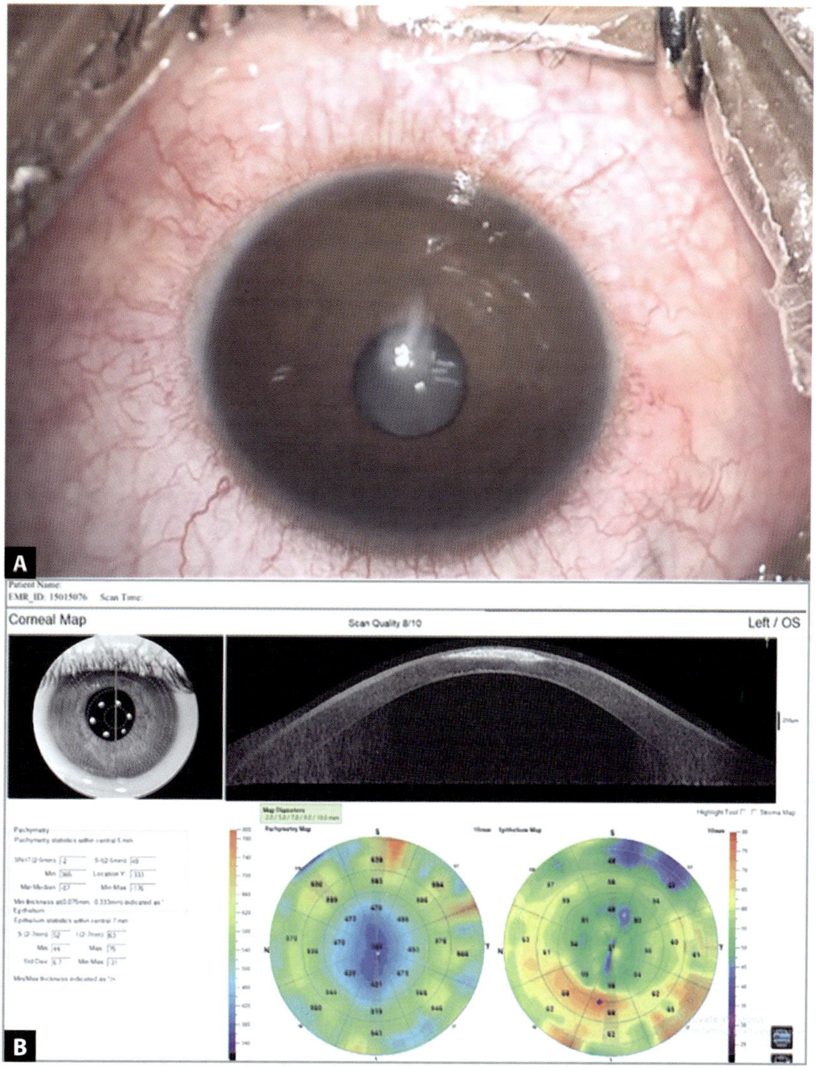

Figs. 4.6 A and B: (A) Superficial stromal scar in a case of keratoconus; (B) ASOCT image of the same eye. (ASOCT: anterior segment optical coherence tomography)

Recent advances in lamellar keratoplasty techniques suggest that OCT assessment of eyes prior to DALK is proving to be a valuable tool. It aids in determining the optimal trephination depth, advocating for a depth as profound as feasible, and enables the identification of scars within the posterior stroma. Specifically in cases of keratoconus with posterior scarring, surgical strategies must be tailored accordingly. While the big bubble technique remains an option, its suitability in such cases may be questioned.

During the execution of DALK procedures targeting superficial scars in keratoconus patients **(Figs. 4.6 A and B)**, the surgical objective is to attain

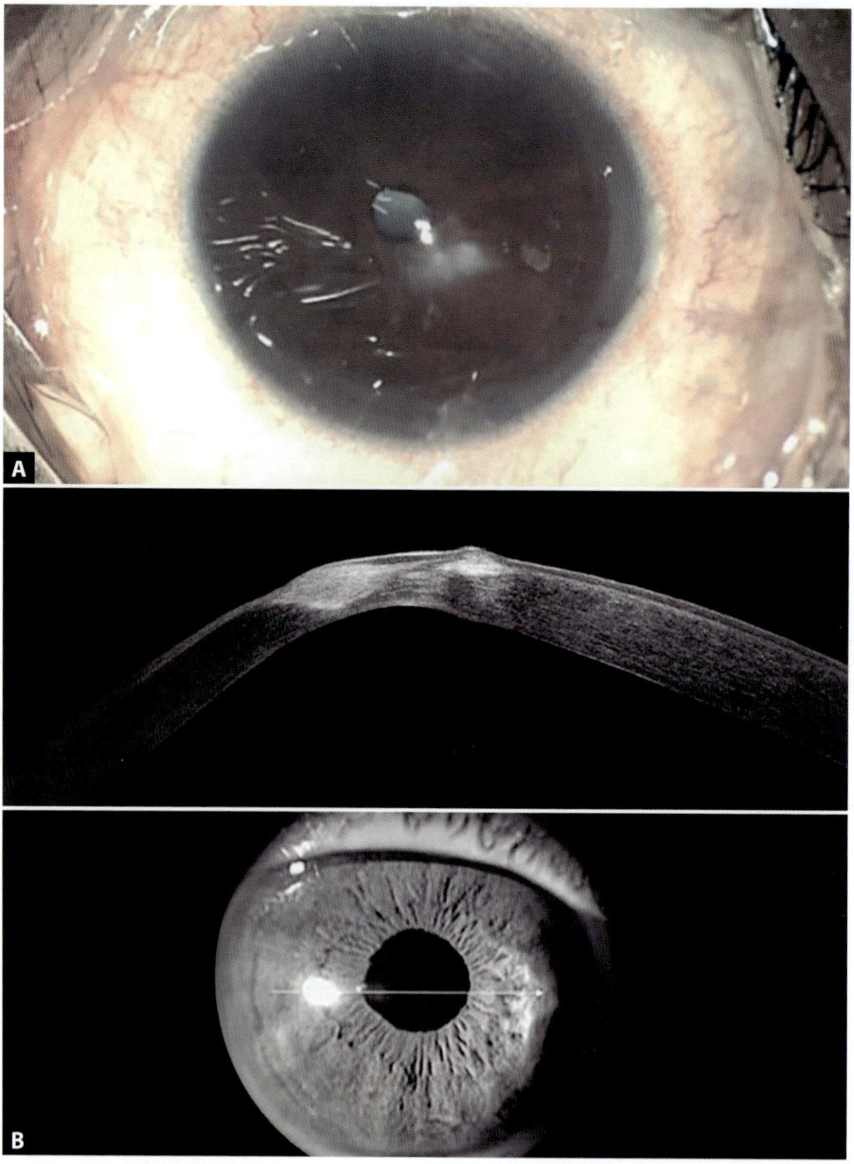

Figs. 4.7 A and B: (A) Deep stromal scar in a case of keratoconus; (B) ASOCT images of the same eye. (ASOCT: anterior segment optical coherence tomography)

a type-1 big bubble, a goal that can be successfully achieved. In cases of deep stromal scars **(Figs. 4.7A and B)**, although type-2 or type-3 big bubble can be achieved, the chances of perforation are high. Therefore, in such cases, dissection with a manual layer-by-layer technique is preferable, as it prevents the chances of perforation intraoperatively and gives better postoperative outcomes. In eyes with healed hydrops **(Figs. 4.8 A and B)**,

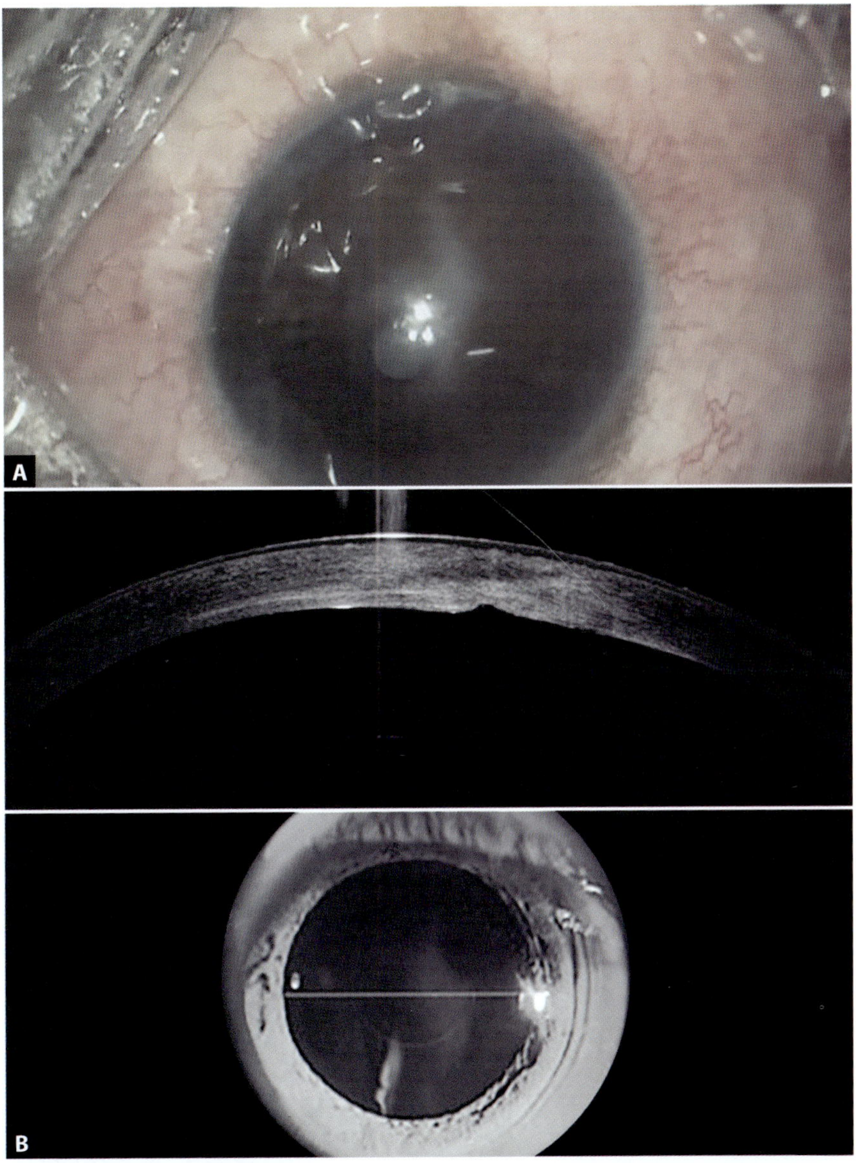

Figs. 4.8 A and B: (A) Healed hydrops scar in a case of keratoconus; (B) ASOCT images of the same eye. (ASOCT: anterior segment optical coherence tomography)

achieving big bubble is not the goal. Intrastromal air is injected to achieve emphysema, which aids in dissection.

Further exploration is warranted to ascertain whether commencing the procedure directly with an alternative lamellar technique or employing the big bubble technique followed by conversion to another lamellar method is preferable. Encouragingly, findings from a 3-year patient follow-up do not advocate for mandatory conversion to penetrating keratoplasty in instances where a type-1 big bubble cannot be achieved. Likewise, there is no compelling evidence supporting the prioritization of penetrating keratoplasty as the initial approach for eyes with posterior stromal scars. These insights mark significant strides in refining and individualizing lamellar keratoplasty procedures, underscoring the importance of precise preoperative assessment and adaptable surgical techniques.[8]

Artificial Corneal Grafts

A growing advancement in vision correction, FALK with bioengineered collagen corneal (LinkCor) implantation stands as a novel approach aimed at enhancing visual quality in cases of anterior stromal opacities **(Figs. 4.9 and 4.10)**.

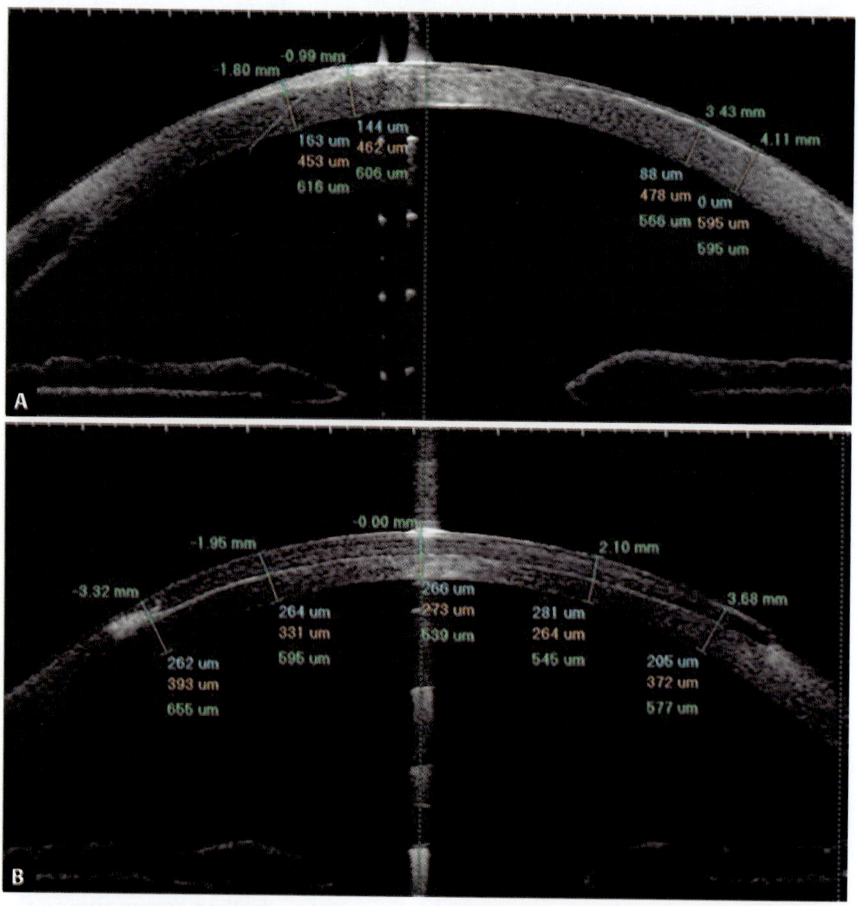

Figs. 4.9A and B: ASOCT images showing (A) corneal scar depth evaluation preoperatively and (B) after implantation of the bioengineered implant using sutureless FALK. (ASOCT: anterior segment optical coherence tomography; FALK: femtosecond laser-assisted anterior lamellar keratoplasty)

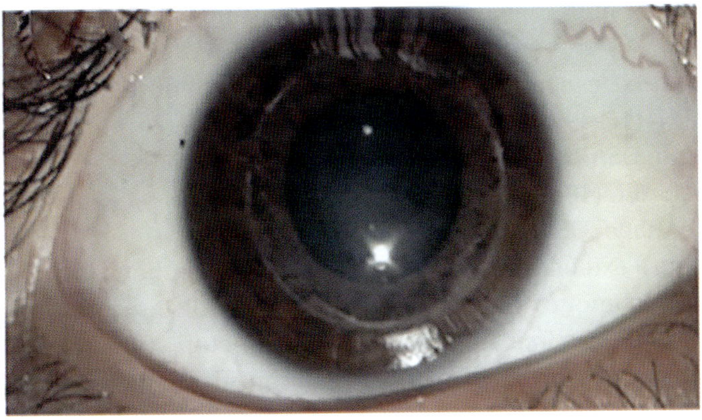

Fig. 4.10: 1-year postoperative photograph of a patient operated for corneal opacity due to corneal dystrophy.

This innovative procedure not only diminishes the reliance on human donor tissue but also mitigates potential complications associated with human donor-related issues and suture-related concerns. It is a promising avenue for improving vision while addressing some of the limitations and challenges associated with traditional treatments.[9]

ADVANCEMENTS IN POSTERIOR LAMELLAR KERATOPLASTY

Role of Bandage Contact Lens in Endothelial Keratoplasty

The placement of a bandage contact lens (BCL) serves a dual purpose in the postoperative phase, not only alleviating pain and discomfort but potentially contributing to lower rates of donor graft detachment and rebubbling. Although the reduction in endothelial cell loss (ECL) observed in patients with a BCL was noted, it was not statistically significant. Nevertheless, the established correlation between low ECL and higher graft survival rates underscores the potential advantages of incorporating a BCL in the postoperative management protocol.[10]

Descemet Stripping Endothelial Keratoplasty/Descemet Stripping Automated Endothelial Keratoplasty

Several authors have introduced numerous modifications throughout the procedures.[11] From the initial steps of harvesting the donor graft to techniques for inserting the donor button and managing air, various claims have been made regarding the superiority of one method over another. These claims often focus on factors such as the percentage loss of endothelial cells, the restoration of good uncorrected visual acuity (UCVA), efficient epithelial healing, and overall patient satisfaction.

Various donor graft thicknesses are available and fall into the four general categories:[12]

1. Nanothin Descemet stripping automated endothelial keratoplasty (DSAEK) (15–49 μm)
2. Ultrathin DSAEK (50–99 μm)
3. Thin DSAEK (100–149 μm)
4. Conventional DSAEK (150–250 μm)

Literature extensively discusses the comparison between manual and automated techniques for donor graft preparation, diverse insertion methods involving tools like Tan's endoglide, endoinjector, endoserter, Macaluso inserter, or Kobayashi–Busin glide, and the consideration of push versus pull techniques. Additionally, the use of an anterior chamber maintainer during donor insertion has also been explored.[13]

Advantages

- Faster visual recovery
- Minimal alteration in corneal topography
- Fewer allograft rejections because there will be lesser antigenic load as only the diseased selected layer of the cornea is replaced

Another development in DSEK/DSAEK is the *triple procedure*, which is the combination of DSEK/DMEK with phacoemulsification with intraocular lens implantation **(Figs. 4.11A and B)**.

This surgical approach is recommended for eyes with decompensated corneas, such as those affected by Fuchs endothelial corneal dystrophy or other related conditions, concurrently presenting with cataracts. The decision to opt for either a combined or staged approach to cataract and transplant surgery hinges on a comprehensive eye examination. Factors considered include the assessment of anterior chamber depth and the condition of the anterior surface of the cornea, impacting the reliable evaluation of keratometry. Additional aspects influencing the decision-making process include the selection of the lens implant, desired refractive outcomes, and the patient's preference regarding whether to undergo a single or dual surgical procedure for each eye.[14]

Ultrathin DSEK

Ultrathin DSEK (UT-DSEK) is a procedure designed to enhance visual outcomes and reduce the risk of immunologic rejection, adopting the positive aspects seen in DMEK while minimizing postoperative complications. Similar to DSEK, UT-DSEK is versatile and suitable for various eye types, even those with complex anatomies or challenges in anterior chamber visualization. Due to progress in tissue-processing techniques, surgeons can now produce thinner grafts **(Figs. 4.12 and 4.13)**, leading to a less-invasive procedure and expediting visual recovery.[15]

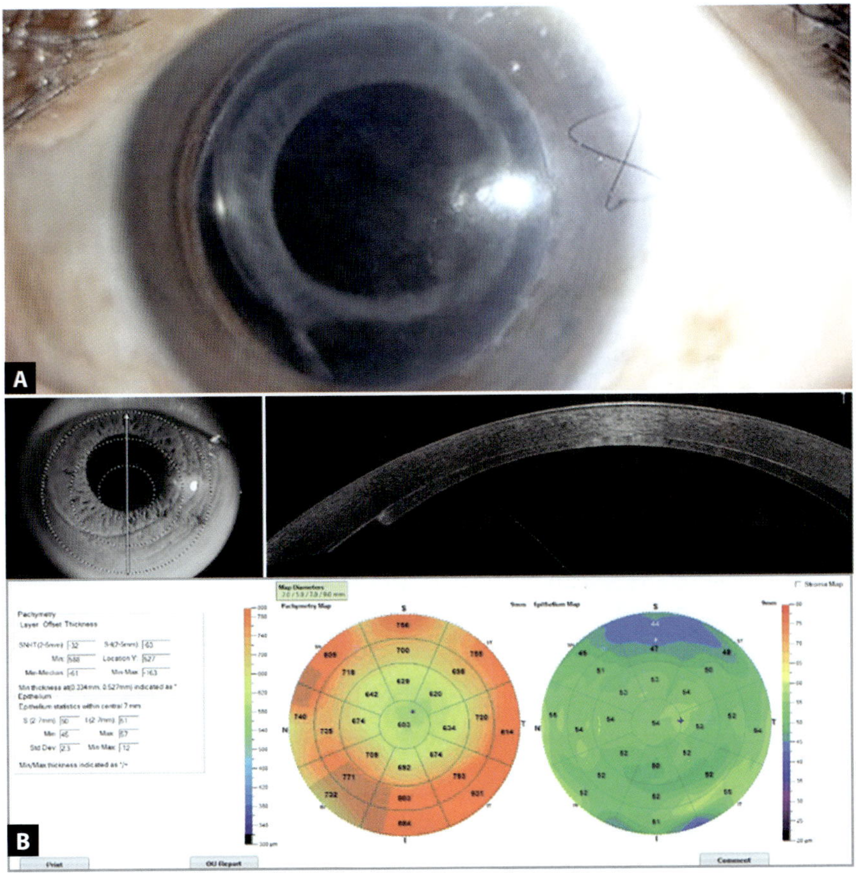

Figs. 4.11A and B: (A) Postoperative image after phacoemulsification with PCIOL placement combined with DSEK. (B) ASOCT image of the same eye. (ASOCT: anterior segment optical coherence tomography; DSEK: Descemet's stripping endothelial keratoplasty; PCIOL: posterior chamber intraocular lens)

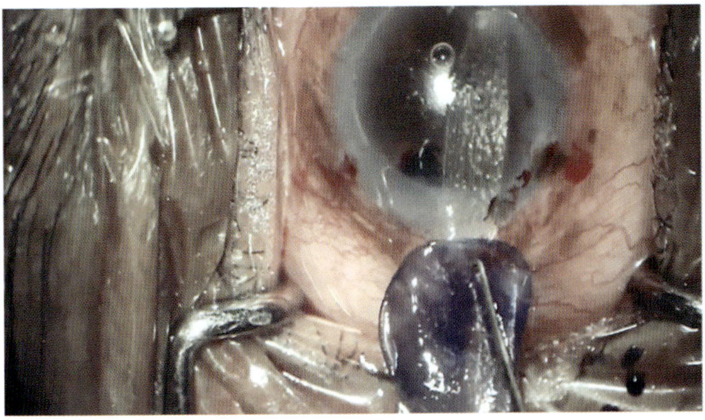

Fig. 4.12: Intraoperative image of placement of donor lenticule in UT-DSEK. (UT-DSEK: ultrathin Descemet's stripping endothelial keratoplasty)

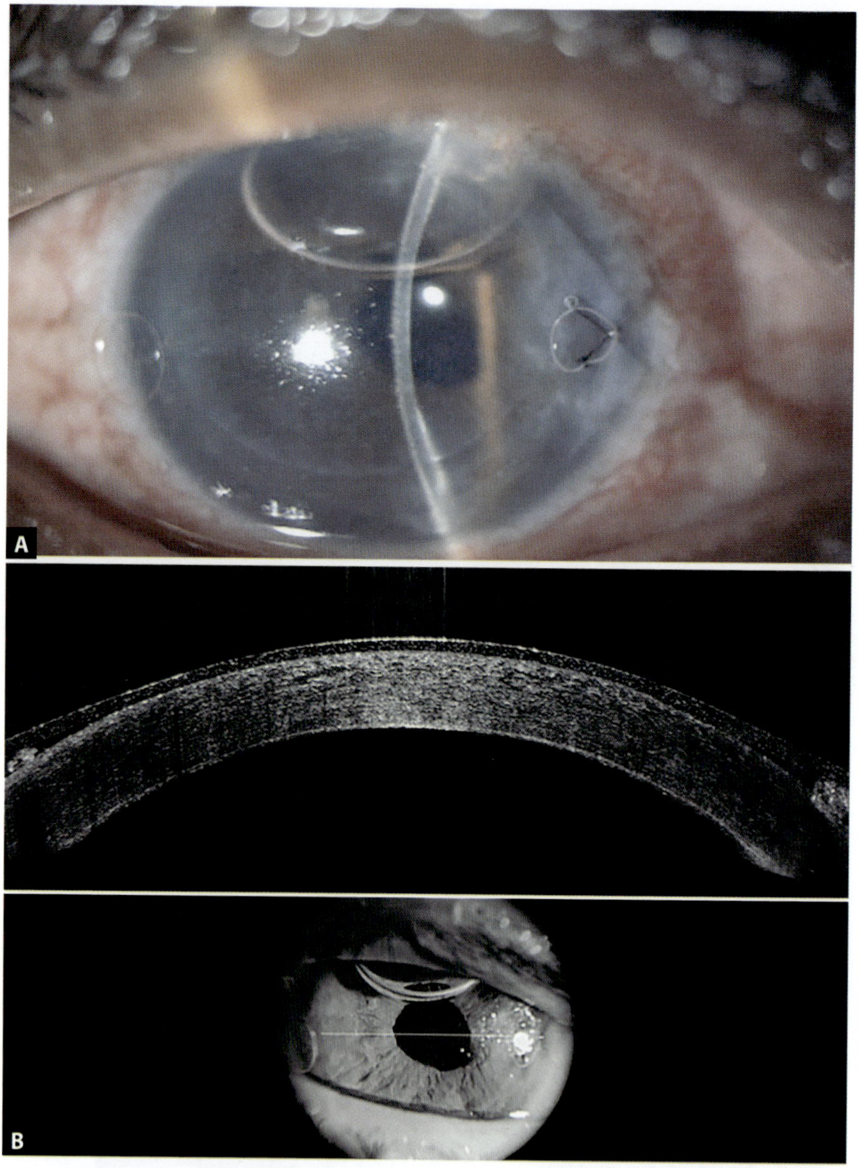

Figs. 4.13A and B: (A) Image of postoperative day 1; (B) ASOCT images of the same eye showing well-apposed ultrathin DSEK lenticule. (ASOCT: anterior segment optical coherence tomography; DSEK: Descemet's stripping endothelial keratoplasty)

Pre-Descemet's Endothelial Keratoplasty

Pre-Descemet's endothelial keratoplasty is a newer variant in the arena of endothelial keratoplasties and it involves the separation of pre-Descemet's layer (PDL) along with DM-endothelium as a donor lenticule. In the spectrum of endothelial keratoplasties, PDEK[16-18] has two major benefits—

the use of younger grafts and tear resistance. On the other hand, DSEK is widely accepted due to it being technically easier as compared to DMEK, which involves isolation of the donor DM-endothelium complex exclusively.

Dua et al.[16] discovered a novel PDL or Dua's layer that is approximately 10 μm in thickness and primarily composed of type-1 collagen bundles. Dua et al. distinctly described the type-1, type-2, and mixed bubble, emphasizing and demonstrating the significance and existence of each.[17]

Donor Graft Preparation

The donor corneoscleral button is placed on the Teflon block with the endothelial side up, and a 30-G needle attached to an air-filled 5-mL syringe is introduced from the edge of the corneal tissue to the mid-periphery. Then the air is injected, and a central, dome-shaped type-1 bubble that characteristically spreads from center to periphery is formed **(Fig. 4.14A)**. The extreme periphery of the bubble is punctured with a side port blade, and trypan blue is injected to stain the graft. After carefully cutting the bubble around its whole periphery with corneal trephine or corneoscleral scissors, the graft is removed and placed onto an injector, making sure that the graft is scrolled the right way up **(Fig. 4.14B)**.

Recipient Bed Preparation

Epithelial debridement can be done in cases with poor visualization or significant corneal edema to enhance the intraoperative visualization. A trocar AC maintainer (ACM) is introduced inside the eye and air is infused into the AC **(Fig. 4.15)**. Descemetorhexis is performed under air with the reverse Sinskey's hook that scrapes off the entire diseased endothelium with

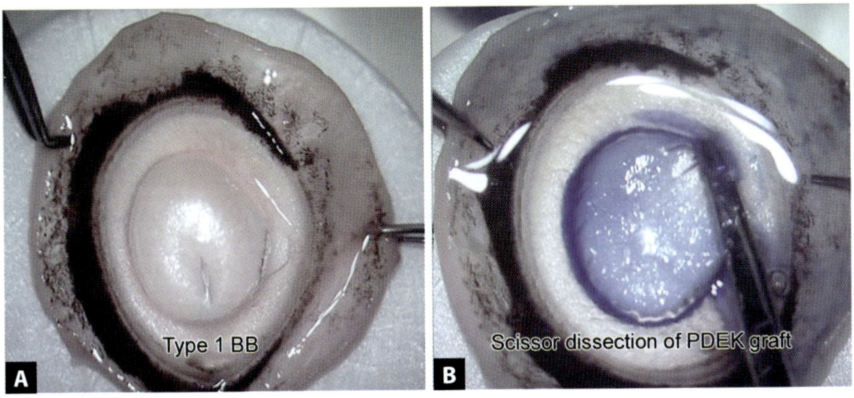

Figs. 4.14A and B: (A) Preparation of donor corneal button in PDEK by injecting air and achieving type-1 bubble; (B) Dissection of donor corneal graft which is stained with trypan blue using corneo-scleral scissors. (BB: big bubble; PDEK: pre-Descemet's endothelial keratoplasty)

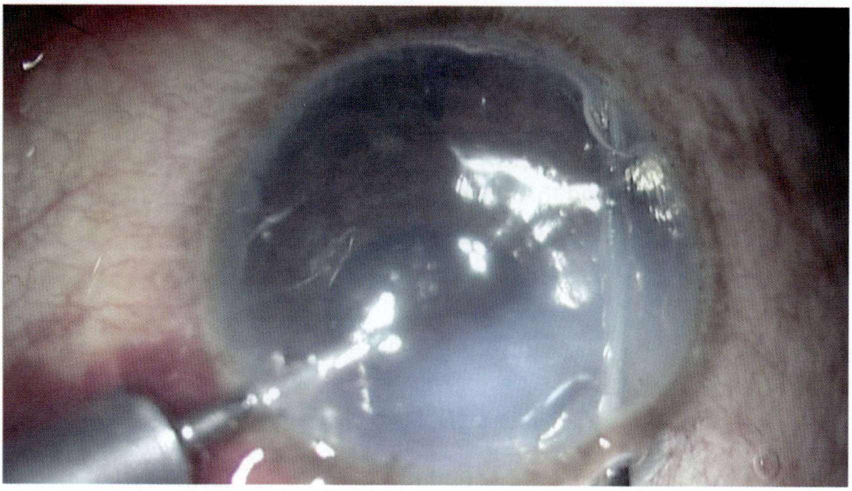

Fig. 4.15: During PDEK in recipient cornea, a trocar AC maintainer is introduced inside the AC and air is infused. Descemetorhexis is performed under air with reverse Sinskey hook. (AC: anterior chamber; PDEK: pre-Descemet's endothelial keratoplasty)

Descemet membrane in the recipient's eye, and then the scrapped complex is removed from the anterior chamber with the help of forceps.

Some techniques and advancements to get the most out of the procedure are given in the following text.

JACOB AIR PUMP-ASSISTED TECHNIQUE

With air continuously flowing into the anterior chamber through an ACM, connected to the air pump present in newer phacoemulsification machines or using the fluid–air exchange system present in posterior vitrectomy systems, the host Descemet membrane is stripped to a diameter 0.5 mm smaller than the graft using the descemetorhexis technique.[19,20] The continuous pressurized air infusion helps not only with descemetorhexis and graft adherence but aids in several other critical processes, including synechiolysis, stopping blood from leaking into AC from incision sites, graft edge unfolding, graft unwrinkling, graft floatation, graft centration, and preventing fluctuations in AC depth **(Fig. 4.16)**. As a result, it makes PDEK with young grafts more reproducible and easier to apply.

ENDOILLUMINATOR-ASSISTED PRE-DESCEMET'S ENDOTHELIAL KERATOPLASTY

The endoilluminator provides a clear overview of the entire graft. The focused light of the light probe can pierce through the edematous cornea and allow better visualization. The endoilluminator-aided approach to such cases is highly feasible, practical, and convenient **(Figs. 4.17A and B)**. It can serve as a

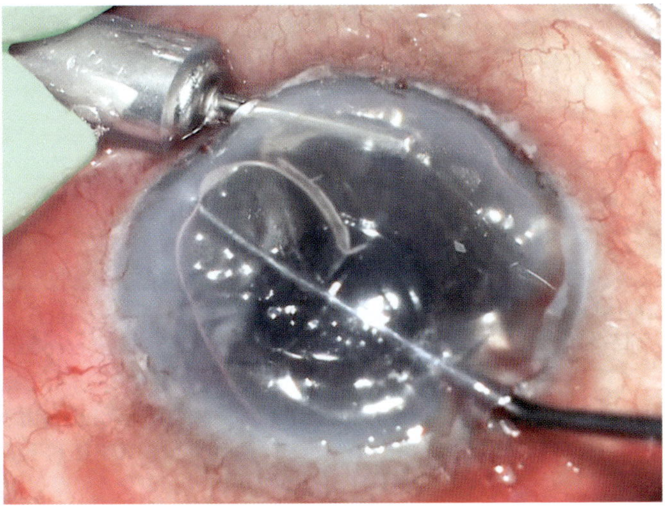

Fig. 4.16: Jacob air pump-assisted technique for descemetorhexis and graft adherence in PDEK. (PDEK: pre-Descemet's endothelial keratoplasty)

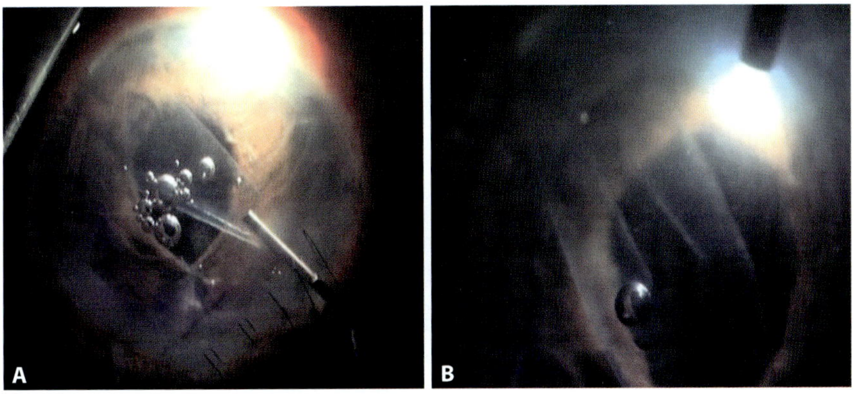

Figs. 4.17A and B: (A) Endoilluminator-assisted PDEK (E-PDEK); (B) Graft orientation easily verifiable. (PDEK: pre-Descemet's endothelial keratoplasty)

smart addition to our surgical armamentarium as patients with concomitant pathology can still get good postoperative vision helping achieve better results both intra- and postoperatively.[21]

USE OF S-STAMP IN PRE-DESCEMET'S ENDOTHELIAL KERATOPLASTY SURGERY

An irreversible letter stamp is a method that is frequently used to identify the orientation of the graft in endothelial keratoplasty grafts, including ultrathin DSAEK grafts, automated endothelial keratoplasty, and DMEK grafts. S, F, and P are a few instances of irreversible letters that can be employed. It is

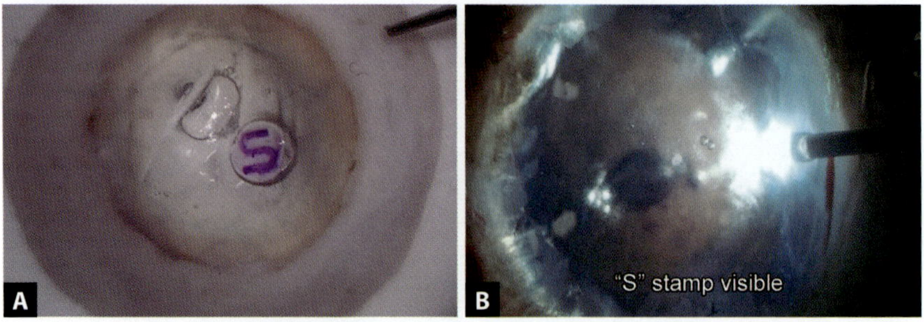

Figs. 18A and B: (A) S-stamp seen on donor tissue graft to identify correct orientation while graft placement; (B) S-stamp visible on graft after adherence.

also possible to indicate the PDEK graft with an S-stamp, which will facilitate the beginner surgeon's adaptation and transfer to PDEK **(Figs. 4.18A and B)**.

A popular method for spotting inverted grafts and correcting their position before floating them up is the S-stamp. Similar to what was previously mentioned, it has been utilized for DMEK grafts for a very long time. Additionally, this eliminates the worry that a transplant may fail during preparation, facilitates improved patient logistics, and eliminates the chance that surgery may need to be postponed in the event of a graft loss. Having premarked, prestained, precut, and preloaded PDEK grafts readily available for use will help PDEK to be rapidly adopted by surgeons. PDEK surgery will enable a far greater number of patients to benefit from these grafts because it is simpler to execute than DMEK surgery, especially in complex eyes.

HOST DESCEMETIC SCAFFOLDING

The descemetorhexis technique is used to remove the host Descemet membrane to a diameter 0.5 mm smaller than the graft. One quadrant or the full 360° surrounding the graft may be stripped, depending on the extent of the modification. Usually, the surgeon makes two opposing quadrants of the host descemtorhexis smaller. With the use of a reverse Sinskey hook, the host Descemet membrane is carefully lifted from beneath the graft and permitted to overlap it in a scaffolding fashion from the posterior aspect. Starting at the free edge of the host Descemet membrane, you can gently pull it out by dragging the reverse Sinskey hook along the graft's margin without actually touching the graft **(Fig. 4.19)**. Under the pressured infusion, graft adhesion is quickly established. Scaffolding maneuvers result in an extra degree of scaffolding or support that provides graft stability and thereby prevents the graft from detaching. This is especially useful if performed at the inferior aspect, where intracameral air does not always support the graft. It is also useful in complex eyes, such as those with aphakia, previous vitrectomy, a broken posterior capsule, etc.

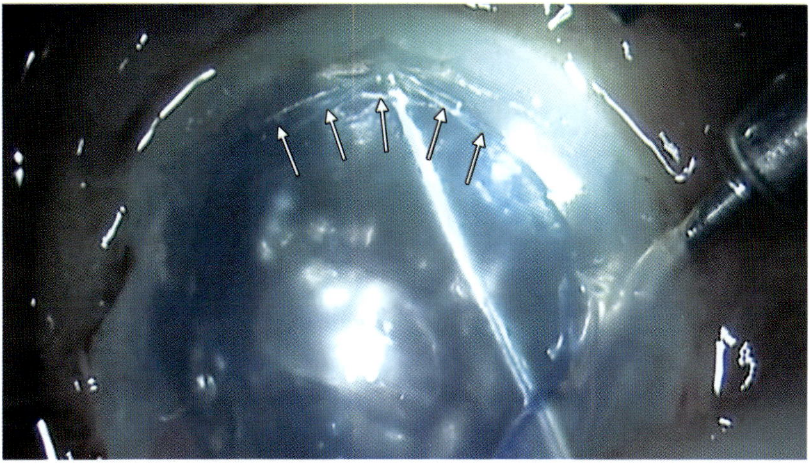

Fig. 4.19: Descemetorhexis using host Descemetic scaffolding technique using reverse Sinskey hook in pre-Descemet's endothelial keratoplasty (PDEK).

Descemetorhexis without Endothelial Keratoplasty

The surgical removal of Descemet membrane without subsequent endothelial transplantation, specifically in the treatment of Fuchs endothelial corneal dystrophy (FECD), has been a subject of both interest and controversy.[22,23] This technique, while not ensuring lasting corneal clarity for all patients, proves beneficial in selected FECD cases, reducing the necessity for endothelial keratoplasty (EK) in these specific scenarios.

Key considerations in the surgical technique include:
- Limiting the size of descemetorhexis (<4 mm)
- Ensuring centration of descemetorhexis
- Avoiding engagement with the stroma
- Opting for the peeling of DM instead of scraping

Indications

Fuchs endothelial corneal dystrophy is diagnosed clinically and on confocal microscopy, particularly in cases with:[24]
- Presence of central guttae as the primary cause of visual symptoms (such as decreased visual acuity, contrast sensitivity, and glare)
- A clear peripheral cornea with an endothelial cell count >1,000 cells/mm^2 on confocal or specular microscopy
- Patients considering endothelial keratoplasty
- Both phakic and pseudophakic individuals

Contraindications

- Advanced corneal stroma edema (haze, bullae, and DM folds)
- Peripheral endothelial cell count <1,000 cells/mm^2

- Presence of secondary corneal pathology
- History of herpes simplex virus or cytomegalovirus keratitis

Descemet Membrane Endothelial Keratoplasty

The final iteration of endothelial keratoplasty came with pure anatomic replacement: DM was removed from the recipient and replaced with only donor DM and no stromal carrier tissue compared to its predecessor DSEK/DSAEK. The first case of this was performed by Melles et al. in 2006 and he named it DMEK.[25-28]

Several variations of the surgical technique of DMEK and different DMEK graft injectors have evolved[29] over the years, yet no standardized protocol has been adopted worldwide for DMEK surgery due to its technical difficulty itself, economic practicalities, and increased postoperative complications compared with those of DSEK or DSAEK.[30] Unlike western world, patients in India also present at a later stage[31] during which stromal scarring starts due to chronic corneal decompensation,[32] resulting in poor visibility for unfolding the DM scroll in the anterior chamber. Another key issue for surgeons is that in DMEK, a total dislocation of tissue will require replacement of tissue, whereas DSEK requires only rebubbling.[33-35] Since there is a dearth of corneal tissues in India, surgeons are worried about the tissue loss and resort to the safer and standard DSEK procedure.

Donor Preparation

Initial scoring: The donor tissue is placed in the well of the cutting block and a 10-mm trephine is used to gently mark the DM (use very minimal pressure so that only the DM and a thin layer of stroma are cut) with the endothelial side facing up **(Fig. 4.20A)**. The marked DM is scored with a Sinskey hook 360° gently without creating any tags or irregularities at the edge of the DM **(Fig. 4.20B)**. The scoring is performed, while the donor tissue and the subsequent graft remain submerged in balanced salt solution (BSS). The tissue is scored 0.5–1 mm central to the limbus, as more peripherally, the stroma and DM are adherent and an edge cannot be created.

Staining: Trypan blue is used to stain the graft only after the initial trephination. First, the storage media in which the graft has been submerged is largely removed with a Weck-cel ophthalmic sponge so that it will not dilute or prevent adequate staining. After staining with the dye for approximately 2 minutes, excess dye is decanted and several drops of the media are again used to fill the donor rim. With this process, scored tissue edges are highlighted in dark blue.

Lifting up the edge and DM stripping: The periphery of the scored endothelial edge is elevated with a blunt Sinskey hook to separate the endothelium–Descemet membrane 360° circumferentially. Once the peripheral tissue is

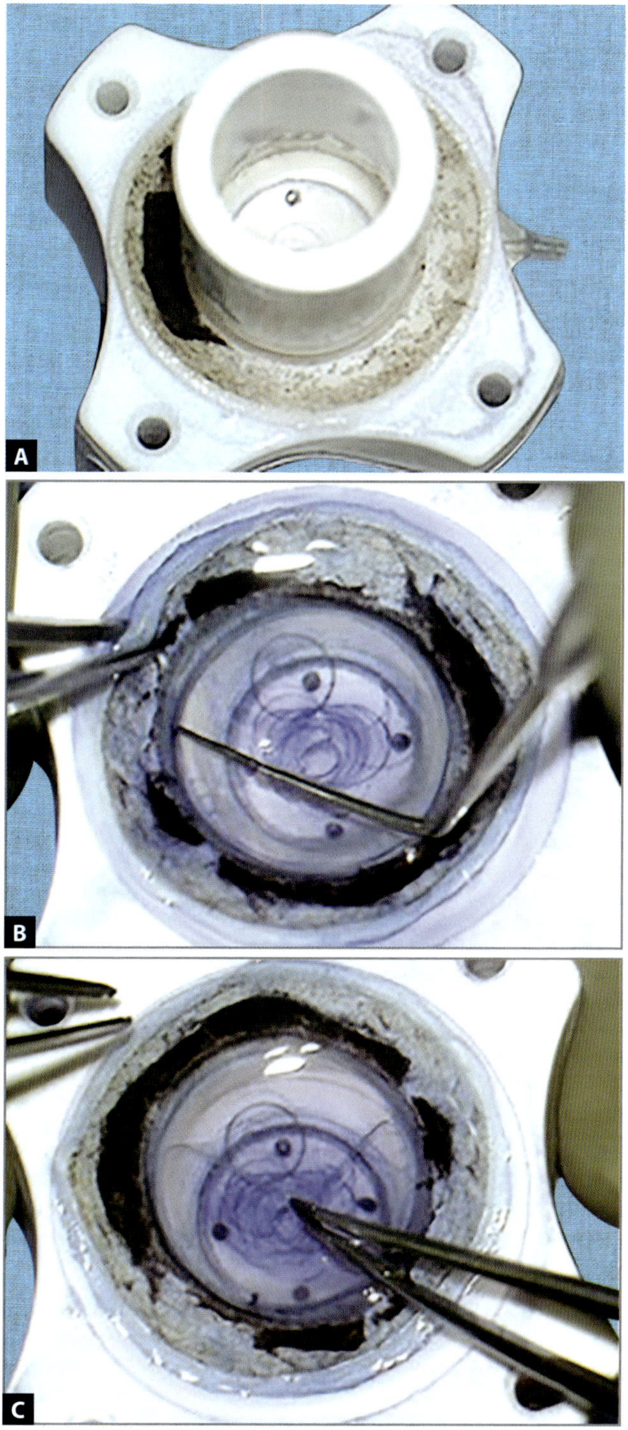

Figs. 4.20A to C

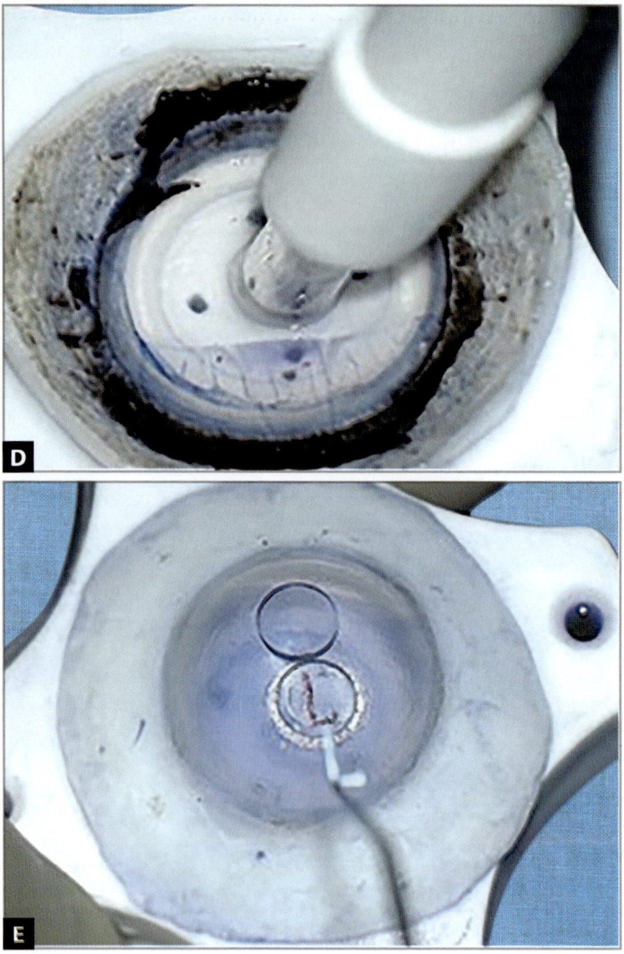

Figs. 20D and E

Figs. 4.20A to E: (A) Donor preparation in DMEK where donor corneal button is placed on Teflon block endothelial side up. A 10-mm trephine is used to gently mark the DM making a thin cut; (B) Marked and stained DM is scored using a Sinskey hook all around from periphery; (C) DM + endothelium complex is stripped using a single pull technique with a smooth curved forceps; (D) After stripping half of DM + endothelium from stroma, 3-mm trephine is used to create a central punch in the donor stroma; (E) "L"-shaped mark is made through the stromal window on donor tissue with endothelium facing down which helps in orientation while graft placement. (DM: Descemet membrane; DMEK: Descemet membrane endothelial keratoplasty)

separated, an edge is grasped with smooth curved forceps and an additional endothelial-Descemet membrane is stripped under BSS using the "single-pull technique" **(Fig. 4.20C)**.

Marking the tissue: After stripping half of the DM from the donor and creating a 3-mm punch in the stroma **(Fig. 4.20D)**, an "L"-shaped mark is made through the stromal window on the DM using a stained "L" stamp with the horizontal arm being shorter and the vertical arm being longer **(Fig. 4.20E)** so that the shorter horizontal arm always comes to the right side of the longer vertical arm when oriented endothelial side down. After this, the DM is replaced back on the stroma.

Trephination: The size of trephine used is determined by the host's underlying corneal pathology and also the horizontal diameter of the cornea. Baron's vacuum punch is used to cut the tissue.

Storage: After trephination to the desired graft size and complete separation of the DMEK tissue, the tissue scrolls with the endothelium facing outward **(Fig. 4.21A)**. The DMEK tissue is then placed in BSS and stained again with trypan blue to allow visualization after insertion.

Preloaded DMEK graft tissues are also available which are prestripped and preloaded into a transport cartridge to be inserted by the surgeon, similar to a preloaded intraocular lens in cataract surgery **(Figs. 4.22A to C)**. DMEK grafts can be stored and shipped for up to 2 days in dextran-containing medium without significant ECL.[36,37]

Recipient Preparation

Removal of epithelium: Epithelium is removed with a blunt spatula prior to the intraocular procedure for better visualization in all the cases.

Wound construction: Paracentesis is made almost parallel to the iris plane in the superior and inferior clear corneal limbus. The main incision is made temporally at 3 o'clock in a uniplanar fashion with a 3-mm keratome at the limbus.

Descemet membrane stripping: A desired-sized trephine is gently pressed on the epithelial side to help in the sizing of the descemetorhexis. The edges of the trephine mark are highlighted with a mark in a dot fashion. Using a reverse Sinskey hook, the recipient DM is scored and gently removed from the stromal bed avoiding any trauma to the overlying stroma. Peripheral iridectomy is done at the 6 o'clock position as peripherally as possible to prevent pupillary block.

Loading: Prototype injector: A regular intraocular lens C-cartridge, IV tubing, and 1-cm^3 syringe is assembled **(Fig. 4.21B)**. The DM scroll, which was previously scored in the storage medium, is then sucked into the DMEK injector using the ''no touch technique" **(Fig. 4.21C)**.

Injection into the anterior chamber: Using our prototype injector, the DM scroll is injected into the anterior chamber at one go **(Fig. 4.23A)**. Once the tissue is injected into the anterior chamber, unscrolling or injecting saline into the anterior chamber should be done only after the application of a

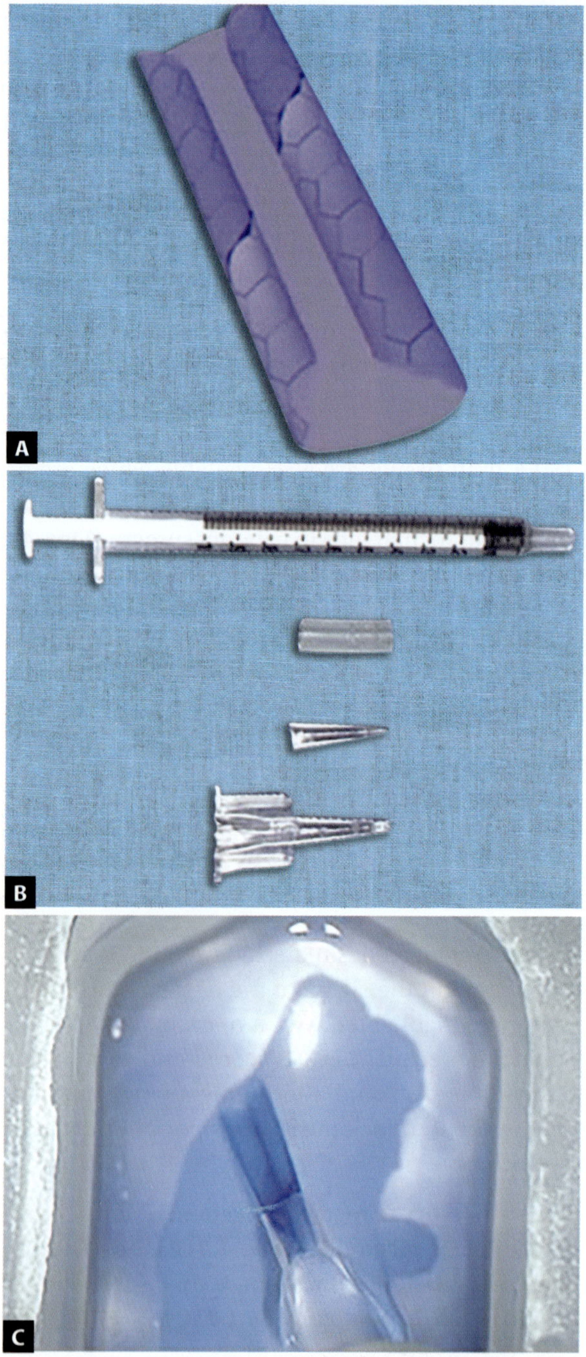

Figs. 21A to C: (A) Folded DMEK graft tissue with endothelial facing outward; (B) Prototype injector, which includes a regular intraocular lens C-cartridge, IV tubing, and 1 cm^3 syringe; (C) Loading of DMEK graft tissue by sucking it into the injector using the no-touch technique. (DMEK: Descemet membrane endothelial keratoplasty)

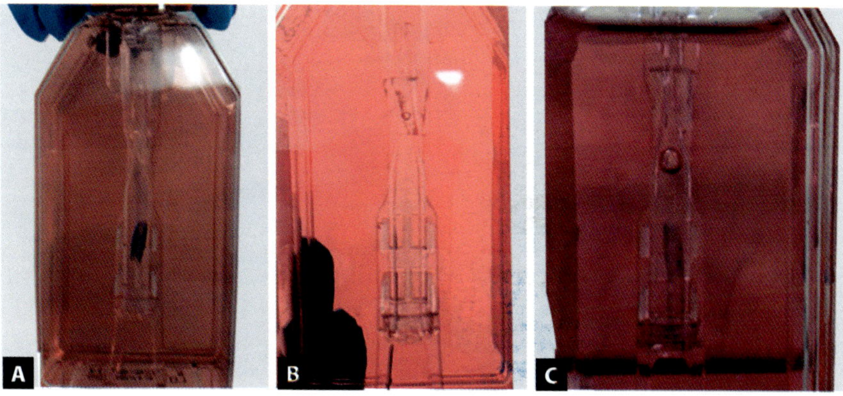

Figs. 22A to C: (A) Culture flask with a trypan blue-stained and preloaded DMEK lamella within a transport cartridge before shipping; (B) Decolored after 48-hour storage and shipping; (C) Restained with trypan blue within the transport cartridge. (DMEK: Descemet membrane endothelial keratoplasty)

single 10-0 nylon on the main tunnel incision to prevent the escape of the scroll from the anterior chamber **(Fig. 4.23B)**.

Unscrolling the Tissue

Saline is injected into the anterior chamber to position the DM scroll. Once the DM scroll is positioned to the desired place and the L mark is seen upright confirming the correct orientation of the graft, we use the "hold and release technique" **(Fig. 4.23C)** in which the far tip of the scroll is held with a hydro canula and the anterior chamber is shallowed from the main tunnel with another hydro cannula. This shallowing is key as the tissue unfolds gently without any tapping or violent maneuvers.

Bubbling

Once unfolded over the iris, the DMEK graft can be easily lifted onto the recipient posterior stroma by positioning an air bubble underneath the graft. A full-chamber air bubble is injected into the anterior chamber which supports the adherence of the graft to the host stroma. No burping of the air was done postoperatively **(Fig. 4.23D)**.

Why DMEK Is Superior?

Descemet membrane endothelial keratoplasty has been shown to have superior visual outcomes when compared to its predecessor DSEK **(Fig. 4.24A to D)**. In multiple studies where patients had DSAEK in one eye and DMEK in the fellow eye, significantly better visual acuity and preference were reported in the DMEK eye.[29-32] 85% reported a better quality of vision

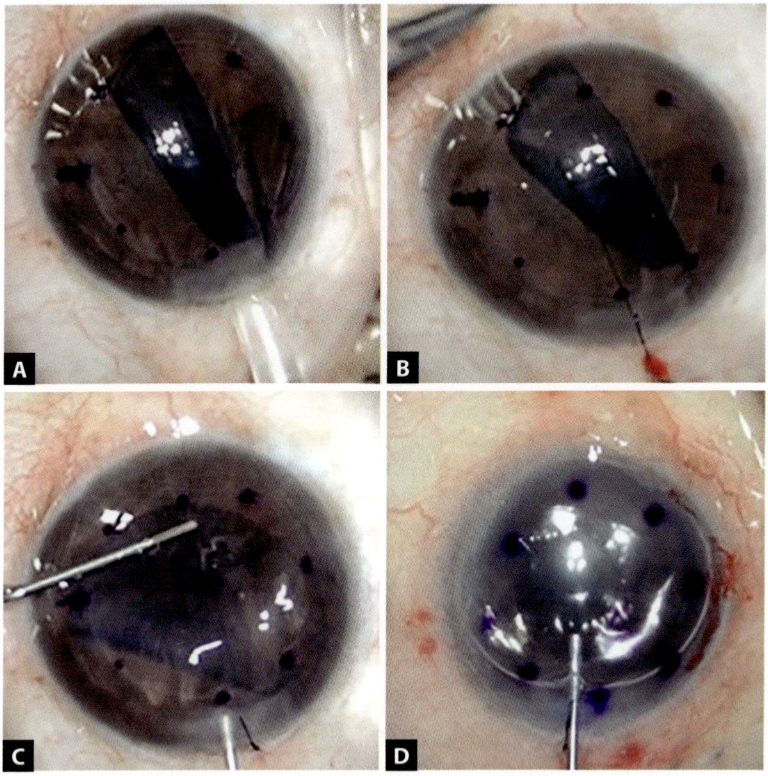

Figs. 23A to D: (A) DM scroll is injected into the anterior chamber (AC) using the prototype injector. (B) The main wound is sutured before any intraocular manipulation to prevent escape of the DM scroll. (C) Unscrolling of the graft tissue done using the "hold and release technique" wherein the far tip of the DM scroll is held with a hydrocannula and AC is shallowed from the main wound using another hydrocannula. (D) Injection of a large air bubble filling the AC facilitating graft–host apposition. (DM: Descemet membrane)

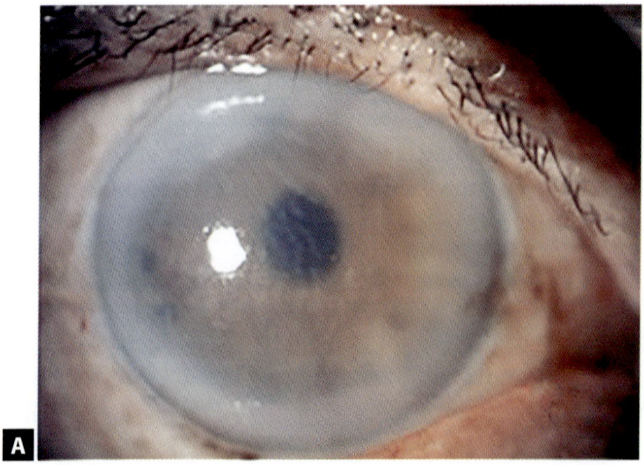

Fig. 24A

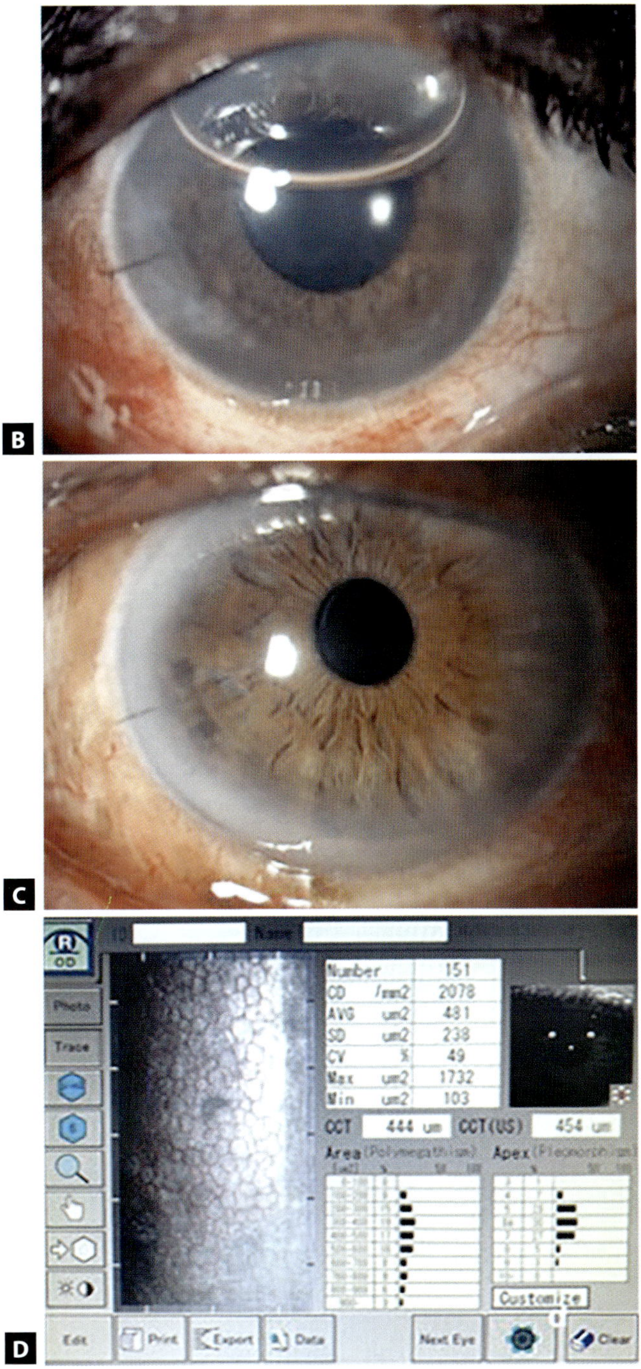

Figs. 24B to D

Figs. 24A to D: DMEK in pseudophakic bullous keratopathy. (A) Preoperative period; (B) immediate postoperative period; (C) 6 months postoperative period; (D) specular count—6 months. (DMEK: Descemet membrane endothelial keratoplasty) in the DMEK eye. ECL at 1 year was 31% in DMEK eyes and 34% in DSAEK eyes.[38,39] DMEK also has a lower immunologic rejection rate and has the advantage of using a smaller incision (2.8 mm) than DSAEK (5 mm).[40] Also, postoperative use of milder steroids will reduce the incidence of glaucoma in these patients.

Future Directions

Descemet membrane endothelial keratoplasty is a relatively new procedure and surgeons continue to develop many new exciting techniques and strategies. The use of real-time intraoperative OCT[41] and FSL[42] with DMEK have recently been discussed. Eye banks will likely continue to play an important role in DMEK surgery, and their involvement with prestripping DMEK tissue decreases tissue wasting by the surgeon during preparation.[43] Enhancing endothelial cell number and viability should remain an important research focus.[44] Descemet membrane endothelial transfer,[45] gene therapy, or Rho-associated kinase inhibitors[46] are particularly exciting areas of research in this area.

Artificial Endothelial Replacement Membrane Implantation (EndoArt, EyeYon Medical, Israel)

Artificial endothelial replacement membrane represents a paradigm shift in the management of corneal endothelial dysfunction. Developed through years of research and innovation, EndoArt is a synthetic membrane designed to mimic the function of the native endothelium, providing a durable and biocompatible solution for restoring corneal clarity **(Fig. 4.25)**.

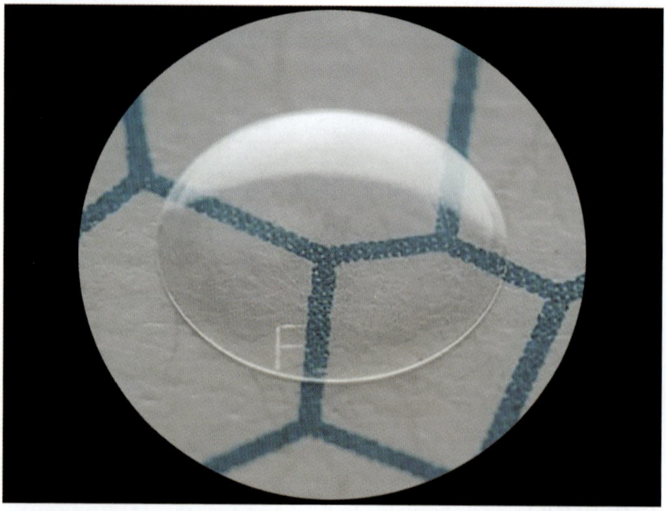

Fig. 4.25: Image of artificial endothelial replacement membrane with the letter "F" used for device orientation.

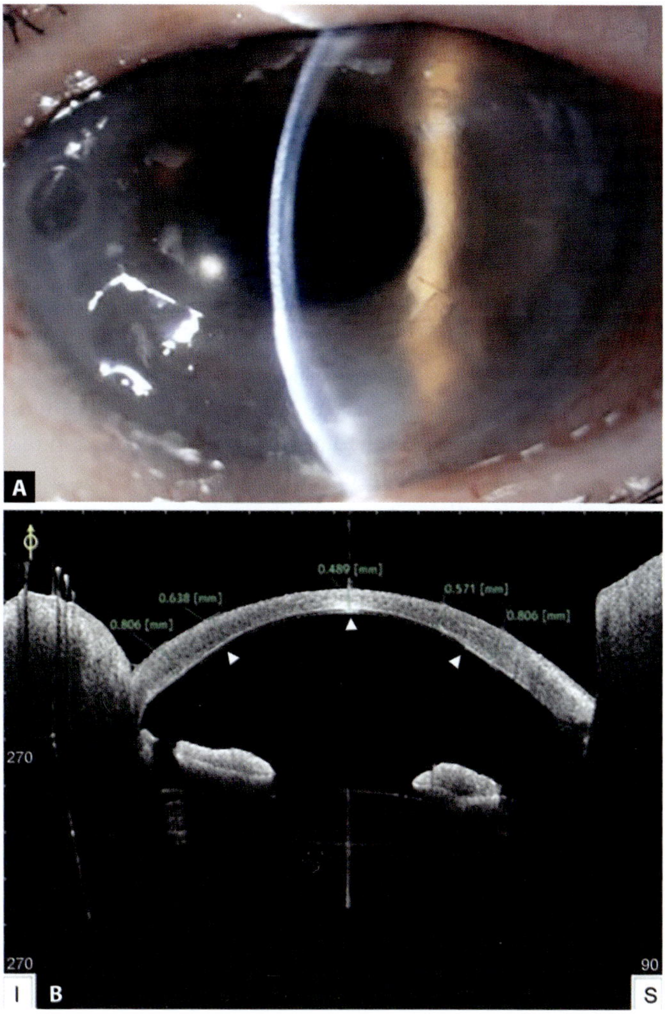

Figs. 4.26A and B: (A) Slit-lamp photograph 6 months after artificial endothelial replacement membrane implantation. The image shows a clear central cornea (5–6 mm diameter) corresponding to the area of the implant. The peripheral cornea is edematous and opaque. (B) ASOCT of the same patient. The ASOCT shows the artificial endothelial replacement membrane well adherent to the posterior corneal surface (arrowheads). The calipers indicate the corneal thickness excluding the implant. (ASOCT: anterior segment optical coherence tomography)

It is composed of an acrylic hydrophilic, flexible material measuring 50 mm in thickness and 6.5 mm in diameter, shaped according to the posterior corneal curvature **(Figs. 4.25 and 4.26)**, engineered to replicate the physiological properties of the endothelial layer. Upon implantation onto the posterior surface of the cornea, it forms a barrier that prevents the influx of fluid into the cornea, effectively reducing corneal edema and improving corneal transparency. Unlike traditional corneal transplantation techniques, it eliminates the need for donor tissue, streamlining the surgical process and reducing the risk of rejection.

There are concerns surrounding the long-term viability of grafts, especially in certain patient populations. Factors such as prior graft failure, bullous keratopathy, glaucoma, and history of complex anterior segment surgeries are known to negatively impact graft survival rates. Studies indicate that there is an overall probability of 14.3% of requiring repeat keratoplasty within 5 years, with the likelihood increasing to 26% in cases where the initial graft has failed.[47] Similar to penetrating keratoplasty (PK), the anticipated survival duration of repeat endothelial keratoplasty diminishes with each subsequent graft procedure. Consequently, as the number of EK surgeries continues to rise globally, the burden of repeat EK procedures is expected to escalate. This issue could be addressed by an artificial endothelial membrane.

Studies have been done showing good outcomes with the use of EndoArt in treating corneal edema in eyes after failed repeat endothelial keratoplasty.[48]

CONCLUSION

The advancements in lamellar keratoplasty underscore the transformative impact of technology, surgical refinements, and collaborative research efforts leading to improved visual outcomes, enhanced graft survival, and potential solutions for corneal blindness worldwide.

ACKNOWLEDGMENTS

We would like to acknowledge Dr Shreyas Ramamurthy, Dr Soosan Jacob, and Dr Amar Agarwal for their contribution in preparing this manuscript.

REFERENCES

1. Sharma B, Dubey A, Prakash G, Vajpayee RB. Bowman's layer transplantation: evidence to date. Clin Ophthalmol Auckl NZ. 2018;12:433-7.
2. Parker JS, Huls F, Cooper E, Graves P, Groeneveld-van Beek EA, Lie J, et al. Technical feasibility of isolated Bowman layer graft preparation by femtosecond laser: a pilot study. Eur J Ophthalmol. 2017;27(6):675-7.
3. Yoo SH, Kymionis GD, Koreishi A, Ide T, Goldman D, Karp CL, et al. Femtosecond laser-assisted sutureless anterior lamellar keratoplasty. Ophthalmology. 2008;115(8):1303-7.
4. Bonfadini G, Moreira H, Jun AS, Campos M, Kim EC, Arana E, et al. Modified femtosecond laser-assisted sutureless anterior lamellar keratoplasty. Cornea. 2013;32(4):533.
5. Nagpal R, Sharma N, Bafna RK, Muraleekrishna M, Vajpayee RB. Tuck-in deep anterior lamellar keratoplasty for the management of post-radial keratotomy keratectasia. J Cataract Refract Surg. 2022;48(8):937.

6. Guindolet D, Nguyen DT, Bergin C, Doan S, Cochereau I, Gabison EE. Double-docking technique for femtosecond laser-assisted deep anterior lamellar keratoplasty. Cornea. 2018;37(1):123.
7. Sandali O, El Sanharawi M, Temstet C, Hamiche T, Galan A, Ghouali W, et al. Fourier-domain optical coherence tomography imaging in keratoconus: a corneal structural classification. Ophthalmology. 2013;120(12):2403-12.
8. Borderie VM, Touhami S, Georgeon C, Sandali O. Predictive factors for successful type 1 big bubble during deep anterior lamellar keratoplasty. J Ophthalmol. 2018:4685406.
9. Khodaparast M, Shahraki K, Jabbarvand M, Shahraki K, Rafat M, Moravvej Z. Sutureless femtosecond laser-assisted anterior lamellar keratoplasty using a bioengineered cornea as a viable alternative to human donor transplantation for superficial corneal opacities. Cornea. 2020;39(9):1184.
10. Sridhar U, Tripathy K. Commentary: recent advances in endothelial keratoplasty and the postoperative use of bandage contact lens. Indian J Ophthalmol. 2021;69(1):81-2.
11. Güell JL, El Husseiny MA, Manero F, Gris O, Elies D. Historical review and update of surgical treatment for corneal endothelial diseases. Ophthalmol Ther. 2014;3(1-2):1-15.
12. Tourabaly M, Chetrit Y, Provost J, Georgeon C, Kallel S, Temstet C, et al. Influence of graft thickness and regularity on vision recovery after endothelial keratoplasty. Br J Ophthalmol. 2020;104(9):1317-23.
13. Khan SN, Shiakolas PS, Mootha VV. Descemet's stripping automated endothelial keratoplasty tissue insertion devices. J Ophthalmic Vis Res. 2015;10(4):461-8.
14. Price FWJ, Price MO. Combined cataract/DSEK/DMEK: changing expectations. Asia-Pac J Ophthalmol. 2017;6(4):388.
15. Busin M, Albé E. Does thickness matter: ultrathin Descemet stripping automated endothelial keratoplasty. Curr Opin Ophthalmol. 2014;25(4):312-8.
16. Dua HS, Faraj LA, Said DG, Gray T, Lowe J. Human corneal anatomy redefined: a novel pre-Descemet's layer (Dua's layer). Ophthalmology. 2013;120(9):1778-85.
17. Agarwal A, Dua HS, Narang P, Kumar DA, Agarwal A, Jacob S, et al. Pre-Descemet's endothelial keratoplasty (PDEK). Br J Ophthalmol. 2014;98(9):1181-5.
18. Agarwal A, Agarwal A, Narang P, Kumar DA, Jacob S. Pre-Descemet endothelial keratoplasty with infant donor corneas: a prospective analysis. Cornea. 2015;34(8):859-65.
19. Jacob S. Use of pressurized air infusion for Pre Descemet's endothelial keratoplasty (PDEK)—The air pump assisted PDEK technique. Open Ophthalmol J. 2018;12:175-80.
20. Jacob S, Narasimhan S, Agarwal A, Agarwal A, Saijimol AI. Air pump-assisted graft centration, graft edge unfolding, and graft uncreasing in young donor graft pre-Descemet endothelial keratoplasty. Cornea. 2017;36(8):1009-13.
21. Jacob S, Agarwal A, Agarwal A, Narasimhan S, Kumar DA, Sivagnanam S. Endoilluminator-assisted transcorneal illumination for Descemet membrane endothelial keratoplasty: enhanced intraoperative visualization of the graft in corneal decompensation secondary to pseudophakic bullous keratopathy. J Cataract Refract Surg. 2014;40(8):1332-6.

22. Kaufman AR, Nosé RM, Pineda R. Descemetorhexis without endothelial keratoplasty (DWEK): proposal for nomenclature standardization. Cornea. 2018;37(4):20-1.
23. Borkar DS, Veldman P, Colby KA. Treatment of Fuchs endothelial dystrophy by Descemet stripping without endothelial keratoplasty. Cornea. 2016;35(10): 1267-73.
24. Moloney G, Petsoglou C, Ball M, Kerdraon Y, Höllhumer R, Spiteri N, et al. Descemetorhexis without grafting for Fuchs endothelial dystrophy-supplementation with topical Ripasudil. Cornea. 2017;36(6):642-8.
25. Melles GRJ, Ong TS, Ververs B, van der Wees J. Preliminary clinical results of Descemet membrane endothelial keratoplasty. Am J Ophthalmol. 2008; 145(2):222-7.
26. Sharma A, Woodman A. Comment on transplantation of Descemet's membrane carrying viable endothelium through a small scleral incision. Cornea. 2002;21(8): 840.
27. Ham L, Balachandran C, Verschoor CA, van der Wees J, Melles GRJ. Visual rehabilitation rate after isolated descemet membrane transplantation: descemet membrane endothelial keratoplasty. Arch Ophthalmol Chic Ill 1960. 2009;127(3):252-5.
28. Ham L, Dapena I, van Luijk C, van der Wees J, Melles GRJ. Descemet membrane endothelial keratoplasty (DMEK) for Fuchs endothelial dystrophy: review of the first 50 consecutive cases. Eye Lond Engl. 2009;23(10):1990-8.
29. Siebelmann S, Janetzko M, König P, Scholz P, Matthaei M, Händel A, et al. Flushing versus pushing technique for graft implantation in Descemet membrane endothelial keratoplasty. Cornea. 2020;39(5):605-8.
30. Gorovoy MS. DMEK complications. Cornea. 2014;33(1):101-4.
31. Basak SK, Basak S, Pradhan VR. Outcomes of Descemet membrane endothelial keratoplasty (DMEK) using surgeon's prepared donor DM-roll in consecutive 100 Indian eyes. Open Ophthalmol J. 2018;12:134-42.
32. Morishige N, Chikama T, Yamada N, Takahashi N, Morita Y, Nishida T, et al. Effect of preoperative duration of stromal edema in bullous keratopathy on early visual acuity after endothelial keratoplasty. J Cataract Refract Surg. 2012;38(2):303-8.
33. Price FW, Price MO. Descemet's stripping with endothelial keratoplasty in 200 eyes: early challenges and techniques to enhance donor adherence. J Cataract Refract Surg. 2006;32(3):411-8.
34. Terry MA, Shamie N, Chen ES, Hoar KL, Friend DJ. Endothelial keratoplasty a simplified technique to minimize graft dislocation, iatrogenic graft failure, and pupillary block. Ophthalmology. 2008;115(7):1179-86.
35. Terry MA, Shamie N, Chen ES, Phillips PM, Shah AK, Hoar KL, et al. Endothelial keratoplasty for Fuchs' dystrophy with cataract: complications and clinical results with the new triple procedure. Ophthalmology. 2009;116(4):631-9.
36. Rickmann A, Wahl S, Hofmann N, Knakowski J, Haus A, Börgel M, et al. Comparison of preloaded grafts for Descemet membrane endothelial keratoplasty (DMEK) in a novel preloaded transport cartridge compared to conventional precut grafts. Cell Tis Ban. 2020;21(2):205-13.
37. Català P, Vermeulen W, Rademakers T, van den Bogaerdt A, Kruijt PJ, Nuijts RMMA, et al. Transport and preservation comparison of preloaded and prestripped-only DMEK grafts. Cornea. 2020;39(11):1407-14.

38. Guerra FP, Anshu A, Price MO, Price FW. Endothelial keratoplasty: fellow eyes comparison of Descemet stripping automated endothelial keratoplasty and Descemet membrane endothelial keratoplasty. Cornea. 2011;30(12):1382-6.
39. Maier AKB, Gundlach E, Gonnermann J, Klamann MKJ, Bertelmann E, Rieck PW, et al. Retrospective contralateral study comparing Descemet membrane endothelial keratoplasty with Descemet stripping automated endothelial keratoplasty. Eye Lond Engl. 2015;29(3):327-32.
40. Veldman PB, Terry MA, Straiko MD. Evolving indications for Descemet's stripping automated endothelial keratoplasty. Curr Opin Ophthalmol. 2014;25(4):306-11.
41. Cost B, Goshe JM, Srivastava S, Ehlers JP. Intraoperative optical coherence tomography-assisted descemet membrane endothelial keratoplasty in the DISCOVER study. Am J Ophthalmol. 2015;160(3):430-7.
42. Jardine GJ, Holiman JD, Galloway JD, Stoeger CG, Chamberlain WD. Eye bank-prepared femtosecond laser-assisted automated Descemet membrane endothelial grafts. Cornea. 2015;34(7):838-43.
43. Terry MA. Endothelial keratoplasty: why aren't we all doing Descemet membrane endothelial keratoplasty? Cornea. 2012;31(5):469-71.
44. Mian SI. Evolution of a revolution in keratoplasty. Curr Opin Ophthalmol. 2014;25(4):298-9.
45. Lam FC, Bruinsma M, Melles GRJ. Descemet membrane endothelial transfer. Curr Opin Ophthalmol. 2014;25(4):353-7.
46. Koizumi N, Okumura N, Ueno M, Kinoshita S. New therapeutic modality for corneal endothelial disease using Rho-associated kinase inhibitor eye drops. Cornea. 2014;33(11):25-31.
47. Zafar S, Wang P, Woreta FA, Aziz K, Makary M, Srikumaran D. Risk factors for repeat keratoplasty after endothelial keratoplasty in the medicare population. Am J Ophthalmol. 2021; 221:287-98.
48. Fontana L, di Geronimo N, Cennamo M, Mencucci R, Versura P, Moramarco A. Early outcomes of an artificial endothelial replacement membrane implantation after failed repeat endothelial keratoplasty. Cornea. 2023;10:1097.

5 CHAPTER

Integrated Intraoperative Optical Coherence Tomography in Anterior Segment Surgeries

Deeksha Thorat, Somasheila I Murthy, Aafreen Bari, Namrata Sharma

ABSTRACT

Intraoperative optical coherence tomography (i-OCT) provides a real-time visualization of the structures of anterior segment and improves the understanding of intraoperative dynamics. These systems provide high-quality images intraoperatively and are added to the surgeon's oculars, with the images visible in real time and the surgeon need not look away from the surgical field. The use of the i-OCT in anterior segment surgeries enhances efficacy and decision-making intraoperatively, especially in anterior lamellar keratoplasty and endothelial keratoplasty. This also has application in other anterior segment surgeries like phacoemulsification for assessing incisions, intralenticular pressures, posterior capsular integrity, and glaucoma filtering surgeries for assessing the angles and thickness of scleral flaps. Intraoperative OCT can be used to establish diagnosis in pediatric patients with cloudy corneas by imaging the anterior segment and angle structures. There are certain limitations to the current i-OCT systems in terms of surgical field tracking, instrument compatibility, and real-time images. Future technological advances hold integration of OCT in surgical microscopes for all ocular surgeries.

Keywords: Optical coherence tomography, keratoplasty, lamellar keratoplasty, endothelial keratoplasty, integrated intraoperative OCT

INTRODUCTION

Optical coherence tomography (OCT) provides a histological cross-sectional image of the ocular tissues and is, therefore, increasingly being used in visualization intraoperatively for anterior segment surgeries for dynamic imaging and instrument interactions.[1] Optical coherence tomography is based on the principle of low coherence interferometry; light interference is achieved by an optical fiber-based interferometer. The light is split up into two beams using a coupler into reference and sample beams. The reference beam is reflected from the mirror and the sample beam is reflected from the tissues. These beams are then combined to create an interference pattern by the coupler and measured by the photodetector.[1]

There are two types of OCT: (1) Time-domain OCT and (2) Fourier-domain OCT (FD-OCT). Time-domain OCT is dependent on the measurement of the time delay of the reflection from the ocular tissue compared with the reflection from the reference mirror. The FD-OCT utilizes either the spectrometer (spectral-domain OCT) or rapidly tuning laser (swept-source OCT). Swept-source OCT has a faster scanning speed compared to spectral-domain OCT.[2]

Intraoperative OCT devices can be either handheld or mounted on the surgical microscope. Microscope-mounted OCT devices provide a control board operated by foot, good quality of image capture, and have to be sterile while in operation but take up a lot of space as compared to hand-held OCT.[3] According to the landmark DISCOVER study, i-OCT demonstrated feasibility with successful imaging in 98% of cases and impacted decision-making in 44% of cases.[1]

APPLICATIONS OF INTEGRATED OPTICAL COHERENCE TOMOGRAPHY FOR ANTERIOR SEGMENT SURGERIES

The integrated OCT provides images intraoperatively in three ways: (1) On a different screen for an OCT image, (2) as an inset into the video recording, and (3) as direct projection into the ocular of the microscope. Currently, the new version A3 of Haag-Streit i-OCT, Haag-Streit group of companies' manufacturer in Lubeck, Germany, superimposes images directly into the ocular of the microscope.[2] With a click on the foot pedal, the surgeon can start the i-OCT module and does not have to look away from the microscope.[4]

Corneal Surgeries

Anterior segment OCT helps by providing the depth of the corneal scars, anterior chamber morphology, and extent of detachment of graft in endothelial keratoplasty, especially in cases with poor anterior chamber view.

Penetrating Keratoplasty

Anterior segment OCT (AS-OCT) helps assess the depth of the corneal scar, the morphology of the anterior chamber, and the presence of posterior synechiae. The depth of the trephination can be assessed with real-time OCT to prevent damage to the intraocular structures. It helps detect iris tissue incarceration into the graft–host junction after passing the sutures. It can also detect Descemet's membrane (DM) detachment during the procedure.[5]

Anterior Lamellar Keratoplasty

In anterior lamellar keratoplasty, intraoperative OCT can help locate the depth of the needle or the cannula ensuring the formation of big bubble and also to assure the residual stromal thickness for manual dissection.[6] It also helps to identify the presence of any residual graft interface fluid, graft apposition, and complications such as double anterior chamber formation.[7] Passing the needle through the graft and host at appropriate thickness poses the challenge of perforation. The needle can be visualized through i-OCT as it traverses through the stroma. The interface can be evaluated for apposition at the end of surgery. The interface fluid can be drained through the interface to prevent the formation of a second anterior chamber **(Fig. 5.1)**.

Endothelial Keratoplasty

Endothelial keratoplasty offers replacement of selective diseased layers of the cornea and facilitates faster visual recovery with a better safety profile when compared to penetrating keratoplasty. The learning curve associated with endothelial keratoplasty is longer due to challenges related to graft orientation and apposition.[1] i-OCT helps in the recognition of complete DM scoring, identifies remnants or tags, and facilitates its removal.

- *Descemet's stripping automated endothelial keratoplasty:* Intraoperative OCT can be used to identify the correct orientation of the graft, visualization of the graft unfolding, and graft positioning **(Fig. 5.2)**. In cases of lenticule manipulation and flipping, i-OCT can assess the correct orientation of the graft helping in identifying the stromal and endothelial side. Moreover, the objective assessment of the presence of residual interface fluid and the impact of corneal sweeping in graft apposition can be done using i-OCT **(Fig. 5.3)**.[8]
- *Descemet's membrane endothelial keratoplasty:* Intraoperative-OCT enables the visualization of graft and host side of the scroll in both clear and opaque corneas. Incorrect attachment of the scroll can cause

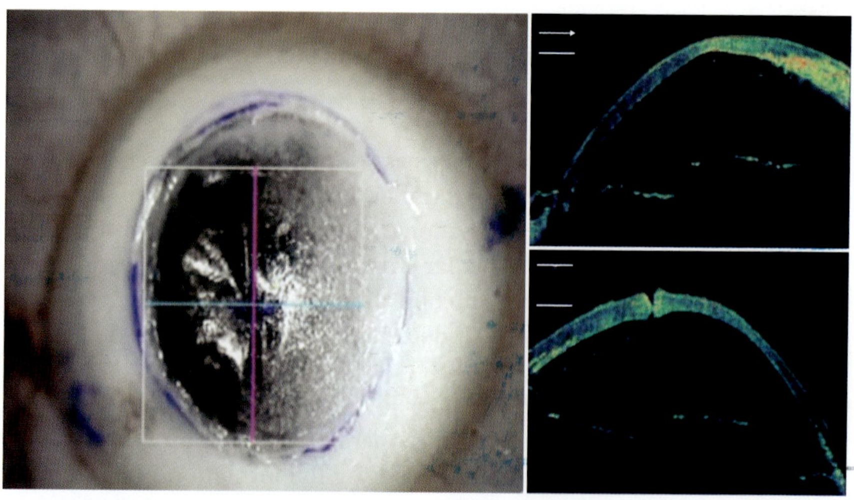

Fig. 5.1: Intraoperative optical coherence tomography-guided deep lamellar keratoplasty showing type 1 big bubble.

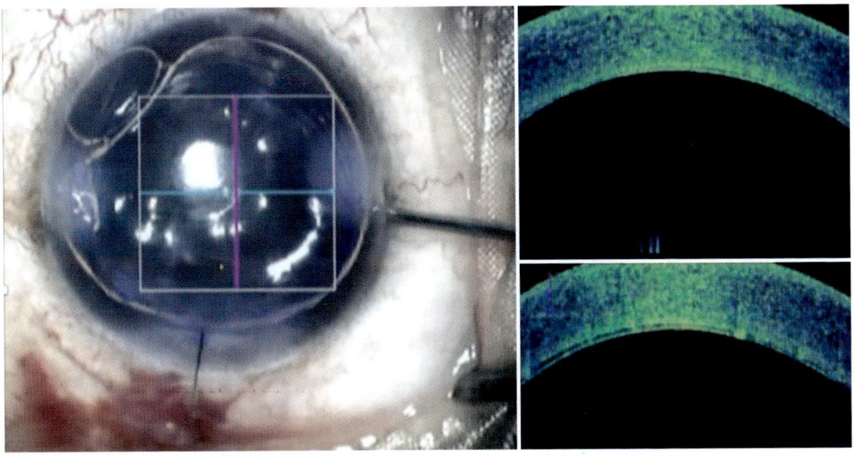

Fig. 5.2: Complete donor apposition as assessed by intraoperative optical coherence tomography at the end of surgery in a case of Descemet's stripping endothelial keratoplasty.

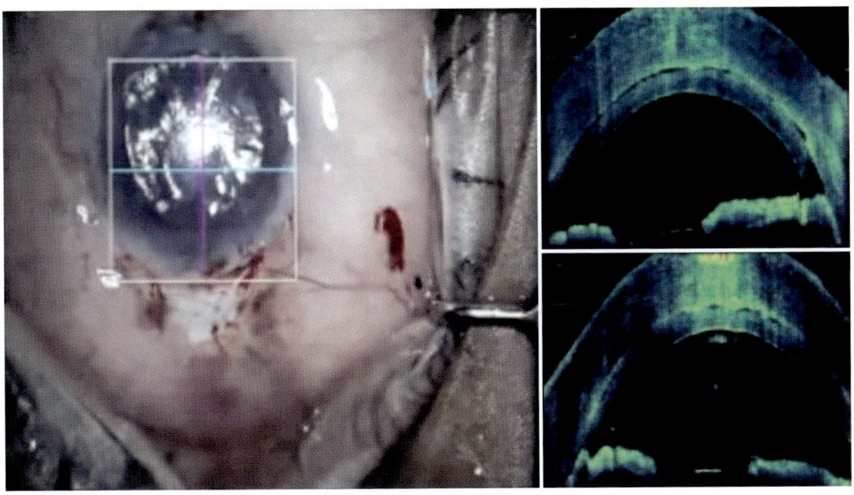

Fig. 5.3: Demonstration of apposition of donor lenticule to the host stroma by intraoperative optical coherence tomography.

primary graft failure. After attachment, i-OCT can be used to identify the orientation and presence of DM folds in the graft.

Ocular Surface Disorders

The role of i-OCT in ocular surface disorders is yet to be completely explored. It is currently being used to identify the depth of fibrotic tissue during pannus dissection. In the future, it can be used to identify neoplastic from non-neoplastic tissues.[9]

In cases of limbal stem cell deficiency, simple limbal transplantation can be planned. The surgery requires complete pannus dissection. i-OCT can be used to assess the thickness of the underlying stroma for thinning to prevent perforation during the procedure.

Phacoemulsification

Visualization of anterior segment dynamics during phacoemulsification helps in planning and assessing the steps of the surgery. i-OCT helps to assess the wound construction, identify the capsular flap during capsulorhexis **(Fig. 5.4)**, and measure the intraocular pressure and wound-site Descemet's membrane detachment.[10] In cases of posterior polar cataracts, it assists in making a judgment regarding the status of the posterior capsule, and a decision about performing hydrodissection can be taken. i-OCT can be used to assess the depth of trenching during nucleotomy.[11] It guides the surgeon to decide if further trenching is required before proceeding with chopping. The OCT can help assess the position of intraocular lens (IOL) at the end of the surgery **(Fig. 5.5)** and clear corneal wound integrity after

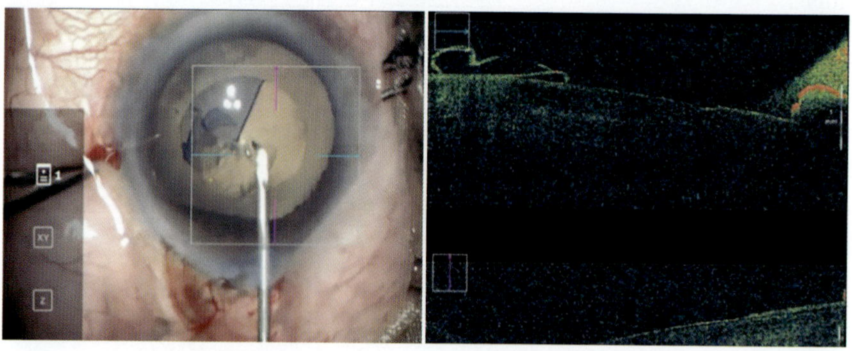

Fig. 5.4: Intraoperative optical coherence tomography demonstrating the capsular flap during capsulorhexis.

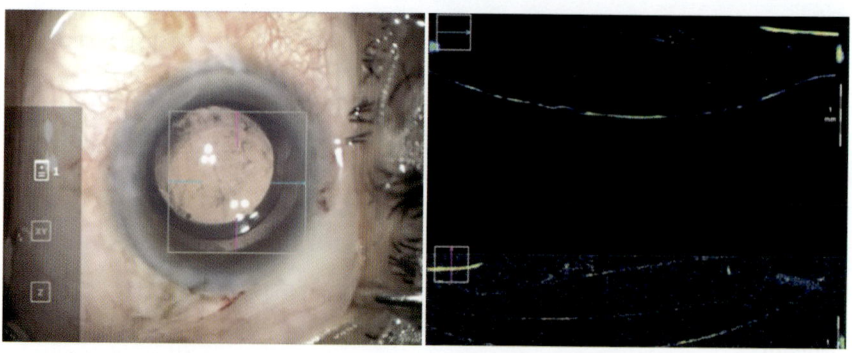

Fig. 5.5: Intraoperative optical coherence tomography demonstrating the gap between IOL and posterior capsule postimplantation in the bag. (IOL: intraocular lens)

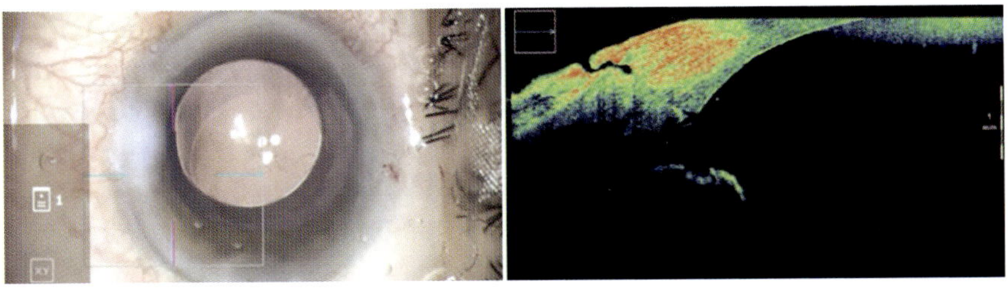

Fig. 5.6: Hydrated wound postoperatively in phacoemulsification surgery with apposed wound and no leak.

stromal hydration **(Fig. 5.6)**. There are a few limitations of the use of OCT intraoperatively like poor view of the posterior capsule in the presence of dense nuclear sclerosis and obscuration or shadowing of the anterior segment structures while using the metallic instruments during surgery.

Refractive Surgeries

The use of i-OCT is suggested in certain modern-day refractive surgeries such as small-incision lenticule extraction and phakic IOL implantation. In small-incision lenticule extraction, OCT helps in identifying the plane of dissection and lenticule edge making sure that no tags or remnants of lenticule are present in the interface.[12] Phakic IOL implantation is a safe and efficacious modality of treating moderate-to-high myopia.[13] It needs the placement of an IOL in the ciliary sulcus anterior to the phakic clear lens. In the case of the lens vaults, that is, the distance between the phakic IOL and the anterior surface of the lens is high, it can cause angle closure glaucoma whereas if the lens vault is low, it can cause deprivation of lens nutrition and early progression of cataractous changes.[1] Traditionally, the lens vault can be assessed in the postoperative period using OCT to decide if phakic IOL explantation is required; however, the vault can be assessed intraoperatively using i-OCT and further decision-making can be made in the same sitting.[14]

Glaucoma Filtering Surgeries

Intraoperative OCT can be used in various glaucoma surgeries such as trabeculectomy, glaucoma drainage device placement, bleb needling, canaloplasty, and goniosynechialysis. Intraoperative OCT helps the surgeon decide the thickness of the flap during trabeculectomy.[15] Release of the goniosynechiae can be done under visualization of i-OCT. This obviates the use of intraoperative gonioscopy, which can be challenging for new surgeons.[16] One of the common complications of trabeculectomy can be bleb fibrosis which needs needling of the bleb. Bleb needling is, otherwise, a blind procedure, but with i-OCT the areas that have adhesions and fibrosis can be identified.[17] In glaucoma drainage devices, placing the tube in the anterior chamber can be challenging due to the extensive synechial closure, complex anterior segment anatomy, small eyes, and shallow anterior chamber. i-OCT helps in the correct placement of the tube in cases of hazy cornea and prevents extrusion and erosion due to the tube. Minimally invasive glaucoma surgeries require accurate passage of microcatheter into the Schlemm canal during canaloplasty; this procedure can be done using i-OCT to prevent complications such as complete penetration.[1]

Pediatric Congenital Corneal Opacities

Children with ocular disorders are often uncooperative for slit-lamp examination; hence, they are examined under anesthesia. However, in the supine position, investigative modalities such as OCT cannot be used to assess the status of the anterior chamber. Anterior segment dysgenesis such as Peters' anomaly, sclerocornea, congenital primary aphakia, and congenital hereditary endothelial dystrophy needs a view of the anterior chamber to decide the further course of action.[18] The clarity of the anatomical structures can be better assessed using OCT than ultrasound biomicroscopy. i-OCT can be used in such cases where corneal opacity precludes the anterior segment view.

Pediatric keratoplasties are complex surgeries, right from planning to execution. i-OCT can be used to perform manual trephination in a guarded manner to prevent full-thickness entry. The anterior chamber can be assessed for the position of iridocorneal or irido-kerato-lenticular adhesions while performing keratoplasty.

LIMITATIONS

There are certain limitations when it comes to incorporating OCT systems into operating microscopes, such as increased surgical time, unstable image acquisition, and low resolution of images. The use of metallic instruments for the surgery limits image acquisition due to shadowing beyond the instruments.[4] Moreover, the current systems of visualization have limited resolution, contrast, and field of view that can lead to missing out on subtle anatomical details. The commercially available microscope-integrated OCTs have a low A-scan rate (usually <40 kHz) with a two-dimensional view of the surgical field; therefore, deriving three-dimensional or volumetric imaging during surgery becomes challenging.[19-21]

CONCLUSION

Intraoperative OCT has introduced an additional visual dimension to ophthalmic surgical interventions. It facilitates improvement in the understanding of changing intraoperative dynamics of anterior segment surgeries. The role of i-OCT in lamellar surgeries, encompassing both anterior lamellar and endothelial keratoplasties, is widely being accepted as it influences surgical decision-making. This in turn improves the surgical outcome. Furthermore, i-OCT has found its utility in phacoemulsification, refractive surgeries, glaucoma surgeries, and ocular surface disorders. Particularly in pediatric cases where preoperative assessments may be challenging, i-OCT assumes paramount importance, offering both diagnostic insights and therapeutic guidance, thereby enhancing the quality of surgical interventions. Ongoing technological advancements are driving the evolution of i-OCT-compatible instruments, automated tracking systems, and real-time volumetric analysis tools, facilitating seamless integration of i-OCT into routine surgical practices.

ACKNOWLEDGMENT

The authors would like to thank Hyderabad Eye Research Foundation, Hyderabad, India, for the support.

REFERENCES

1. Titiyal JS, Kaur M, Nair S, Sharma N. Intraoperative optical coherence tomography in anterior segment surgery. Surv Ophthalmol. 2021;66(2):308-26.
2. Price FW. Intraoperative optical coherence tomography: game-changing technology. Cornea. 2021;40(6):675-8.
3. Ehlers JP, Dupps WJ, Kaiser PK, Goshe J, Singh RP, Petkovsek D, et al. The Prospective Intraoperative and Perioperative Ophthalmic ImagiNg with Optical CoherEncE TomogRaphy (PIONEER) study: 2-year results. Am J Ophthalmol. 2014;158(5):999-1007.
4. Ray R, Barañano DE, Fortun JA, Schwent BJ, Cribbs BE, Bergstrom CS, et al. Intraoperative microscope-mounted spectral domain optical coherence tomography for evaluation of retinal anatomy during macular surgery. Ophthalmology. 2011;118(11):2212-17.
5. Hong J, Yang Y, Cursiefen C, Mashaghi A, Wu D, Liu Z, et al. Optimising keratoplasty for Peters' anomaly in infants using spectral-domain optical coherence tomography. Br J Ophthalmol. 2017;101(6):820-27.
6. Sarnicola V, Toro P. Blunt cannula for descemetic deep anterior lamellar keratoplasty. Cornea. 2011;30(8):895-98.
7. Steven P, Le Blanc C, Lankenau E, Krug M, Oelckers S, Heindl LM, et al. Optimising deep anterior lamellar keratoplasty (DALK) using intraoperative online optical coherence tomography (iOCT). Br J Ophthalmol. 2014;98(7):900-904.
8. Sharma N, Sharma VK, Arora T, Singh KR, Agarwal T, Vajpayee RB. Novel technique for Descemet membrane remnant stripping in hazy cornea during DSAEK. Cornea. 2016;35(1):140-2.
9. Zakaria N, Ní Dhubhghaill S, Taal M, Berneman Z, Koppen C, Tassignon MJ. Optical coherence tomography in cultivated limbal epithelial stem cell transplantation surgery. Asia Pac J Ophthalmol (Phila). 2015;4(6):339-45.
10. Titiyal JS, Kaur M, Ramesh P, Shah P, Falera R, Bageshwar LMS, et al. Impact of clear corneal incision morphology on incision-site Descemet membrane detachment

in conventional and femtosecond laser-assisted phacoemulsification. Curr Eye Res. 2018;43(3):293-9.

11. Das S, Kummelil MK, Kharbanda V, Arora V, Nagappa S, Shetty R, et al. Microscope integrated intraoperative spectral domain optical coherence tomography for cataract surgery: uses and applications. Curr Eye Res. 2016;41(5):643-52.
12. Urkude J, Titiyal JS, Sharma N. Intraoperative optical coherence tomography-guided management of cap-lenticule adhesion during SMILE. J Refract Surg. 2017;33(11):783-6.
13. Chen H, Liu Y, Niu G, Ma J. Excimer laser versus phakic intraocular lenses for myopia and astigmatism: a meta-analysis of randomized controlled trials. Eye Contact Lens. 2018;44(3):137-43.
14. Matarazzo F, Day AC, Fernandez-Vega Cueto L, Maurino V. Vertical implantable collamer lens (ICL) rotation for the management of high vault due to lens oversizing. Int Ophthalmol. 2018;38(6):2689-92.
15. Heindl LM, Siebelmann S, Dietlein T, Hüttmann G, Lankenau E, Cursiefen C, et al. Future prospects: assessment of intraoperative optical coherence tomography in ab interno glaucoma surgery. Curr Eye Res. 2015;40(12):1288-91.
16. Kumar RS, Jariwala MU, Sathidevi VA, Venugopal JP, Puttaiah NK, Balu R, et al. A pilot study on feasibility and effectiveness of intraoperative spectral-domain optical coherence tomography in glaucoma procedures. Transl Vis Sci Technol. 2015;4(2):2.
17. Dada T, Angmo D, Midha N, Sidhu T. Intraoperative optical coherence tomography guided bleb needling. J Ophthalmic Vis Res. 2016;11(4):452-4.
18. Siebelmann S, Bachmann B, Matthaei M, Horstmann J, Dietlein T, Lappas A, et al. Microscope-integrated intraoperative optical coherence tomography in examination of pediatric patients under anesthesia. Ophthalmology. 2018;115(9):785-92.
19. Binder S, Falkner-Radler CI, Hauger C, Matz H, Glittenberg C. Feasibility of intrasurgical spectral-domain optical coherence tomography. Retina. 2011;31(7):1332-36.
20. Ehlers JP, Goshe J, Dupps WJ, Kaiser PK, Singh RP, Gans R, et al. Determination of feasibility and utility of microscope-integrated optical coherence tomography during ophthalmic surgery: the DISCOVER study RESCAN results. JAMA Ophthalmol. 2015;133(10):1124-32.
21. Ehlers JP, Srivastava SK, Feiler D, Noonan AI, Rollins AM, Tao YK. Integrative advances for OCT-guided ophthalmic surgery and intraoperative OCT: microscope integration, surgical instrumentation, and heads-up display surgeon feedback. PLoS One. 2014;9(8):105224.

6 CHAPTER

Advances in Medical Management of Glaucoma

R Ramakrishnan, Madhavi Ramanatha Pillai, Devendra Maheshwari

ABSTRACT

Glaucoma is an etiologically complex disorder characterized by progressive loss of retinal ganglion cells and their axons. Medical management of glaucoma revolves around lowering intraocular pressure (IOP), which is the only modifiable risk factor. However, despite the lowering of IOP, many patients continue to have progressive visual field loss. A deeper understanding of the cellular, molecular, and genetic levels of ocular changes associated with glaucoma has paved the way for the development of newer medications. The introduction of Rho-kinase inhibitors which have alternative mechanisms of action has been a turning point in the world of medical management. Sustained drug delivery systems, nanotechnology, and other upcoming medications such as latanoprostene bunod and adenosine receptor agonists are other potential options. Stem cell therapy and specific gene silencing are promising options in the pipeline. This chapter aims to give an overview of the new medications and future trends that hope to bring a revolutionary change in the medical management of glaucoma.

Keywords: Rho-kinase inhibitors, adenosine receptor agonists, latanoprostene bunod, punctal plugs, nanoparticles, sustained release

INTRODUCTION

Glaucoma is the leading cause of irreversible blindness worldwide and it is estimated to affect 111.8 million people by 2040.[1,2] For the majority of adult-onset glaucomas, medical management is the initial course of treatment.[3] The only modifiable risk factor identified is intraocular pressure (IOP) and the medical management strategy depends on lowering IOP.[4-7] However, the disease pathogenesis is multifold and complex and despite achieving a target IOP, it may still progress.[8-10] This has led to the search for medications focusing on different mechanisms and neuroprotection.[11,12]

Medical management of glaucoma has come a long way since the 1800s **(Figs. 6.1 and 6.2)** with substantial advancements occurring in recent years.[12,13] This chapter will provide an extensive overview of the

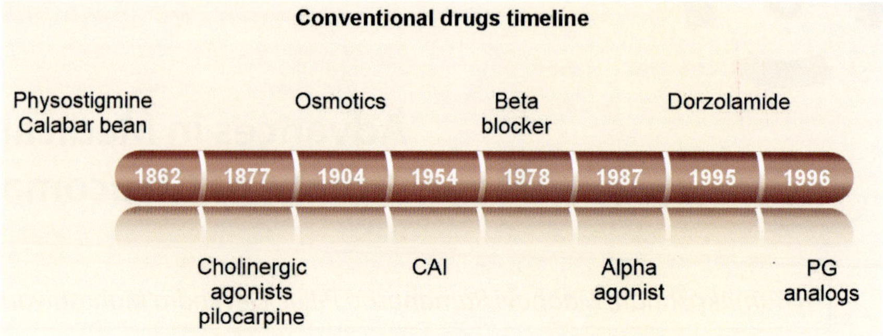

Fig. 6.1: Timeline of conventional drugs in glaucoma. (CAI: carbonic anhydrase inhibitors; PG: prostaglandin)

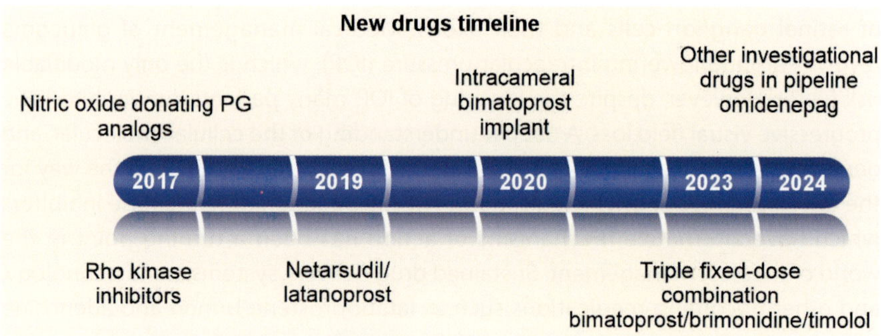

Fig. 6.2: Timeline of new drugs in glaucoma. (PG: prostaglandin)

newer medications, sustained drug delivery systems, as well as potential medications in the pipeline **(Table 6.1)**.

RHO-KINASE INHIBITORS

The Rho family (Rho A, B, and C) is a small group of guanosine triphosphate (GTP) binding proteins. It aids in regulation of cell structure, motility, division, and apoptosis. The Rho kinases (ROCK 1 and ROCK 2) are the members of the Rho family. These cytoskeletally active agents are found to regulate trabecular outflow.[14-16]

Rho-kinase inhibitors act by increasing the ability of the Schlemm's canal endothelial cells to form pores, thereby increasing aqueous outflow and decreasing outflow resistance. It is thought to induce smooth muscle fiber relaxation in the trabecular meshwork and, as a result, increases the outflow.[17,18]

In India, there are two commercially available formulations of Rho-kinase inhibitors that target ROCK 1 and ROCK 2 receptors: Ripasudil and netarsudil.[19]

- Ripasudil hydrochloride hydrate 0.4% (Glanatec®) was first approved in Japan for use in primary open-angle glaucoma (POAG) and ocular

TABLE 6.1: Summary of newer medications.

Drug	*Mechanism of action*	*IOP lowering mechanism*	*Status*	*Indication*	*IOP reduction*
Netarsudil mesylate	• Rho-kinase inhibition • NET-EN inhibition	• Increased trabecular outflow • Decreased episcleral venous pressure	Launched—2018	POAG, OHT	From a baseline IOP of 22.5–22.6 mm Hg to 17.9–18.8 mm Hg
Ripasudil hydrochloride	Rho-kinase inhibition	Increased trabecular outflow	Launched—2017 in Japan	POAG, OHT	IOP reduction by 2.6 mm Hg at trough and 3.7 mm Hg at peak
Latanoprostene bunod	NO donor	Increased trabecular outflow	Launched—2017	POAG, OHT	IOP reductions of up to 9 mm Hg
Omidenepag isopropyl	Prostaglandin EP2 agonist	Increased uveoscleral outflow	NCT03691662 (launched in Japan phase III in the USA)	POAG, OHT	At week 6 ranged from -7.11 ± 0.45 to -7.25 ± 0.49 mm Hg
Brinzolamide/brimonidine/timolol Triple FD	CAI + α-agonist + β-blocker	• Decreased aqueous production • Enhanced uveoscleral outflow	Launched in 2023		IOP reduction 10.532 ± 0.189 mm Hg at 12 weeks

(CAI: carbonic anhydrase inhibitor; FD: fixed dose; IOP: intraocular pressure; NET: norepinephrine transporter; NO: nitric oxide; OHT: ocular hypertension; POAG: primary open-angle glaucoma) hypertension (OHT). In a twice-daily dosage, it reduces IOP at trough by 2.6 mm Hg and peak by 3.7 mm Hg.[20-22] Randomized controlled trials (RCTs) have shown an additive effect with timolol. The additive effect was 0.9 mm Hg at the trough and 1.6 mm Hg at the peak. When combined with latanoprost, there was no significant difference compared to placebo at trough; at peak, ripasudil resulted in an additional 1.4 mm Hg reduction.[23] It is available as a 0.4% solution applied twice daily. The most common side effects **(Fig. 6.3)** reported are conjunctival hyperemia around 76%, allergic conjunctivitis (20%), and blepharitis (21%).[24] In real-world settings, the frequency of hyperemia is underreported with a postmarketing surveillance showing that only 4% had conjunctival hyperemia.[25] Other adverse drug reactions associated with ripasudil, such as allergic conjunctivitis, blepharitis, eye pruritus, and punctate keratitis, were not high.[26,27] Rarely reported adverse events include reduced blood pressure, constipation, and headache.[26]

Many small-scale studies have shown the utility of ripasudil in secondary glaucoma, including uveitic and exfoliation glaucoma.[28,29] Additionally, in mouse or rabbit models, ripasudil has been proven to mitigate excessive scarring in vitro and following glaucoma filtration surgery.[30] A recent retrospective study has shown that ripasudil is safe and effective after bleb needling procedures maintaining IOP for 12 weeks.[31] An RCT on the effect of postoperative use of ripasudil after trabeculectomy in uveitic glaucoma showed a statistically significant association between ripasudil use and IOP reduction at 3 months postoperatively.[32]

- Netarsudil (Rhopressa®) was approved for use in the USA to treat open-angle glaucoma and OHT as a once-daily formulation in late 2017.[33]

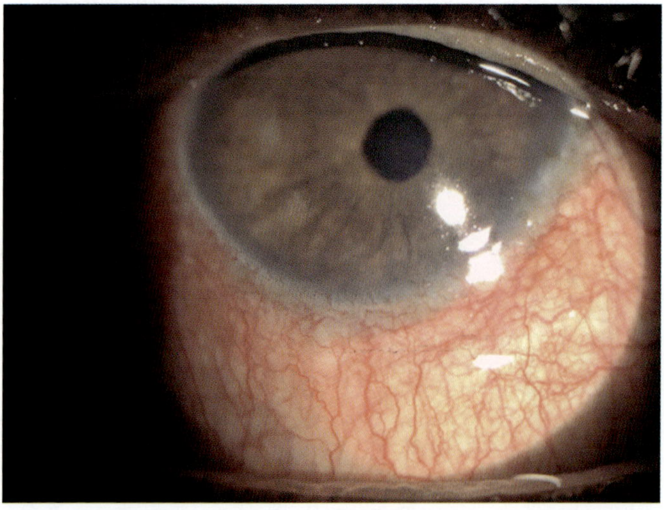

Fig. 6.3: Conjunctival hyperemia induced by Rho-kinase inhibitors.

It is a Rho-kinase inhibitor and inhibitor of norepinephrine transport and belongs to a class of amino-isoquinoline amide Rho kinase inhibitors. Apart from lowering outflow resistance, it has also been shown to decrease aqueous humor production and to decrease episcleral venous pressure. These latter mechanisms of IOP reduction are unique for netarsudil and may be related to the norepinephrine transporter inhibitory activity.[34,35] It is available as 0.02% eye drops, and the dose is once daily.

In a double-masked RCT, netarsudil was found to be noninferior to latanoprost, when IOP was ≤26 mm Hg. At higher IOP ≥26 and <36 mm Hg, it could not meet the noninferiority criteria. Conjunctival hyperemia was the most frequently reported adverse event, and it occurred more frequently when using netarsudil than when using latanoprost.[36]

Adverse events reported with netarsudil include conjunctival hyperemia (50–53%), perilimbal conjunctival microhemorrhages (13–17%), and cornea verticillata (9–15%). All the adverse effects are usually reversed after stopping medications.[37] Many reports are available on the occurrence of reticular corneal edema **(Fig. 6.4)** with netarsudil which causes diminution of vision.[38,39]

A fixed-dose combination of netarsudil with latanoprost (FCNL) was shown to have higher IOP reduction when compared to monotherapy in MERCURY 1 and 2 trials. **Table 6.2** summarizes the trials involving ripasudil and netarsudil.

Rho-kinase inhibitors by their different mechanisms of action are important adjuncts to the current medical management of glaucoma. However, long-term compliance may be affected by a high incidence of conjunctival hyperemia.

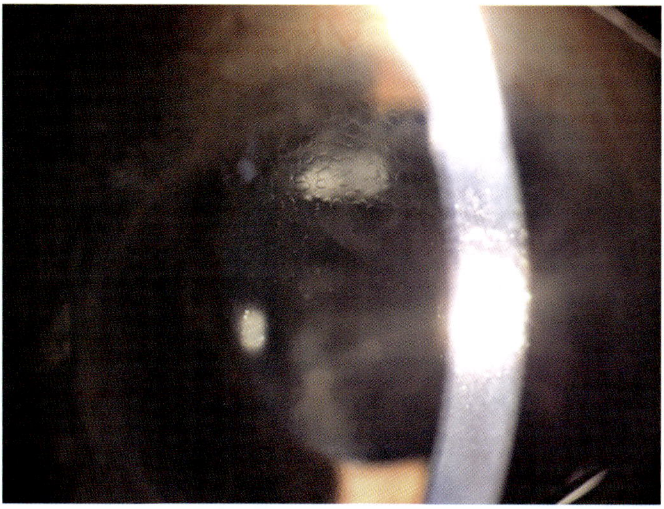

Fig. 6.4: Reticular corneal epithelial edema in a patient on netarsudil.

TABLE 6.2: Summary of clinical trials involving netarsudil and ripasudil.

Drug	*Study type*	*Indication*	*Number of patients*	*Follow-up*	*Conclusion*
Ripasudil	RCT	POAG, OHT	210	8 weeks	The ideal dosage was determined to be K 115 0.4% BD
Ripasudil phase 3	Nonrandomized	POAG, OHT, PXFG	388	1 year	IOP reduction and a tolerable safety profile when used in combination or monotherapy
Ripasudil with timolol phase 3	RCT	POAG, OHT	208	8 weeks	Additive IOP reduction at peak and trough when combined with timolol
Ripasudil with latanoprost	RCT	POAG, OHT	205	8 weeks	When combined with latanoprost additive IOP lowering at peak
Netarsudil[36]	RCT, double-masked	POAG, OHT	224	28 days	Latanoprost was more effective than AR-13324 0.02% by about 1 mm Hg
ROCKET 1 Netarsudil phase 3	RCT, double-masked	POAG, OHT	411	3 months	Netarsudil 0.02% was safe, well tolerate, and effective
ROCKET 2 Netarsudil phase 3	RCT, double-masked	POAG, OHT	756	12 months	In the subgroup of patients with IOP <25 mm Hg, netarsudil was statistically noninferior to timolol 0.05%
Netarsudil + Latanoprost—fixed combination phase 2[40]	RCT, Double-masked	POAG, OHT	298	28 days	When compared to individual components, the combination of FDC AR-13324 0.02% and latanoprost 0.005% results in a statistically superior ocular hypotensive effect
Mercury 1–2 fixed-drug combination of netarsudil and latanoprost—pooled data[41]	RCT	POAG, OHT	1,468	3 months	Netarsudil/latanoprost FDC once daily resulted in a statistically significant decrease in mean IOP

(FDC: fixed-dose combination; IOP: intraocular pressure; OHT: ocular hypertension; POAG: primary open-angle glaucoma; PXFG: pseudoexfoliation glaucoma; RCT: randomized controlled trial)

LATANOPROSTENE BUNOD

Latanoprostene bunod (LBN) ophthalmic solution 0.024% (Vyzulta™) is a prostaglandin $F_{2\alpha}$ analog approved in the USA for the reduction of IOP in an open-angle glaucoma or OHT. It donates nitric oxide (NO) and lowers IOP by increasing aqueous humor outflow through the uveoscleral pathway (mediated by latanoprost acid) and through the trabecular meshwork pathway (mediated by NO).[42]

When different concentrations of LBN and latanoprost 0.005% were compared, the VOYAGER study showed that LBN (0.024%) reduced IOP more than latanoprost 0.005% while having similar side effects.[42] The CONSTELLATION study found that LBN (0.024%) significantly reduced both diurnal and nocturnal IOP when compared to timolol 0.5%.[43] According to the results of the APOLLO and LUNAR studies, timolol 0.5% was noninferior to LBN 0.024%. The JUPITER study assessed the long-term safety profile of LBN over a 52-week period of observation. The most frequently reported side effects were conjunctival hyperemia (17%), eyelash growth (16%), irritation (11%), pain (10%), and iris pigmentation (10%).[44-47]

The dosage of LBN is once daily at bedtime. It is unknown at this time how safe the medication is during pregnancy and lactation. Animal studies have shown adverse effects with systemic administration during embryogenesis.[48]

TRIPLE FIXED-DOSE COMBINATIONS

Most often, target IOP cannot be achieved by a single medication alone, and multiple medications are frequently used to prevent disease progression.[49] Fixed-drug combinations reduce costs, improve treatment adherence, minimize medication washout, and lower exposure to preservatives, thereby reducing adverse effects.[50-53]

A triple fixed-dose combination (FDC) of bimatoprost/brimonidine/timolol was introduced in India in 2023.

Studies have shown a superior IOP lowering efficacy of the triple FDC while maintaining a better safety and tolerability profile.[54,55] A study conducted in India showed an IOP lowering of 10.532 ± 0.189 mm Hg at 12 weeks. 92.2% of the patients reported no adverse events. This has the potential to improve patient adherence and quality of life.[56]

SUSTAINED DRUG DELIVERY SYSTEMS

For glaucoma patients, medication noncompliance poses a significant challenge. They frequently report experiencing difficulties administering drops and adhering to the regimen of eye drops.

In the past two decades, sustained drug delivery systems have been developed to reduce the need for chronic medication **(Table 6.3)**.

TABLE 6.3: Sustained drug delivery systems for glaucoma.

Device	*Drug*	*Site*	*Status*	*Indication*	*IOP reduction*
Bimatoprost sustained-release	Bimatoprost	Anterior chamber	Phase III	OHT, OAG	At month 24, mean IOP reduction from baseline was 7.5, 7.3, 7.3, and 8.9 mm Hg in eyes treated with bimatoprost SR 6, 10, 15, and 20 µg, respectively
Bimatoprost ring	Bimatoprost	Fornix	Phase II	OHT, OAG	A mean reduction from baseline IOP of −3.2 to −6.4 mm Hg
Travoprost punctum plug	Travoprost	Puncta	Phase III	OHT, OAG	The IOP reduction from baseline was 6.2 (23%), 5.4 (21%), and 7.5 mm Hg (28%) at 8 AM, 10 AM, and 4 PM, respectively
iDose TR	Travoprost	Anterior chamber	Phase III	OHT, OAG	Mean IOP reduction from baseline was 7.4 or 7.8 mm Hg in 24 months
Latanoprost-eluting contact lens	Latanoprost	Cornea	Phase I	OHT, OAG	CLHI lowered IOP by 10.5 ± 1.4, 11.1 ± 4, and 10 ± 2.5 mm Hg on days 3, 5, and 8, respectively

(IOP: intraocular pressure; OAG: open-angle glaucoma; OHT: ocular hypertension)

Introduced in 1975, Ocusert was the first sustained pilocarpine implant. Its low tolerability led to its removal from the market.

- Durysta™ is a sustained-release biodegradable bimatoprost implant. It administers drugs intracamerally using the NOVADUR drug delivery system. A 28-gauge, single-use, prefilled applicator is used to inject the implant into the anterior chamber. The biodegradable drug delivery system hydrolyzes to produce water and carbon dioxide. Both the 10 and 15 µg doses of durysta were found to be noninferior to timolol 0.5% in the Artemis 1 trial. There were no adverse events related to skin hyperpigmentation growth of eyelashes or periorbital fat atrophy. The main concern was the decrease in corneal endothelial cell density (CECD). In phase 3 trials, 3.6% of eyes in the 10 µg group and 10.3% of eyes in the 15 µg group needed implant removal due to corneal edema and loss of endothelial cells.[57] Ongoing trials are looking at new regimens of administration that will prevent corneal endothelial cell loss.[58]
- Bimatoprost ocular ring (BIM ring) is a polypropylene and silicon ring impregnated with bimatoprost (diameters ranging from 24 to 29 mm) designed for insertion between the upper and lower fornices. It continuously emits bimatoprost for up to 6 months and needs replacement after that. The rate of drug elution decreases with time, ranging from 35 µg/day on the day of insertion to 6 µg/day at 6 months. Over a 6-month period, it was found that the IOP reduction was equivalent to 0.03% topical drops of bimatoprost, with mucinous discharge as the major side effect. The results of phase 3 trials are awaited, and the device is not currently Food and Drug Administration (FDA) approved for clinical use.[59] Contact lenses are another attractive option for drug delivery due to patient familiarity and long hours of use. The use of micelle-laden contact lenses for delivery of glaucoma medications is currently undergoing animal studies, and initial results are promising.[60]
- Travoprost punctum plugs (OTX-TP, Ocular Therapeutix, Inc.) are undergoing phase 2 clinical trials. Travoprost impregnated in a polyethylene glycol resorbable hydrogel rod is inserted into the upper or lower punctum. Within the hydrogel rod, travoprost particles are encapsulated in polylactic acid microparticles. This hydrolyzes with time to provide sustained release of travoprost over 90 days. To help with visualization, fluorescein is also impregnated into the rod. Both the OTX TP group and the timolol 0.5% group demonstrated a significant reduction in IOP, with the OTX TP group showing a reduction of 4.5–5.7 mm Hg and the timolol group showing a reduction of 6.4–7.6 mm Hg. A major concern was the retention of the plugs and the adverse events reported were foreign body sensation (38.5%), itching (15.4%), and increased tearing (3.8%). The tolerability of the implant improved with time.[61]
- Intracameral travoprost-eluting inserts (iDose TR, Glaukos) are in the pipeline. Implantation is similar to iStent, although the travoprost-eluting

stent is larger than the iStent inject W. The iDose is inserted through the main corneal incision and placed in the trabecular meshwork. Its drug-eluting membrane is reported to produce a treatment effect for 36 months or potentially longer. When all of the travoprost is released, the implant is intended to be taken out and replaced. This titanium-based implant showed a mean IOP reduction of 7.4 or 7.8 mm Hg from baseline within the first 24 months.[62]

NANOTECHNOLOGY

Another rapidly developing method of drug delivery is nanotechnology. Nanoparticles vary from 1 to 100 nm in size. Drugs are attached to different nanoparticles that are able to get past biological barriers and reach the target site directly. Successful animal studies have been conducted using subconjunctival injection of polymer microparticles loaded with dorzolamide, supraciliary injection of microspheres loaded with brimonidine, and intravitreal injection of nanosponges loaded with brimonidine, travoprost, and bimatoprost.[63]

ADENOSINE RECEPTOR AGONISTS

Adenosine receptors (A1, A2A, A2B, and A23) are linked to the G protein, which is activated by the nucleoside adenosine. It causes the extracellular matrix to be remodeled and the cell volume to shrink in human trabecular meshwork cells, increasing the trabecular outflow facility. Trabodenoson is an A1 receptor-selective adenosine derivative. Topical application was well tolerated without clinically important ocular and systemic side effects. Its IOP-lowering effect was dose-dependent with a mean change of 4 mm Hg from baseline.[64,65]

PROSTANOID RECEPTOR AGONIST

Omidenepag isopropyl (OMDI) is a selective prostanoid EP2 receptor agonist that lowers IOP by promoting uveoscleral and trabecular outflows. Clinically significant IOP reductions and good tolerance were observed in phase 1 trials.[66] In POAG and OHT, over a 4-week period, phase 3 trials published from Japan demonstrated the noninferiority of OMDI at 0.002% compared to latanoprost at 0.005%. Conjunctival hyperemia (24.5%), increased corneal thickness (11.7%), and photophobia (4.3%) were the most frequently reported side effects. There was an observed mean increase in central corneal thickness of 15 μm (2.7%); the underlying mechanism remains unclear. Japan currently has approval to use this medication.[67]

SMALL INTERFERENCE RNA

Ribonucleic acid (RNA) interference, or small interference RNA (siRNA), is a relatively new technique for selectively silencing genes.[68] A siRNA called

SYL040012 was created with the specific goal of silencing the β_2 adrenergic receptor (ADRB2) at the ciliary body, which in turn lowers the production of aqueous humor. Studies using SYL040012 animal models have demonstrated a good safety profile and a notable decrease in IOP.[68]

NEUROPROTECTION

Glaucoma is a chronic neurodegenerative disease that causes retinal ganglion cell (RGC) death in a progressive manner. The quest for non-IOP-dependent neuroprotection continues. Exposure to neurotoxic substances such as glutamate and NO, loss of internal trophic factors, intracellular destructive process, and loss of cellular self-repair process are the cellular processes that result in RGC death. The goal of neuroprotective therapy is to maintain visual function by balancing the signals that indicate cellular death and survival.[69]

Memantine

Memantine is an antagonist of the *N*-methyl-D-aspartate (NMDA) receptor that stops calcium influx-induced cell death. Retinal ganglion cells are toxic to high glutamate levels, and the NMDA receptor's excitotoxicity mediates the ensuing cell death by producing an excess of intracellular calcium. Based on standard automated perimetry and optic disk photography findings, memantine 10 and 20 mg daily doses did not prevent or slow the progression of glaucoma, according to 4-year follow-up results from two multicenter RCTs with patients with POAG.[70,71]

Brimonidine

Animal models have shown that brimonidine has an IOP-independent neuroprotective effect. Antiapoptotic factors are upregulated, glutamate-induced excitotoxicity is modulated, NO synthetase is inhibited, and glial activity is inhibited as part of the proposed mechanism. Studies comparing OHT patients treated with brimonidine versus those treated with timolol revealed a significant reduction in retinal nerve fiber layer loss.[72-74]

Neurotrophins

Neurotrophic factors are critical for the survival of cells. Neuroprotectants under clinical investigation include brain-derived neurotrophic factor (BDNF), ciliary neurotrophic factor, glial cell line-derived neurotrophic factor, and nerve growth factor (NGF). It has been demonstrated that valproic acid induces neuroprotection by activating the TrkB (BDNF-tropomyosin receptor kinase) pathway. Epilepsy was traditionally treated with this. In a rat model of glaucoma, the protective effect of topical application of NGF drops on RGCs has been shown. In a small number of patients with advanced glaucoma, it has also shown improvement in visual fields, contrast sensitivity, and electrophysiological tests. The safe administration of these molecules at the targeted site of action, inadequate knowledge of pharmacokinetics, and uncertainty regarding the long-term effects are the main areas of concern.[75,76]

GENE THERAPY

Research on gene therapy for glaucoma is still in its early stages. The development of gene therapy has been hampered by the numerous chromosome loci linked to POAG, difficulties transferring genes to their intended sites, and the potential for mutagenesis. A protein found in the ciliary body called aquaporin 1 helps move water across membranes, which is how aqueous is produced. It has been observed that in animal models, disrupting aquaporin 1 through CRISPR Cas9 RNA gene therapy lowers intracranial pressure. Treatments that target a gene involved in a physiological process, as opposed to a particular gene mutation, may be broadly applicable.[77,78]

In mouse models, a novel adeno-associated virus (AAV) gene therapy targeting the BDNF has been proven effective in treating glaucoma. By upregulating tropomyosin-related receptor kinase B, intravitreal injection of AAV2 vectors increased both the amount of BDNF produced and the length of time that BDNF was active.[79]

STEM CELL THERAPY

The goal of stem cell therapy is to potentially regenerate and repopulate retinal ganglion cells (RGCs) in order to restore vision that has been lost due to glaucoma. Neurotrophins, which are released by mesenchymal stem cells, help cells survive and can regenerate RGCs. Preclinical studies have validated this. It might also be involved in the trabecular meshwork's cell-based functional restoration. According to available data, the anterior trabecular meshwork and Schwalbe's ring contain adult stem cell populations. These stem cells can be grown in vitro to promote tissue regeneration and are crucial for tissue repair. It has been reported that transplanting trabecular meshwork cells derived from induced pluripotent stem cells (iPSCs) restores aqueous humor flow in mouse models. The role of stem cells in glaucoma management needs further clinical validation.[80,81]

CONCLUSION

Advances in drugs and drug delivery are helping ophthalmologists to optimize glaucoma care, improve treatment adherence, achieve better efficacy, safety, and stability, and improve patients' overall quality of life.

REFERENCES

1. Allison K, Patel D, Alabi O. Epidemiology of glaucoma: the past, present, and predictions for the future. Cureus. 2020;12(11):e11686.

2. Tham Y-C, Li X, Wong TY, Quigley HA, Aung T, Cheng C-Y. Global prevalence of glaucoma and projections of glaucoma burden through 2040: a systematic review and meta-analysis. Ophthalmology. 2014;121(11):2081-90.
3. European Glaucoma Society Terminology and Guidelines for Glaucoma, 5th Edition. Br J Ophthalmol. 2022;105(1):1-169.
4. Leidl MC, Choi CJ, Syed ZA, Melki SA. Intraocular pressure fluctuation and glaucoma progression: what do we know? Br J Ophthalmol. 2014;98(10):1315-19.
5. Quigley HA, Enger C, Katz J, Sommer A, Scott R, Gilbert D. Risk factors for the development of glaucomatous visual field loss in ocular hypertension. Arch Ophthalmol. 1994;112(5):644-9.
6. Leske MC, Connell AM, Wu SY, Hyman LG, Schachat AP. Risk factors for open-angle glaucoma. The Barbados Eye Study. Arch Ophthalmol. 1995;113(7):918-24.
7. Tielsch JM, Katz J, Sommer A, Quigley HA, Javitt JC. Hypertension, perfusion pressure, and primary open-angle glaucoma. A population-based assessment. Arch Ophthalmol. 1995;113(2):216-21.
8. Burgoyne CF, Downs JC, Bellezza AJ, Suh JK, Hart RT. The optic nerve head as a biomechanical structure: a new paradigm for understanding the role of IOP-related stress and strain in the pathophysiology of glaucomatous optic nerve head damage. Prog Retin Eye Res. 2005;24(1):39-73.
9. Fechtner RD, Weinreb RN. Mechanisms of optic nerve damage in primary open angle glaucoma. Surv Ophthalmol. 1994;39(1):23-42.
10. Yücel YH, Zhang Q, Weinreb RN, Kaufman PL, Gupta N. Atrophy of relay neurons in magno- and parvocellular layers in the lateral geniculate nucleus in experimental glaucoma. Invest Ophthalmol Vis Sci. 2001;42(13):3216-22.
11. Vishwaraj CR, Srinivasan K, Rengaraj SA, Premanand, Tripathi S. Neuroprotection in glaucoma. Indian J Ophthalmol. 2022;70(2):380-5.
12. Liu P, Wang F, Song Y, Wang M, Zhang X. Current situation and progress of drugs for reducing intraocular pressure. Ther Adv Chronic Dis. 2022;13: 20406223221140392.
13. Latimer K, Pendleton C, Martinez A, Subramanian PS, Quiñones-Hinojosa A. Insight into glaucoma treatment in the early 1900s: Harvey Cushing's 1905 Operation. Arch Ophthalmol. 2012;130(4):510-13.
14. Tanna AP, Johnson M. Rho kinase inhibitors as a novel treatment for glaucoma and ocular hypertension. Ophthalmology. 2018;125(11):1741-56.
15. Harrison BA, Almstead ZY, Burgoon H, Gardyan M, Goodwin NC, Healy J, et al. Discovery and development of LX7101, a dual LIM-kinase and ROCK inhibitor for the treatment of glaucoma. ACS Med Chem Lett. 2015;6(1):84-88.
16. Li G, Mukherjee D, Navarro I, Ashpole NE, Sherwood JM, Chang J, et al. Visualization of conventional outflow tissue responses to Netarsudil in living mouse eyes. Eur J Pharmacol. 2016;787:20-31.
17. Thieme H, Nuskovski M, Nass JU, Pleyer U, Strauss O, Wiederholt M. Mediation of calcium-independent contraction in trabecular meshwork through protein kinase C and Rho-A. Invest Ophthalmol Vis Sci. 2000;41(13):4240-46.
18. Rao PV, Deng PF, Kumar J, Epstein DL. Modulation of aqueous humor outflow facility by the Rho kinase-specific inhibitor Y-27632. Invest Ophthalmol Vis Sci. 2001;42(5):1029-37.
19. Wang J, Wang H, Dang Y. Rho-kinase inhibitors as emerging targets for glaucoma therapy. Ophthalmol Ther. 2023;12(6):2943-57.

20. Tanihara H, Inoue T, Yamamoto T, Kuwayama Y, Abe H, Araie M, et al. K-115 Clinical Study Group. Phase 1 clinical trials of a selective Rho kinase inhibitor, K-115. JAMA Ophthalmol. 2013;131(10):1288-95.
21. Tanihara H, Inoue T, Yamamoto T, Kuwayama Y, Abe H, Araie M, et al. 'K-115' Clinical Study Group. Phase 2 randomized clinical study of a Rho kinase inhibitor, in primary open-angle glaucoma and ocular hypertension. Am J Ophthalmol. 2013;156(4):731-36.
22. Tanihara H, Kakuda T, Sano T, Kanno T, Gunji R. Safety and efficacy of ripasudil in Japanese patients with glaucoma or ocular hypertension: 12-month interim analysis of ROCK-J, a post-marketing surveillance study. BMC Ophthalmol. 2020;20(1):275-76.
23. Tanihara H, Inoue T, Yamamoto T, Kuwayama Y, Abe H, Suganami H, et al. Additive intraocular pressure-lowering effects of the Rho kinase inhibitor Ripasudil (K-115) combined with timolol or latanoprost: a report of 2 randomized clinical trials. JAMA Ophthalmol. 2015;133(7):755-761.
24. Kusuhara S, Nakamura M. Ripasudil hydrochloride hydrate in the treatment of glaucoma: safety, efficacy, and patient selection. Clin Ophthalmol. 2020;14:1229-36.
25. Tanihara H, Kakuda T, Sano T, Kanno T, Imada R, Shingaki W, et al. Safety and efficacy of Ripasudil in Japanese patients with glaucoma or ocular hypertension: 3-month interim analysis of ROCK-J, a post-marketing surveillance study. Adv Ther. 2019;36:333-43.
26. Saito H, Kagami S, Mishima K, Mataki N, Fukushima A, Araie M. Long-term side effects including blepharitis leading to discontinuation of ripasudil. J Glaucoma. 2019;28:289-93.
27. Inoue K, Okayama R, Shiokawa M, Ishida K, Tomita G. Efficacy and safety of adding Ripasudil to existing treatment regimens for reducing intraocular pressure. Int Ophthalmol. 2018;38:93-8.
28. Kusuhara S, Katsuyama A, Matsumiya W, Nakamura M. Efficacy and safety of Ripasudil, a Rho-associated kinase inhibitor, in eyes with uveitic glaucoma. Graefes Arch Clin Exp Ophthalmol. 2018;256:809-14.
29. Matsumura R, Inoue T, Matsumura A, Tanihara H. Efficacy of Ripasudil as a second-line medication in addition to a prostaglandin analog in patients with exfoliation glaucoma: a pilot study. Clin Drug Investig. 2017;37:535-39.
30. Ko JA, Komatsu K, Minamoto A, Kondo S, Okumichi H, Hirooka K, et al. Effects of Ripasudil, a rho-kinase inhibitor, on scar formation in a mouse model of filtration surgery. Curr Eye Res. 2023;48:826-35.
31. Mizuno Y, Komatsu K, Tokumo K, Okada N, Onoe H, Okumichi H, et al. Safety and efficacy of the Rho-kinase inhibitor (Ripasudil) in bleb needling after trabeculectomy: a prospective multicenter study. J Clin Med. 2023;13(1):75.
32. Mimura T, Noma H, Inoue Y, Kawashima M, Kitsu K, Mizota A. Early postoperative effect of ripasudil hydrochloride after trabeculectomy on secondary glaucoma: a randomized controlled trial. Open Ophthalmol J [online]. 2022;16(1). Available from: http://dx.doi.org/10.2174/18743641-v16-e2206201. [Last accessed 20 May 2024].
33. Batra M, Gupta S, Nair AB, Dhanawat M, Sandal S, Morsy MA. Netarsudil: a new ophthalmic drug in the treatment of chronic primary open angle glaucoma and ocular hypertension. Eur J Ophthalmol. 2021;31:2237-44.

34. Wang R-F, Williamson JE, Kopczynski C, Serle JB. Effect of 0.04% AR-13324, a ROCK, and norepinephrine transporter inhibitor, on aqueous humor dynamics in normotensive monkey eyes. J Glaucoma. 2015;24:51-4.
35. Kiel JW, Kopczynski CC. Effect of AR-13324 on episcleral venous pressure in Dutch belted rabbits. J Ocul Pharmacol Ther. 2015;31:146-51.
36. Bacharach J, Dubiner HB, Levy B, Kopczynski CC, Novack GD; AR-13324-CS202 Study Group. Double-masked, randomized, dose-response study of AR-13324 versus latanoprost in patients with elevated intraocular pressure. Ophthalmology. 2015;122:302-7.
37. Serle JB, Katz LJ, McLaurin E, Heah T, Ramirez-Davis N, Usner DW, et al. Two phase 3 clinical trials comparing the safety and efficacy of netarsudil to timolol in patients with elevated intraocular pressure: Rho kinase elevated IOP treatment trial 1 and 2 (ROCKET-1 and ROCKET-2). Am J Ophthalmol. 2018;186:116-27.
38. Moumneh K, Sheybani A, Fellman RL, Godfrey DG, Grover DS. Reticular corneal edema or corneal honeycombing in eyes treated with netarsudil: a case series. J Glaucoma. 2020;29:607-10.
39. LoBue SA, Moustafa GA, Vu A, Amin M, Nguyen T, Goyal H. Transient reticular cystic corneal epithelial edema with topical netarsudil: a case series and review. Cornea. 2021;40:1048-54.
40. Lewis RA, Levy B, Ramirez N, Kopczynski CC, Usner DW, Novack GD, et al. Fixed-dose combination of AR-13324 and latanoprost: a double-masked, 28-day, randomised, controlled study in patients with open-angle glaucoma or ocular hypertension. Br J Ophthalmol. 2016;100:339-44.
41. Asrani S, Bacharach J, Holland E, McKee H, Sheng H, Lewis RA, et al. Fixed-dose combination of netarsudil and latanoprost in ocular hypertension and open-angle glaucoma: pooled efficacy/safety analysis of phase 3 MERCURY-1 and -2. Adv Ther. 2020;37:1620-31.
42. Weinreb RN, Ong T, Scassellati Sforzolini B, Vittitow JL, Singh K, Kaufman PL; VOYAGER study group. A randomised, controlled comparison of latanoprostene bunod and latanoprost 0.005% in the treatment of ocular hypertension and open angle glaucoma: the VOYAGER study. Br J Ophthalmol. 2015;99(6):738-45.
43. Liu JHK, Slight JR, Vittitow JL, Scassellati Sforzolini B, Weinreb RN. Efficacy of latanoprostene bunod 0.024% compared with timolol 0.5% in lowering intraocular pressure over 24 hours. Am J Ophthalmol. 2016;169:249-57.
44. Weinreb RN, Scassellati Sforzolini B, Vittitow J, Liebmann J. Latanoprostene bunod 0.024% versus timolol maleate 0.5% in subjects with open-angle glaucoma or ocular hypertension: the APOLLO study. Ophthalmology. 2016;123:965-73.
45. Medeiros FA, Martin KR, Peace J, Scassellati Sforzolini B, Vittitow JL, Weinreb RN. Comparison of latanoprostene bunod 0.024% and timolol maleate 0.5% in open-angle glaucoma or ocular hypertension: the LUNAR study. Am J Ophthalmol. 2016;168:250-9.
46. Weinreb RN, Liebmann JM, Martin KR, Kaufman PL, Vittitow JL. Latanoprostene bunod 0.024% in subjects with open-angle glaucoma or ocular hypertension: pooled phase 3 study findings. J Glaucoma. 2018;27:7-15.
47. Kawase K, Vittitow JL, Weinreb RN, Araie M; JUPITER study group. Long-term safety and efficacy of latanoprostene bunod 0.024% in Japanese subjects with open-angle glaucoma or ocular hypertension: The JUPITER study. Adv Ther. 2016;33:1612-27.

48. VYZULTA (latanoprostene bunod ophthalmic solution) 0.024%, for topical ophthalmic use: Bausch & Lomb Inc. [online] Updated 2 Nov 2017. Available from https://www.accessdata.fda.gov/drugsatfda_docs/label/2017/207795Orig1s000lbl.pdf. [Last accessed 25 May 2024].
49. Kass MA, Heuer DK, Higginbotham EJ, Johnson CA, Keltner JL, Miller JP, et al. The ocular hypertension treatment study: a randomized trial determines that topical ocular hypotensive medication delays or prevents the onset of primary open-angle glaucoma. Arch Ophthalmol. 2002;120(6):701-830.
50. Higginbotham EJ. Considerations in glaucoma therapy: fixed combinations versus their component medications. Clin Ophthalmol. 2010;4:1-9.
51. Holló G, Topouzis F, Fechtner RD. Fixed-combination intraocular pressure-lowering therapy for glaucoma and ocular hypertension: advantages in clinical practice. Expert Opin Pharmacother. 2014;15(12):1737-47.
52. Konstas AG, Schmetterer L, Costa VP, Holló G, Katsanos A, Denis P, et al. Current and emerging fixed combination therapies in glaucoma: a safety and tolerability review. Expert Opin Drug Saf. 2020;19(11):1445-60.
53. Machen L, Razeghinejad R, Myers JS. Fixed-combination topical anti-hypertensive ophthalmic agents. Expert Opin Pharmacother. 2020;21(10):1269-82.
54. Belfort R Jr., Paula JS, Lopes Silva MJ, Della Paolera M, Kim T, Chen MY, et al. Fixed-combination bimatoprost/brimonidine/timolol in glaucoma: a randomized, masked, controlled, phase III Study conducted in Brazil. Clin Ther. 2020;42(2):263-75.
55. Hartleben C, Parra JC, Batoosingh A, Bernstein P, Goodkin M. A masked, randomized, phase 3 comparison of triple fixed-combination bimatoprost/brimonidine/timolol versus fixed-combination brimonidine/timolol for lowering intraocular pressure. J Ophthalmol. 2017;4586763.
56. Menon MG, Goodkin ML. Triple fixed-combination bimatoprost/brimonidine/timolol in glaucoma and ocular hypertension in India: a multicenter, open-label, phase 3 study. Clin Ophthalmol. 2022;16:3559-69.
57. Medeiros FA, Walters TR, Kolko M, Coote M, Bejanian M, Goodkin ML, et al. Phase 3, randomized, 20-month study of bimatoprost implant in open-angle glaucoma and ocular hypertension (ARTEMIS 1). Ophthalmology. 2020;127:1627-41.
58. U.S. National Library of Medicine; Clinical trial-NCT04647214. 18-month prospective efficacy and safety study of bimatoprost intracameral implant (DURYSTA). [online] Last Updated 10 June 2024. Available from: https://classic.clinicaltrials.gov/ct2/show/NCT04647214 [Last accessed 15 June 2024].
59. Brandt JD, DuBiner HB, Benza R, Sall KN, Walker GA, Semba CP, et al. Long-term safety and efficacy of a sustained-release bimatoprost ocular ring. Ophthalmology. 2017;124:1565-6.
60. Xu J, Ge Y, Bu R, Zhang A, Feng S, Wang J, et al. Co-delivery of latanoprost and timolol from micelles-laden contact lenses for the treatment of glaucoma. J Control Release. 2019;305:18-28.
61. Perera SA, Ting DS, Nongpiur ME, Chew PT, Aquino MCD, Sng CC, et al. Feasibility study of sustained-release travoprost punctum plug for intraocular pressure reduction in an Asian population. Clin Ophthalmol. 2016;10:757-64.
62. Kesav NP, Young CEC, Ertel MK, Seibold LK, Kahook MY. Sustained-release drug delivery systems for the treatment of glaucoma. Int J Ophthalmol. 2021;14:148-159.

63. Occhiutto ML, Maranhão RC, Costa VP, Konstas AG. Nanotechnology for medical and surgical glaucoma therapy: a review. Adv Ther. 2020;37:155-99.
64. Chen J, Runyan SA, Robinson MR. Novel ocular antihypertensive compounds in clinical trials. Clin Ophthalmol. 2011;5:667-77.
65. Myers JS, Sall KN, DuBiner H, Slomowitz N, McVicar W, Rich CC, et al. A dose-escalation study to evaluate the safety, tolerability, pharmacokinetics, and efficacy of 2 and 4 weeks of twice-daily ocular trabodenoson in adults with ocular hypertension or primary open-angle glaucoma. J Ocul Pharmacol Ther. 2016;32:555-62.
66. Aihara M, Lu F, Kawata H, Tanaka Y, Yamamura K, Odani-Kawabata N, et al. Pharmacokinetics, safety, and intraocular pressure-lowering profile of omidenepag isopropyl, a selective, nonprostaglandin, prostanoid EP2 receptor agonist, in healthy Japanese and Caucasian volunteers (Phase I study). J Ocul Pharmacol Ther. 2019;35:542-50.
67. Aihara M, Lu F, Kawata H, Iwata A, Odani-Kawabata N, Shams NK. Omidenepag isopropyl versus latanoprost in primary open-angle glaucoma and ocular hypertension: The phase 3 AYAME study. Am J Ophthalmol. 2020;220:53-63.
68. Martínez T, González MV, Roehl I, Wright N, Pañeda C, Jiménez AI. In vitro and in vivo efficacy of SYL040012, a novel siRNA compound for treatment of glaucoma. Mol Ther. 2014;22:81-91.
69. Schwartz M, Yoles E. Neuroprotection: a new treatment modality for glaucoma? Curr Opin Ophthalmol. 2000;11:107-11.
70. Sucher NJ, Lipton SA, Dreyer EB. Molecular basis of glutamate toxicity in retinal ganglion cells. Vision Res. 1997;37:483-93.
71. Weinreb RN, Liebmann JM, Cioffi GA, Goldberg I, Brandt JD, Johnson CA, et al. Oral memantine for the treatment of glaucoma: design and results of 2 randomized, placebo-controlled, phase 3 studies. Ophthalmology. 2018;125:1874-85.
72. Chrysostomou V, Rezania F, Trounce IA, Crowston JG. Oxidative stress and mitochondrial dysfunction in glaucoma. Curr Opin Pharmacol. 2013;13:12-5.
73. Krupin T, Liebmann JM, Greenfield DS, Ritch R, Gardiner S. Low-pressure glaucoma study group. A randomized trial of brimonidine versus timolol in preserving visual function: results from the low-pressure glaucoma treatment study. Am J Ophthalmol. 2011;151:671-81.
74. Sena DF, Lindsley K. Neuroprotection for treatment of glaucoma in adults. Cochrane Database Syst Rev. 2017;1(1):CD006539.
75. Rocco ML, Soligo M, Manni L, Aloe L. Nerve growth factor: early studies and recent clinical trials. Curr Neuro Pharmacol. 2018;16:1455-65.
76. Kimura A, Namekata K, Guo X, Harada C, Harada T. Neuroprotection, growth factors and BDNF-TrkB signalling in retinal degeneration. Int J Mol Sci. 2016;17:1584.
77. Wilson AM, Di Polo A. Gene therapy for retinal ganglion cell neuroprotection in glaucoma. Gene Ther. 2012;19:127-36.
78. Wu J, Bell OH, Copland DA, Young A, Pooley JR, Maswood R, et al. Gene therapy for glaucoma by ciliary body aquaporin 1 disruption using CRISPR-Cas9. Mol Ther. 2020;28:820-9.
79. Osborne A, Khatib TZ, Songra L, Barber AC, Hall K, Kong GYX, et al. Neuroprotection of retinal ganglion cells by a novel gene therapy construct

that achieves sustained enhancement of brain-derived neurotrophic factor/tropomyosin-related kinase receptor-B signaling. Cell Death Dis. 2018; 9:1007.

80. Harrell CR, Fellabaum C, Arsenijevic A, Markovic BS, Djonov V, Volarevic V. Therapeutic potential of mesenchymal stem cells and their secretome in the treatment of glaucoma. Stem Cells Int. 2019;7869130.
81. Sun H, Zhu Q, Guo P, Zhang Y, Tighe S, Zhu Y. Trabecular meshwork cells are a valuable resource for cellular therapy of glaucoma. J Cell Mol Med. 2019;23:1678-86.

7 CHAPTER

Management of Noninfectious Uveitis

Dipankar Das, Jessica Basumatary, Himanshu Garkoti, Rajendra Prakash Maurya

ABSTRACT

Noninfectious uveitis (NIU) is an inflammatory condition of the uveal tract occurring as a result of autoimmune or autoinflammatory processes. It can lead to devastating consequences including blindness, if appropriate therapy is not introduced in time. Since the 1950s, corticosteroids have played a major role in the management of NIU; however, research continues to grow in this field as chronic usage of steroids can result in multiple ocular and systemic side effects. Steroid-sparing immunosuppressives are gradually being employed to achieve long-term control of inflammation. Recent developments in the understanding of the ocular immune system have resulted in the identification of various proinflammatory cytokines and other mediators of inflammation. This information has led to the introduction of a new class of drugs, the biological response modifiers. Posterior uveitis such as Behçet's disease responds well to biologics and adalimumab is increasingly being used in pediatric juvenile idiopathic arthritis-related uveitis.

Keywords: Noninfectious uveitis, biological response modifiers, biologics in NIU, anti-TNF-α, adalimumab, tocilizumab, JAK inhibitors

INTRODUCTION

Uveitis is defined as the inflammation of uvea, the vascular coat of the eyeball. The etiology can be broadly categorized into two groups, infectious and noninfectious. Experiments on animal models like experimental autoimmune uveitis (EAU) and experimental autoimmune anterior uveitis (EAAU) have shed light on the role of autoimmunity in causing noninfectious uveitis (NIU). However, recent trends have shown a steady rise in autoinflammatory diseases. These disorders are caused by gene mutations that cause the innate immune system to malfunction in the absence of high titers of autoantibodies or T-cell responses.[1] Therefore, NIU is a result of a dysregulation in the body's immune system and inflammatory mechanisms causing tissue damage most likely in the setting of infectious, genetic, epigenetic, and environmental triggers. These findings strongly advocate the use of anti-inflammatory agents in the treatment of NIU.

Since the discovery of corticosteroids for the treatment of rheumatoid arthritis (RA) in the 1950s, it has remained the first-line therapy for most systemic and ocular inflammatory diseases. Corticosteroids can be delivered topically, orally, and locally to the targeted site. However, long-term usage of corticosteroids can result in severe sight-threatening complications like cataract and glaucoma, as well as osteoporosis, weight gain, diabetes, hypertension, hirsutism, avascular necrosis of long bones, and growth retardation in children, to name a few.

The understanding of uveitis, particularly at the molecular level, has grown steadily over the decades. The fine balance between anti-inflammatory cytokines like interleukin 6 (IL6), tumor necrosis factor α (TNF-α), IL1, IL17, IL12, IL22, IL23, interferon γ (IFN-γ), and anti-inflammatory cytokines like IL10, transforming growth factor β (TGF-β), IL35, IL27, etc., is essential in maintaining the proper functioning of the body's immune system. Having this information in our armamentarium, researchers have been able to develop new drug formulations targeting these specific molecules that downregulate or upregulate the immune system.

IMMUNOSUPPRESSIVE AGENTS FOR NONINFECTIOUS UVEITIS

The steroid-sparing immunosuppressive drugs can be classified into two groups: Nonbiologics and biological agents **(Flowchart 7.1)**. The common nonbiologic agents used to treat NIU are described in **Table 7.1**.

BIOLOGICAL THERAPIES

The target molecules for biologics are the cytokines and their receptors that cause an exaggerated immune response in the absence of appropriate microbiological triggers. These drugs are manufactured by the recombinant DNA technology and include anti-inflammatory cytokines and antibodies to inflammatory cytokines or their receptors. The widely used biologic agents for treating NIU are described in **Table 7.2**.

Tumor Necrosis Factor-α Inhibitor

- *Adalimumab* is a fully human, monoclonal antibody against TNF-α which is a proinflammatory cytokine. The efficacy of this drug in treating NIU has clearly been demonstrated in the VISUAL I study, which was a multicenter, randomized, placebo-controlled trial. The median time to treatment failure in the study participants who received adalimumab was 24 weeks, whereas it was 13 weeks in the placebo group. Although the risk of severe infection was similar in both groups, the adalimumab

Flowchart 7.1: Immunosuppressives in noninfectious uveitis.

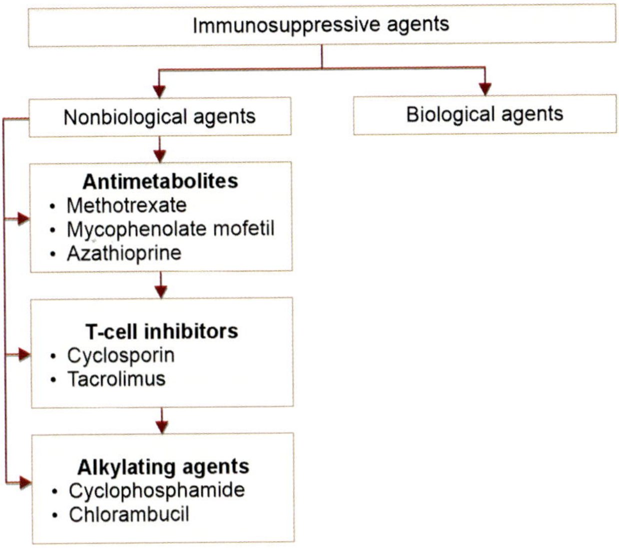

group encountered one case of active tuberculosis (TB), one of latent TB, a lupus-like reaction, one case of secondary malignancy, and one case of demyelinating illness. The efficacy of the drug was further demonstrated in the follow-up VISUAL II and VISUAL III trials.

In the current scenario, Adalimumab is frequently used in the treatment of juvenile idiopathic arthritis (JIA)-associated uveitis. The SYCAMORE[2] is a landmark study that evaluated the safety and efficacy of adding adalimumab in active JIA previously treated with methotrexate. 60 children were enrolled in this multicenter, randomized placebo-controlled trial. The adalimumab group was less likely to have treatment failure and could achieve freedom from corticosteroids as compared to the control group which did not receive adalimumab. The ADJUVITE trial also studied adalimumab in treating JIA and obtained similar results.[3]

- *Infliximab* is a chimeric human-mouse monoclonal antibody against TNF-α. In 1998, it was approved by the Food and Drug Administration (FDA) for Crohn's disease. It has shown a considerable measure of success in treating posterior uveitis in Behçet's disease, refractory to other treatments.[4,5] Several studies have also demonstrated its effectiveness in treating pediatric JIA-related uveitis.[6-8] The major side effects associated with this drug are reactivation of latent TB, lupus-like reaction, and thromboembolism. Infliximab can also be considered as a first- or second-line agent in other NIU refractory to conventional treatment.[9]
- *Golimumab* is a fully human, monoclonal antibody against TNF-α. It has more affinity for TNF-α than adalimumab.[10] In the GO-EASY study, the

TABLE 7.1: Nonbiologics used in NIU management.

Drugs	*Mechanism of action*	*Dose*	*Monitoring*	*Side effects*
Methotrexate (folic acid analog)	Inhibits DNA replication by inhibiting the enzyme dihydrofolate reductase (DHF-R)	7.5–25 mg/week PO, IM, or SC; concomitantly start folic acid 1 mg PO daily	CBC, DLC (TLC, platelet counts), CMP, creatinine, LFT	• Category X, nausea, stomatitis, fatigue, interstitial pneumonitis, cytopenia, and hepatotoxicity • *Antidote:* Leucovorin
Mycophenolate mofetil	Inhibits DNA replication by inhibiting inosine monophosphate dehydrogenase enzyme	500–1,500 mg PO bid	CBC, DLC, CMP, LFT	GI irritation, vomiting, nausea, diarrhea, myelosuppression, hepatotoxicity, leukopenia, drug allergy, flu-like symptoms, palpitations, and epistaxis
Azathioprine (imidazole analog and precursor of 6-mercaptopurine)	It is incorporated into replicating DNA and thus interferes with the DNA replication process	1–3 mg/kg PO daily	CBC, DLC (TLC, platelet counts), CMP, creatinine, serum TPMT level	Category D, allergic reactions, GI disturbances, infection, hepatotoxicity, oral ulcers, hair loss, fatigue, and myelosuppression
Cyclosporine	It is a calcineurin inhibitor which inhibits T-cell receptor transduction and downregulates IL2 action	2.5–10 mg/kg/day divided every 12 hours	CBC, DLC, CMP	• *Early:* Paresthesia and headache • *Chronic:* Hirsutism, neurotoxicity, gingivitis, and metabolic abnormalities • *Severe:* Systemic HTN associated with nephrotoxicity
Tacrolimus		0.1–0.3 mg/kg/day divided every 12 hours	CBC, DLC, CMP, BP, FBS, baseline EKG	HTN, hypomagnesemia, hyperkalemia, neurologic symptoms, DM, tremor, and CKD
Cyclophosphamide	Alkylates the purines in DNA and RNA causing impaired DNA replication	1–3 mg/kg PO daily	Baseline creatinine, CBC, DLC, CMP, urinalysis	Gonadal dysfunction, myelosuppression, leukopenia, hemorrhagic cystitis/bladder cancer (high water intake recommended), and secondary malignancies
Chlorambucil	Inhibits DNA replication by alkylation	0.1–0.2 mg/kg PO daily	CBC, DLC, CMP	Myelosuppression, aplastic anemia, secondary malignancy, infection, and sterility

(BP: blood pressure; bid: twice a day; CBC: complete blood count; CKD: chronic kidney disease; CMP: comprehensive metabolic panel; DLC: differential leukocyte count; DM: diabetes mellitus; GI: gastrointestinal; HTN: hypertension; IM: intramuscular; IV: intravenous; NIU: noninfectious uveitis; PO: per oral; TPMT: thiopurine methyltransferase)

TABLE 7.2: Biological agents used in NIU management.

Class	*Drug*	*Dose*	*Side effects*
TNF-α inhibitor	Adalimumab	80 mg SC on day 0, then 40 mg on day 7, then every 14 days	• Reactivation of TB, lupus-like reaction, demyelinating illness (CNS demyelination must be ruled out before starting therapy), thromboembolism, and malignancy • Etanercept causes endogenous uveitis
	Infliximab	Loading dose of 3–5 mg/kg IV on weeks 0, 2, and 6 and then maintenance therapy with 3–10 mg/kg IV every 8 weeks	
	Golimumab	50 mg SC monthly	
	Etanercept	50 mg SC weekly	
IL1 inhibitor	Anakinra	100 mg SC daily	Flu-like symptoms, neutropenia, bacterial and viral infections, and hepatoxicity
	Canakinumab	150 mg SC every 8 weeks	
	Gevokizumab	30 or 60 mg IV or SC every 4 weeks	
IL2 receptor inhibitor	Daclizumab	1–2 mg/kg IV or SC every 2–4 weeks	Fulminant, liver failure, encephalitis, and meningoencephalitis
IL6 receptor inhibitor	Tocilizumab	4–8 mg/kg IV every 4 weeks or 162 mg SC every 1–2 weeks	Neutropenia, opportunistic infections, hepatoxicity, allergic reaction, GI disorders, malignancies, and paradoxical exacerbation of uveitis
IL17 inhibitor	Secukinumab	300 mg SC every 2–4 weeks or 10 mg/kg IV every 2 weeks or 30 mg/kg IV every 4 weeks	GI distress, hypersensitivity reaction, and infections
B-cell inhibitor	Rituximab	1,000 mg IV on days 0 and 14 and then 500–1,000 mg every 6 months as needed	Pneumonia, UTI, reactivation of prior varicella zoster, and HBV infections
T-cell inhibitor	Abatacept	Loading dose of 500–1000 mg IV and then 125 mg SC weekly	Infection and GI distress
Interferons	IFN-α 2a	3–6 million units SC daily followed by tapering as needed	Flu-like symptoms, hepatoxicity, skin rashes, systemic or ocular sarcoidosis, depression, and IFN retinopathy
	IFN-α 2b	2 million units/m^2 of BSA 3 times/week followed by tapering as needed	
JAK inhibitors	Tofacitinib	5 mg orally twice daily	Hyperlipidemia, nephrotoxicity, hepatotoxicity, neutropenia, Herpes (HSV, VZV) infections, and GI distress

(BSA: body surface area; CNS: central nervous system; GI: gastrointestinal; HBV: hepatitis B virus; HSV: herpes simplex virus; IFN: interferon; IV: intravenous; SC: subcutaneous; TB: tuberculosis; UTI: urinary tract infection; VZV: varicella-zoster virus) rate of occurrence and disease activity of acute anterior uveitis decreased significantly in patients being treated with golimumab for ankylosing spondylitis.[11] Golimumab can be considered as a treatment option in patients not responding to other TNF-α inhibitors.

- *Etanercept* is a fusion protein comprising the Fc fragment of immunoglobulin G (IgG) and p75 subunit of the TNF receptor that binds to both TNF-α and TNF-β. It is frequently used, with some measure of success in the treatment of RA, ankylosing spondylitis, and psoriatic arthritis. However, its use in the setting of uveitis has largely been limited owing to the paradoxical pro-inflammatory nature of the drug that causes frequent flare-up of uveitis.[12,13] The present recommendation is to avoid it in uveitic practice.

Interleukin-1 Inhibitor

High levels of inflammatory cytokine, IL1, have been demonstrated in the aqueous humor of patients with active uveitis.[12] Some of the IL1 inhibitors are listed as follows:

- *Anakinra* blocks IL1 activity by competitively binding to its receptor. Currently, this is the only drug that has been approved for the treatment of neonatal-onset multisystem inflammatory disease (NOMID).[14]
- *Canakinumab* is a human monoclonal antibody against IL1β.

  Both of these drugs have been used with variable measures of success in treating monogenic auto-inflammatory-related uveitic conditions like Blau syndrome.[4,14] Side effects include flu-like symptoms, neutropenia, bacterial and viral infections, and transient increase in liver enzymes.
- *Gevokizumab* is another drug that inhibits the activity of IL1β. However, its efficacy in treating ocular inflammation is doubtful. The EYEGUARD-B study[15] analyzed the efficacy of gevokizumab in Behçet's disease and concluded that even though the drug was well tolerated and preserved the visual acuity, it did not significantly reduce the risk of occurrence of ocular exacerbations, which was the primary endpoint of the clinical trial. Further research is needed to establish its efficacy.

Interleukin 2 Receptor Inhibitor

Daclizumab is a recombinant humanized monoclonal antibody that targets the IL-2 receptor α subunit found in lymphocytes. The drug was initially introduced for the treatment of multiple sclerosis. Several studies[16,17] have shown that the administration of the drug resulted in a significant reduction in inflammation in NIU. However, in 2018, it was discontinued due to multiple reports of fulminant liver failure and central nervous system inflammation including encephalitis and meningoencephalitis.[14]

Interleukin 6 Receptor Inhibitor

- *Tocilizumab* is a recombinant human monoclonal antibody that acts by blocking the receptor of IL6. It has been approved by the FDA for the treatment of JIA, RA, and giant cell arteritis (GCA) refractory to TNF-α therapies. Its safety, efficacy, and tolerability were studied in the STOP uveitis randomized clinical trial. The drug is particularly useful in reducing the central macular thickness in patients with recalcitrant macular edema secondary to uveitis.[18,19]
- *Sarilumab* binds to the α subunit of the IL6 receptor and blocks it. It is a humanized monoclonal antibody. Its efficacy in reducing vitreous haze in posterior NIU was demonstrated in the SATURN study.[20]

  Side effects of IL6 inhibitors are neutropenia, opportunistic infections, increase in liver enzymes, allergic reaction, gastrointestinal (GI) disorders, malignancies, and paradoxical exacerbation of uveitis.[21]

Interleukin 17 Inhibitor

Secukinumab is a monoclonal antibody against IL17A. It is approved for the treatment of plaque psoriasis, psoriatic arthritis, and ankylosing spondylitis. Its potential in treating NIU requires further research. However, studies have shown that a higher dose of intravenous administration can maintain remission in chronic uveitis rather than the standard subcutaneous administration.[22]

Interleukin 23 Inhibitor

Guselkumab and *Ustekinumab* are IL23 inhibitors. The efficacy of these two drugs in NIU is still under evaluation.

B-CELL INHIBITOR

Rituximab is a chimeric murine-human monoclonal antibody against CD20 B cells. It is currently employed for the treatment non-Hodgkin's lymphoma, chronic lymphocytic leukemia, granulomatosis with polyangiitis (GPA), and RA. It can be used as a first- or second-line agent in antineutrophilic cytoplasmic antibody (ANCA) associated retinal vasculitis and scleritis.[9] Adverse events include pneumonia, urinary tract infections (UTIs), and reactivation of prior varicella-zoster and hepatitis B virus (HBV) infection.

T-CELL INHIBITOR

Abatacept is a fusion protein comprising the Fc portion of human IgG and the extracellular domain of cytotoxic T lymphocyte activation-4 (CTLA-4). It prevents T-cell activation by inhibiting CD80/CD86 molecules on antigen-presenting cells. It is used for the treatment of JIA and RA. While its use in uveitis is still off-label, it can be used in refractory cases not responding to anti-TNF-α drugs.[4] Studies on Abatacept in uveitis have demonstrated variable results.

Interferons

Interferons (IFNs) are important regulators of both innate and adaptive immune systems. They are essentially cytokines produced by T cells, macrophages, monocytes, and dendritic cells in response to infection and tumor growth. IFN-α is used for the treatment of hepatitis B and C infections, high-risk melanomas, and even refractory Behçet's disease. TNF exerts its immunomodulatory function via multiple pathways. It reduces neutrophil recruitment by downregulating IL17, increases the concentration of T regulator cells (Treg) in the periphery, and inhibits the natural killer (NK) cells. While IFN-α and IFN-β are immunosuppressors, IFN-γ has both pro-inflammatory and anti-inflammatory properties.[23,24] In relation to NIU, the use of IFN is currently limited to Behçet-related uveitis and multiple sclerosis. Side effects include flu-like symptoms, elevated liver enzymes, skin rashes, development of systemic or ocular sarcoidosis,[25,26] and depression due to reduced dopamine function. IFN retinopathy has been described as the presence of cotton wool spots and retinal hemorrhages in the posterior pole which disappear with reducing the dose.[12,27]

Janus Kinase Inhibitors

Janus kinases (JAKs) are a group of molecules through which multiple cytokines exert their functions, and hence, the inhibitors of these molecules have a role in the treatment of immune-mediated diseases.

- *Tofacitinib* is an inhibitor of JAK1 and JAK3. It has high oral bioavailability[14] which is of particular advantage when treating pediatric cases. It is currently used for the treatment of RA and inflammatory bowel diseases. It is the only biological agent available in oral form and, hence, is less expensive than other injectable biologics. Herpes infection of skin has been reported in many cases with the use of this drug.
- *Baricitinib* is an inhibitor of JAK1 and JAK2.

Multiple studies have been conducted to evaluate the safety and efficacy of these two drugs as potential therapies in refractory JIA-associated uveitis.[28-30]

NEWER DRUG DELIVERY SYSTEMS

- *Intravitreal corticosteroid:*
  - *Dexamethasone implant* is an extended-release, biodegradable implant that is injected into the vitreous cavity via the pars plana route using a 22-gauge device **(Fig. 7.1)**. The HURON study[31] evaluated

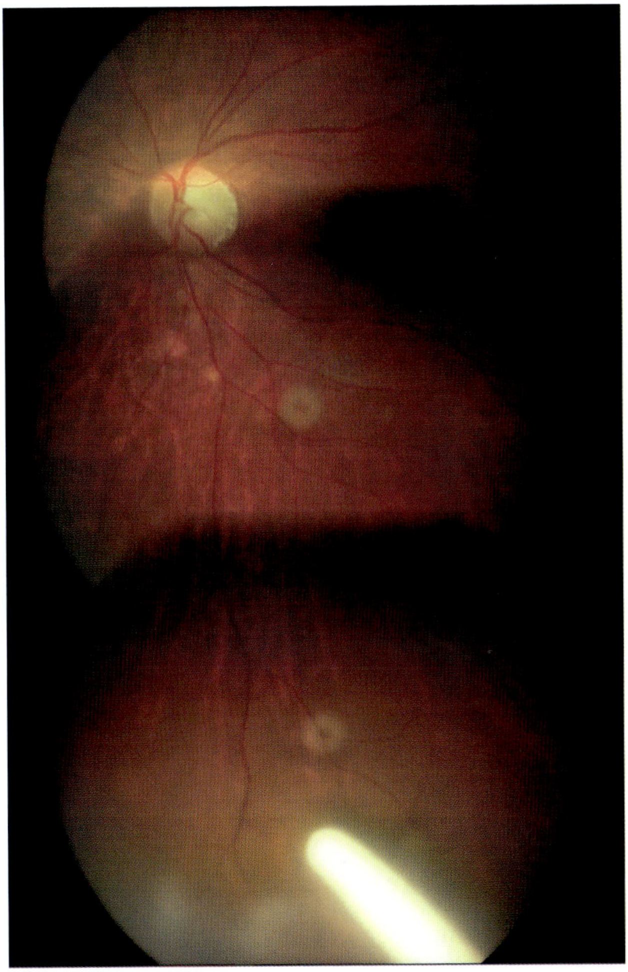

Fig. 7.1: A dexamethasone 0.7 mg implant (Ozurdex) in the vitreous cavity of a patient with intermediate uveitis.

the safety and efficacy of two doses (0.35 and 0.70 mg) of intravitreal dexamethasone implant in intermediate and posterior NIU and concluded that there was significant control of inflammation and improvement in visual acuity persisting for up to 6 months.

- *Fluocinolone acetonide implant* for the treatment of NIU was evaluated in the multicenter uveitis steroid treatment (MUST) trial.[32] The visual outcomes, between the implant group and the group receiving combined oral steroid and immunomodulator therapy, were comparable. Moreover, the implant group demonstrated a faster resolution of inflammation. However, after 7 years, there was a decline in the visual acuity of patients in the implant group possibly due to loss of efficacy of the implant.

Intravitreal steroid implants should be used with caution because even though there is good control of inflammation, side effects like steroid-induced cataract and glaucoma are very common with their use.

- *Intravitreal methotrexate* is indicated in the treatment of primary vitreoretinal lymphoma. Even though its potential use in the treatment of NIU is still at a nascent stage, several studies have documented good control of inflammation with improvement in visual acuity and resolution of uveitic macular edema after its use.[33,34] Intravitreal rituximab is also given in vitreoretinal lymphomas.
- *Suprachoroidal drug delivery* is a novel approach to drug delivery systems in the management of NIU. The suprachoroidal space (SCS) is a potential space between the sclera and the choroid which remains collapsed in the physiological state because of the intraocular pressure and the collagen fibers that attach the sclera to the choroid. Drugs can be delivered into this space by creating an external surgical incision in the sclera (sclerotomy) followed by the insertion of a cannula to reach the target site or by using a microneedle which is less invasive. Studies on animal models have demonstrated a greater baseline concentration of the drug in target tissue with SCS injection when compared to the intravitreal route along with faster clearance of the drug. Although this approach can deliver favorable outcomes in treating NIU, serious challenges associated with this technique include the risk of suprachoroidal hemorrhage, inadvertent globe perforation and endophthalmitis, retinal detachment, choroidal tears, scleral ectasia, and wound abscess.[14,35]

OCULAR GENE THERAPY

Ocular gene therapy using adeno-associated virus (AAV) and lentivirus vectors encoded with anti-inflammatory molecules is currently being studied in animal models. Gene therapy offers the possibility of long-term control of uveitis with a single treatment without side effects.[14,28]

CONCLUSION

Chronic uveitis is a debilitating illness that can severely affect a patient's quality of life. While corticosteroids have remained the mainstay for the treatment of NIU for several decades, there has been a gradual shift in this approach. Although their use is currently limited to cases refractory to standard therapy, the indications of biologics continue to grow. Novel therapies targeting specific molecules in the inflammatory cascade will revolutionize the management of NIU. They can, however, cause severe immune suppression. Therefore, these therapies should be given after thorough consultation with rheumatologists, especially in India because of the high prevalence of TB in our country.

ACKNOWLEDGMENTS

We would like to acknowledge the help and assistance of Dr Pradip Kumar Sharma, DM, Rheumatologist, Apollo Excel Care Centre, Guwahati, Assam, India; Dr Ankit Patawary, DM, Rheumatologist, Medicity Hospital, Guwahati, Assam, India; and Dr Gayatri Bharali, MD, Physician, Sri Sankaradeva Nethralaya, Guwahati, Assam, India.

REFERENCES

1. Forrester JV, Kuffova L, Dick AD. Autoimmunity, autoinflammation and infection in uveitis. Am J Ophthalmol. 2018;189:77-85.
2. Ramanan AV, Dick AD, Jones AP, McKay A, Williamson PR, Compeyrot-Lacassagne S, et al. Adalimumab plus methotrexate for uveitis in juvenile idiopathic arthritis. N Engl J Med. 2017;376(17):1637-46.
3. Quartier P, Baptiste A, Despert V, Allain-Launay E, Koné-Paut I, Belot A, et al. ADJUVITE: a double-blind, randomised, placebo-controlled trial of adalimumab in early onset, chronic, juvenile idiopathic arthritis-associated anterior uveitis. Ann Rheum Dis. 2018;77(7):1003-11.
4. Gamalero L, Simonini G, Ferrara G, Polizzi S, Giani T, Cimaz R. Evidence-based treatment for uveitis. Isr Med Assoc J. 2019;21(7):475-9.
5. Sfikakis PP, Kaklamanis PH, Elezoglou A, Katsilambros N, Theodossiadis PG, Papaefthimiou S, et al. Infliximab for recurrent, sight-threatening ocular inflammation in Adamantiades-Behçet disease. Ann Intern Med. 2004; 140(5):404.
6. Kahn P, Weiss M, Imundo LF, Levy DM. Favorable response to high-dose infliximab for refractory childhood uveitis. Ophthalmology. 2006;113(5):860-64.
7. Rajaraman R, Kimura Y, Li S, Haines K, Chu D. Retrospective case review of pediatric patients with uveitis treated with infliximab. Ophthalmology. 2006;113(2):308-14.
8. Richards JC, Tay-Kearney M, Murray K, Manners P. Infliximab for juvenile idiopathic arthritis-associated uveitis. Clin Experiment Ophthalmol. 2005;33(5):461-8.
9. Thomas AS. Biologics for the treatment of noninfectious uveitis: current concepts and emerging therapeutics. Curr Opin Ophthalmol. 2019;30(3):138-50.
10. Mérida S, Palacios E, Navea A, Bosch-Morell F. New immunosuppressive therapies in uveitis Treatment. Int J Mol Sci. 2015;16(8):18778-95.
11. Van Bentum RE, Heslinga SC, Nurmohamed MT, Gerards AH, Griep EN, Koehorst CBJM, et al. Reduced occurrence rate of acute anterior uveitis in ankylosing spondylitis treated with golimumab—the GO-EASY study. J Rheumatol. 2019;46(2):153-9.
12. Gaggiano C, Sota J, Gentileschi S, Caggiano V, Grosso S, Tosi GM, et al. The current status of biological treatment for uveitis. Expert Rev Clin Immunol. 2020;16(8):787-811.
13. Kakkassery V, Mergler S, Pleyer U. Anti-TNF-α treatment: a possible promoter in endogenous uveitis? Observational report on six patients: occurrence of uveitis following etanercept treatment. Curr Eye Res. 2010;35(8):751-6.
14. Singh RB, Sinha S, Saini C, Elbasiony E, Thakur S, Agarwal A. Recent advances in the management of non-infectious posterior uveitis. Int Ophthalmol. 2020; 40(11):3187-207.

15. Tugal-Tutkun I, Pavesio C, De Cordoue A, Bernard-Poenaru O, Gül A. Use of Gevokizumab in patients with Behçet's disease uveitis: an international, randomized, double-masked, placebo-controlled study and open-label extension study. Ocul Immunol Inflamm. 2018;26(7):1023-33.
16. Nussenblatt RB, Fortin E, Schiffman R, Rizzo L, Smith J, Van Veldhuisen P, et al. Treatment of noninfectious intermediate and posterior uveitis with the humanized anti-Tac mAb: a phase I/II clinical trial. Proc Natl Acad Sci. 1999;96(13):7462-6.
17. Nussenblatt R, Peterson J, Foster C, Rao N, See R, Letko E, et al. Initial evaluation of subcutaneous daclizumab treatments for noninfectious uveitis: a multicenter noncomparative interventional case series. Ophthalmology. 2005;112(5):764-70.
18. Sepah YJ, Sadiq MA, Chu DS, Dacey M, Gallemore R, Dayani P, et al. Primary (Month-6) outcomes of the STOP-uveitis study: evaluating the safety, tolerability, and efficacy of tocilizumab in patients with noninfectious uveitis. Am J Ophthalmol. 2017;183:71-80.
19. Mesquida M, Molins B, Llorenç V, Hernández MV, Espinosa G, Sainz De La Maza M, et al. Twenty-four month follow-up of tocilizumab therapy for refractory uveitis-related macular edema. Retina. 2018;38(7):1361-70.
20. Heissigerová J, Callanan D, De Smet MD, Srivastava SK, Karkanová M, Garcia-Garcia O, et al. Efficacy and safety of sarilumab for the treatment of posterior segment noninfectious uveitis (SARIL-NIU). Ophthalmology. 2019;126(3):428-37.
21. Wendling D, Dernis E, Prati C, Frisch E, Delbosc B. Onset of inflammatory eye disease under tocilizumab treatment for rheumatologic conditions: a paradoxical effect? J Rheumatol. 2011;38(10):2284.
22. Letko E, Yeh S, Foster CS, Pleyer U, Brigell M, Grosskreutz CL. Efficacy and safety of intravenous secukinumab in noninfectious uveitis requiring steroid-sparing immunosuppressive therapy. Ophthalmology. 2015;122(5):939-48.
23. Liu X, Diedrichs-Möhring M, Wildner G. The role of IFN-alpha in experimental and clinical uveitis. Ocul Immunol Inflamm. 2019;27(1):23-33.
24. Lin P, Suhler EB, Rosenbaum JT. The future of uveitis treatment. Ophthalmology. 2014;121(1):365-76.
25. Alazemi S, Campos MA. Interferon-induced sarcoidosis. Int J Clin Pract. 2005;60(2):201-11.
26. Doycheva D, Deuter C, Stuebiger N, Zierhut M. Interferon-alpha-associated presumed ocular sarcoidosis. Graefes Arch Clin Exp Ophthalmol. 2009;247(5):675-80.
27. Plskova J, Greiner K, Forrester JV. Interferon-α as an effective treatment for noninfectious posterior uveitis and panuveitis. Am J Ophthalmol. 2007;144(1):55-61.
28. Chu CJ, Barker SE, Dick AD, Ali RR. Gene therapy for noninfectious uveitis. Ocul Immunol Inflamm. 2012;20(6):394-405.
29. Maccora I, Land P, Miraldi Utz V, Angeles-Han ST. Therapeutic potential of JAK inhibitors in juvenile idiopathic arthritis-associated uveitis. Expert Rev Clin Immunol. 2023;19(7):689-92.
30. Miserocchi E, Giuffrè C, Cornalba M, Pontikaki I, Cimaz R. JAK inhibitors in refractory juvenile idiopathic arthritis-associated uveitis. Clin Rheumatol. 2020;39(3):847-51.

31. Lowder C. Dexamethasone intravitreal implant for noninfectious intermediate or posterior uveitis. Arch Ophthalmol. 2011;129(5):545.
32. Multicenter Uveitis Steroid Treatment Trial Research Group; Kempen JH, Altaweel MM, Holbrook JT, Jabs DA, Sugar EA. The multicenter uveitis steroid treatment trial: rationale, design, and baseline characteristics. Am J Ophthalmol. 2010;149(4):550-61.
33. Taylor SRJ, Habot-Wilner Z, Pacheco P, Lightman S. Intravitreal methotrexate in uveitis. Ophthalmology. 2012;119(4):878-79.
34. Taylor SRJ, Habot-Wilner Z, Pacheco P, Lightman SL. Intraocular methotrexate in the treatment of uveitis and uveitic cystoid macular edema. Ophthalmology. 2009;116(4):797-801.
35. Naftali Ben Haim L, Moisseiev E. Drug delivery via the suprachoroidal space for the treatment of retinal diseases. Pharmaceutics. 2021;13(7):967.

8 CHAPTER

Polymerase Chain Reaction in Uveitis

Anshukita, L Dhanurekha, A R Anand, Jyotirmay Biswas

ABSTRACT

The invention of polymerase chain reaction (PCR) has opened new horizons in not only the field of molecular biology but also in the field of ophthalmology based on its ability to detect deoxyribonucleic acid (DNA) segments of the pathogenic microorganisms from ocular fluids and paraffin-embedded section of ocular tissues. PCR has greatly aided and improved our ability in establishing a definitive and early diagnosis of infectious uveitis. This chapter deals with the principles of PCR and its application in infectious uveitis.

Keywords: Polymerase chain reaction, uveitis, infectious uveitis, ocular fluids, DNA

INTRODUCTION

Polymerase chain reaction (PCR) is a newer molecular diagnostic tool that is used for amplification of the deoxyribonucleic acid (DNA) segment of interest from a DNA template. This technique was first described in its definitive form by Karry Mullis in 1985. He was awarded the Nobel Prize for the same in chemistry in 1993.

Uveitis is the inflammation of the uvea, the pigmented vascular middle layer of the eye, which comprises the iris, ciliary body, and choroid.[1] Although uveitis can be caused by a number of infectious agents such as viruses, bacteria, parasites, and fungi, the most common among them are herpes simplex virus (HSV), cytomegalovirus (CMV), varicella zoster virus (VZV), *Mycobacterium tuberculosis, Treponema pallidum, Toxoplasma gondii,* and *Toxocara.*

The use of the PCR test as a diagnostic modality in infectious uveitis has been on an incline owing to its high sensitivity and specificity and the ability to identify the suspected causative microorganism from a small amount of intraocular fluid. The development of PCR has also led to the identification of newer organisms as the causative agents of uveitic entities.[2,3]

PRINCIPLE OF POLYMERASE CHAIN REACTION

The principle of PCR is based on the fact that the strands of the extracted DNA get separated at a very high temperature (~95°C) due to the breakage of the hydrogen bonds between the nucleotides of the DNA. An enzyme called DNA polymerase enzyme directs the synthesis of DNA from deoxynucleotide substrates on a single-stranded DNA template and amplifies a billion copies of DNA of interest from extracted DNA, thus generating a large number of specific DNA sequences from a given clinical sample.

The prerequisites of PCR are a DNA template, a heat-stable DNA polymerase enzyme (Taq polymerase), primers, and four deoxyribonucleoside triphosphates (dNTPs) in excess in a buffer solution. This mixture is subjected to several thermal cycles in an apparatus containing tubes of these mixtures.[4,5]

STAGES OF POLYMERASE CHAIN REACTION

There are three stages in PCR:

1. Stage of denaturation
2. Annealing of primers
3. Stage of elongation

Stage of Denaturation

The stage of denaturation is the first step of PCR in which the two strands of DNA are separated by raising the temperature of the mixture between 94 and 96°C (called the denaturation temperature). The hydrogen bonds in the DNA break at a temperature higher than 80°C, and thus the double-stranded DNA helix gets denatured and produces single-stranded DNA **(Fig. 8.1)**.

Annealing of Primers

The next step of PCR is annealing of primers. In this step, the mixture is cooled down at a temperature of 40–70°C. The primers, short- and single-strand sequences complementary to target DNA regions, flank the DNA segment of interest for amplification. There is reformation of the broken hydrogen bonds at this temperature leading to the hybridization of complementary DNA segment.[4,5]

Elongation Stage

The elongation of the double-stranded DNA occurs at a temperature of 70–80°C. This stage requires a heat-stable polymerase enzyme (Taq-polymerase). The Taq polymerase enzyme binds to primed single-stranded DNAs in the mixture and catalyzes the process of replication using the dNTPs. After 20–40 cycles, an analyzable amount of DNA (about 0.1 μg) can be synthesized.

After the last stage, the samples are incubated for some time at 72°C.

Polymerase chain reaction is a very rapid procedure and can be completed in just 2–3 hours.[4]

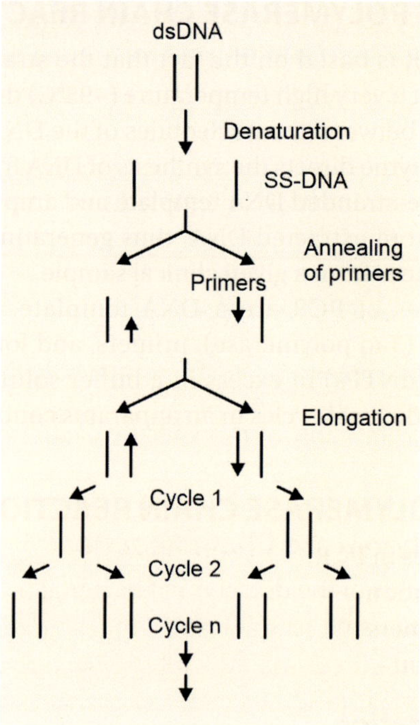

Fig. 8.1: Line diagram of polymerase chain reaction.

DETECTION OF POLYMERASE CHAIN REACTION PRODUCTS

The products of PCR are detected by agarose gel electrophoresis where the ethidium bromide (EtBr) incorporated in agarose gel is used to visualize the bands under ultraviolet transillumination.[4]

TYPES OF POLYMERASE CHAIN REACTIONS

Conventional Polymerase Chain Reaction

Conventional PCR includes the identification of single-target pathogens like *M. tuberculosis*, *T. gondii*, HSV, VZV, and CMV.

It is a time-consuming procedure that requires multiple transfers of reagents, samples, and tubes. Once the PCR products are obtained, gel electrophoresis is carried out for the analysis of the same.

Real-time Polymerase Chain Reaction

Real-time PCR, also known as quantitative PCR, can be used to determine the level of disease burden by determining the pathogen load. By quantifying the amount present, real-time PCR helps to determine if the pathogen is likely a contaminant or active in the disease process.

In real-time PCR, both the amplification and detection occur in a single step, and thus there is no need of processing of the sample after the amplification step. This reduces the time required for the analysis of the sample. The intensity of oligonucleotide probes tagged with fluorescent dye correlates with the amount of the DNA product.[5] When used together, qualitative and quantitative PCR can help to identify and confirm a causative infectious agent.[6]

Nested Polymerase Chain Reaction

Nested PCR is a variant of PCR in which the products of PCR undergo two successive rounds of amplification using two sets of primers. This decreases the chances of amplification of nonspecific segments and increases the sensitivity of PCR.[5]

Broad-range Polymerase Chain Reaction

Broad-range PCR helps in the detection of bacterial or fungal genomic DNA in a given sample by using primers and probes targeting those regions in DNA that are conserved among most of the bacterial and fungal species. This technique can be used to detect the presence of bacteria and fungi in the sample but is unable to identify the strain or species of the organism.[3] 16S ribosomal DNA (bacterial ribosomal DNA gene) or 18S/28S rDNA (fungal ribosomal DNA) genes were being used previously for qualitative broad-range PCR performed with ocular fluid samples of the patients of uveitis and endophthalmitis.[7-9] Nowadays, quantitative measurements of the concerned DNA in the form of copy numbers are made possible by using real-time PCR primers and probes for bacterial 16S rDNA and fungal 18S or 28S rDNA amplification.[3,10-12]

Comprehensive Polymerase Chain Reaction

Comprehensive PCR is a recent development using a combination of multiplex PCR and real-time PCR for diagnosing infectious uveitis.[13] In a few laboratories, multiplex PCR assay is used to screen for infectious genomes of all the human herpes viruses (HHV1-8) and ocular toxoplasma (*T. gondii* B1 gene), and then the quantitative real-time PCR is carried on to measure the copy numbers in the sample positive for the microbes, in order to confirm its pathogenic role.[14,15] If the copy number measured by the real-time PCR assay is high, it is indicative of active replication of the organism in the eye. A negative result in comprehensive PCR can also help to exclude various common infectious etiologies of intraocular inflammation, thus guiding us toward further management of the disease by starting corticosteroids or immunosuppressants as per requirement.[3]

Multiplex Polymerase Chain Reaction

Multiplex PCR is used in simultaneous identification of specific genomic DNA from different pathogens such as viruses, bacteria, fungi, and parasites in a single-closed tube reaction.

In multiplex PCR, multiple primer sets are used in a single PCR mixture to produce amplified products of different sizes specific for different DNA sequences, thus targeting multiple genes in a single run and, hence, reducing the overall time taken and use of reagents.[5]

It can be performed in either conventional (qualitative) mode or real-time (quantitative) mode.

Multiplex Solid Phase Polymerase Chain Reaction Strip Kit

This is a new comprehensive PCR strip kit that consists of a 12-tube multiplex PCR strip coated with probes (6FAM, HEX, and Cy5) and primers that target the genomic DNA of 24 common pathogens responsible for infectious eye diseases, namely HSV1, HSV2, VZV, EBV, CMV, HHV6, HHV7, HHV8, human T-lymphotropic virus/human T-cell leukemia virus type 1 (HTLV-1), adenovirus, *M. tuberculosis, Propionibacterium acnes, T. pallidum, Candida albicans, Candida glabrata, C. krusei*, Fusarium, *Aspergillus*, Toxocara, *T. gondii, Chlamydia trachomatis*, Acanthamoeba, bacterial 16S rDNA, and fungal 28S rDNA, as well as internal controls such as glyceraldehyde 3-phosphate dehydrogenase and TATA-binding protein. Thus, a single easy-to-use assay can be used to detect common ocular infectious agents within a span of few hours, making this kit quite useful.[3]

METAGENOMIC GENE SEQUENCING

Metagenomic gene sequencing (MGS) is a newer molecular technique that helps in a comprehensive analysis of genes of all organisms present in a given clinical sample. This technique is expected to have the potential to improve diagnostic yield as it is bias-free and has the theoretical potential to detect all the pathogens present in a clinical sample.

The advantage of MGS is that we can infer the phenotypic behavior of a pathogen by applying the sequence information from MGS.[16]

POLYMERASE CHAIN REACTION IN INFECTIOUS UVEITIS

Polymerase chain reaction has emerged as a useful tool to diagnose or rule out infectious etiology of uveitis. Although PCR has been proved to be instrumental in establishing diagnosis in all types of infectious uveitis, its maximum utilization can be seen in cases of uveitis involving the posterior segment and panuveitic entities.

Studies have reported quite a high prevalence of infectious uveitis in India (25–31%) which can even result in blindness in severe cases.[17-19] Blindness, as a result of severe infectious uveitis, can be prevented to an extent if we are able to identify the causative pathogen at the earliest followed by appropriate antimicrobial therapy. PCR can be a great tool in this regard as it allows early detection of small quantities of DNA or RNA of the suspected pathogens infecting the uveal tract from the analysis of the ocular fluid sample and is highly sensitive and specific.[13,20,21]

Diagnosis of uveitis is largely clinical, based on the history, clinical presentation, and examination findings **(Fig. 8.2A)**. Establishing a definitive etiology in uveitis is a daunting task, sometimes due to similarities in presenting features of both infectious and noninfectious uveitis or that caused by different pathogens as well. Also, uveitis patients may either lack pathognomonic clinical features or those features can be masked by a miotic pupil or media opacities. Taking these factors into account, making a diagnosis based on clinical presentation and examination alone can

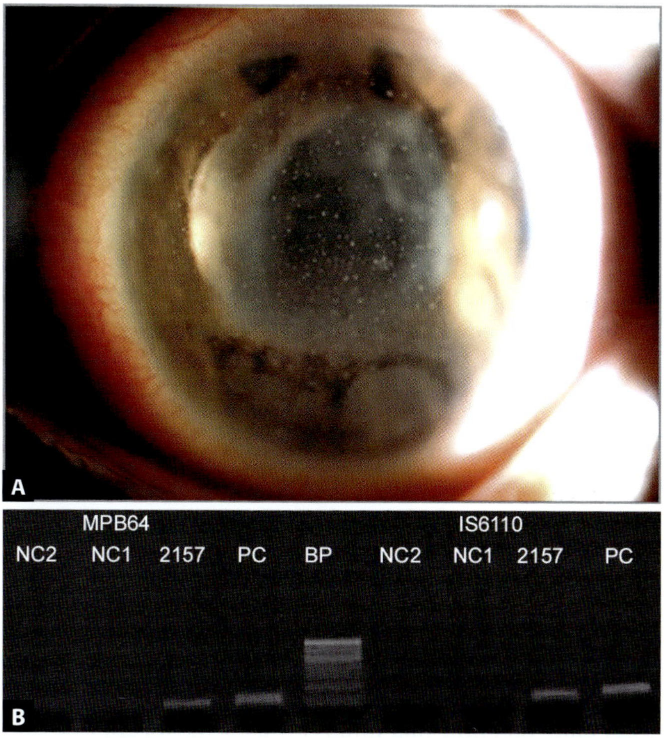

Figs. 8.2A and B: (A) Slit-lamp image showing mutton fat keratic precipitates over the corneal endothelium; (B) Agarose gel electrophotogram showing II round amplified products of PCR targeting *MPB64* and *IS6110* genes of *Mycobacterium tuberculosis* complex genome. [NC 1—Reagent control I round—Negative, NC 2—Negative control II round—Negative, 2157—Aqueous aspirate—positive, PC—Positive control (M. *tuberculosis* H37RV DNA)—positive, BP—Molecular Weight Marker (100 bp Ladder)]. (PCR: polymerase chain reaction)

be difficult sometimes and we can even land up with misdiagnoses and mistreatments of the patients.[22] Owing to the possible severe outcomes of infectious uveitis, establishing an accurate diagnosis and early treatment becomes all the more important.

There are a number of tests that can be used in clinching the diagnosis of uveitis including serology. But serology can itself be misleading sometimes as it requires a certain window period for the serology to become positive and in such cases, we can miss the diagnosis if the patient presents before that particular window period. Incorrect diagnoses could delay the administration of targeted treatment, thereby resulting in visual impairment, the use of drugs with undesirable side effects, and the occurrence of uveitis-related complications.[23]

In such a scenario, PCR can play an important role as it picks up even the tiniest amount of DNA of the suspected organism from the ocular fluids, viz. aqueous and vitreous humors.

Early identification of the causative infectious agent enables us to start adequate antimicrobial therapy early in the disease course which in turn helps in preventing ocular complications as well.

Polymerase chain reaction has proved to be a useful diagnostic tool for infectious uveitis, with high sensitivity and relatively rapid results, as compared to gold standards like culture.[24-27]

SAMPLE COLLECTION IN POLYMERASE CHAIN REACTION

In a patient of uveitis, the most common site of sample collection for performing PCR is aqueous humor from the anterior segment and vitreous humor from the posterior segment of the eye.

Anterior chamber tap: 100–200 μL of aqueous humor is collected by the anterior chamber tap, either in the outpatient department or during intraocular surgery.

In the outpatient department setting, the ocular surface is anesthetized with a topical anesthetic agent (oxybuprocaine hydrochloride) and then sterilized with 0.5% povidone-iodine. Aqueous humor is collected using a 30-gauge needle attached to a tuberculin syringe.

Vitreous tap: Vitreous humor can be collected during vitreous/retinal surgery. For quantitative or semiquantitative PCR, undiluted vitreous is collected with dry vitrectomy before the intraocular irrigation is started.[28]

POLYMERASE CHAIN REACTION IN OCULAR TUBERCULOSIS

India is endemic for tuberculosis and ocular tuberculosis is one of the clinical presentations of extrapulmonary tuberculosis. The diagnosis of ocular tuberculosis is a challenge due to the absence of lung involvement in many cases and the nonfeasibility of conventional methods to detect *M. tuberculosis* in the eye. There has been an increase in the use of PCR in detection of *M. tuberculosis* in the last decade. The sensitivity and specificity of PCR in detection of ocular tuberculosis are 88% and 71%, respectively.[29] Nested PCR can be used to detect the *M. tuberculosis* genomes MPB64 and IS6110 **(Fig. 8.2B)**. Using both the genomes for detection of *M. tuberculosis* has shown to increase the sensitivity and specificity of PCR to even up to 95–100% in some cases.[30,31] Real-time or quantitative PCR can be used to detect the copy numbers of tubercular bacteria to know the actual disease burden.

POLYMERASE CHAIN REACTION IN ACUTE RETINAL NECROSIS

Acute retinal necrosis (ARN) is an inflammatory vision-threatening disease that is characterized by necrotizing retinitis of peripheral retina **(Fig. 8.3A)** and is usually caused by direct infection of the viruses of Herpesviridae family including VZV, HSV, CMV, or rarely Epstein–Barr virus (most common being VZV).[32]

A rapid diagnosis and early commencement of treatment play a key role in the management of ARN. Anterior chamber paracentesis or vitreous tap for PCR for detection of VZV, HSV, and CMV viruses should be performed in all such cases **(Figs. 8.3B and C)**. However, we should not wait for the PCR results and empirical treatment should be started without any delay in all ARN cases.[33,34]

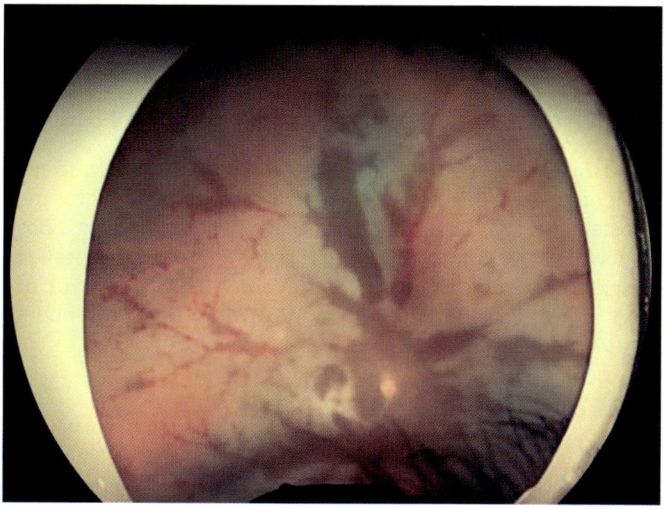

Fig. 8.3A

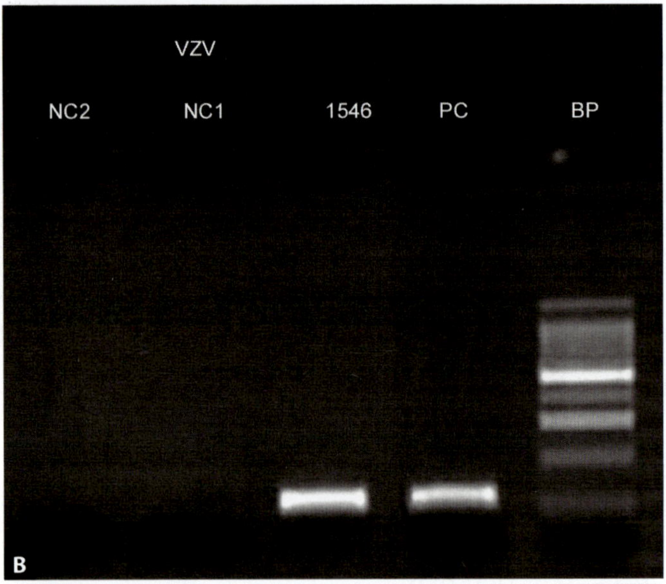

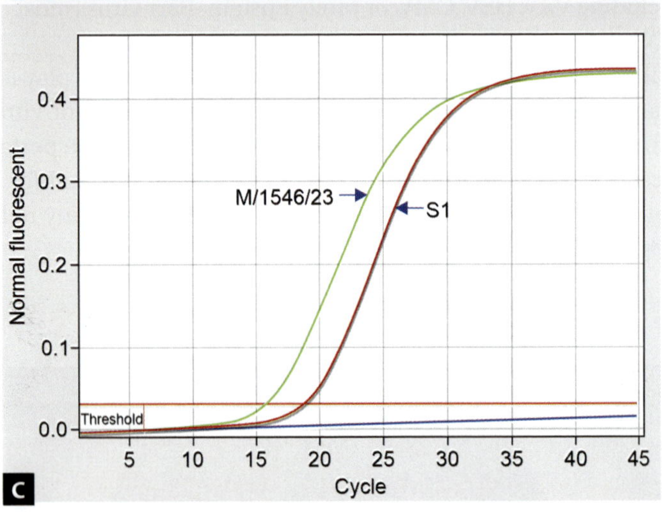

Figs. 8.3A to C: (A) Right-eye OPTOS image showing mild disk pallor, sclerosed vessels with 360° peripheral retinal necrosis with active vasculitis; (B) PCR for the detection of varicella-zoster virus (VZV) DNA targeting *ORF-63* region showing a positive result [blue arrow shows positive control (PC)]; and (C) Real-time PCR for varicella-zoster virus DNA performed on aqueous aspirate. S1: Standard—10,000 copies/μL of VZV DNA. M/1546/23: AH sample 85,400.1 copies/μL of VZV DNA. (DNA: deoxyribonucleic acid; PCR: polymerase chain reaction)

POLYMERASE CHAIN REACTION IN VIRAL ANTERIOR UVEITIS

Viral anterior uveitis is most commonly caused by VZV, HSV **(Fig. 8.4)**, CMV, and rubella virus. A study conducted in South India on isolated viral anterior

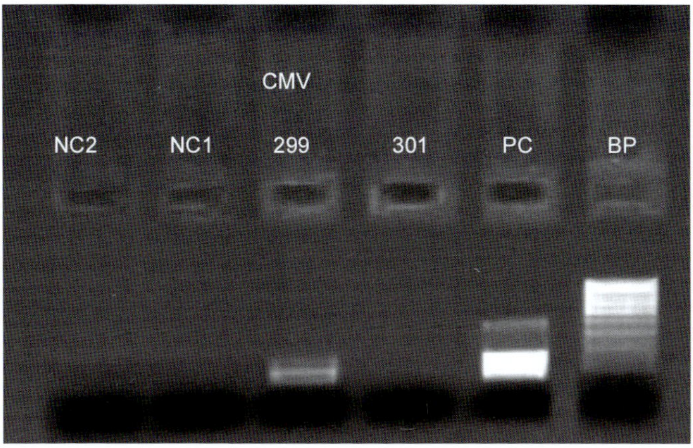

Fig. 8.4: A 59-year-old man had chronic uveitis with pigmented KPs. IOP 40 mm Hg. AC tap done. Real-time PCR for HSV-1 positive. (CMV: cytomegalovirus; HCV-1: hepatitis C virus; HSV: herpes simplex virus; IOP: intraocular pressure; KPs: keratic precipitates; PCR: polymerase chain reaction)

uveitis revealed that most of the cases of viral anterior uveitis (two-thirds) were positive for VZV, 19.4% were positive for HSV-1, and 8.3% were positive for CMV on PCR of anterior chamber aspirate.[35]

POLYMERASE CHAIN REACTION IN OCULAR TOXOPLASMOSIS

Diagnosis of ocular toxoplasmosis is mainly based on clinical features. PCR for detecting *T. gondii* can be performed as an adjunctive investigation for confirming the clinical diagnosis. However, PCR for ocular toxoplasmosis is usually less sensitive as compared to other uveitic entities like viral retinitis.[17]

POLYMERASE CHAIN REACTION IN ENDOPHTHALMITIS

Polymerase chain reaction can prove to be instrumental in identification of pathogens in cases of suspected endophthalmitis. Broad-range PCR test using 16S and 18S RNA for detection of bacterial and fungal genomic DNA has been used in cases of endophthalmitis.[8,17]

LIMITATIONS OF POLYMERASE CHAIN REACTION

- False positivity
- False negativity
- Requirement for technical expertise

False Positives and False Negatives in Polymerase Chain Reaction

Polymerase chain reaction usually has very low false-positive rates when performed on ocular fluids. Contamination of the sample can result in false-positive results. Few practical measures can be followed to prevent contamination like UV light application to the working chamber and cabinets, devising flow line in the inspection room, adequate sterilization with frequent change of gloves by the technicians, and proper training of the staff involved in the process.[28]

On the contrary, failure to collect samples in acute stages of disease, specimen degradation, and polymorphism can be various reasons behind false-negative results in PCR.[36]

An effective way to reduce false-positive and false-negative burdens is the use of positive and negative controls in the laboratory.[17]

CONCLUSION

Polymerase chain reaction has emerged as a newer and effective molecular diagnostic tool in uveitis, especially in case of uveitis where early and precise diagnosis followed by adequate treatment is the key to management. It has given us an edge over the conventional methods like culture and sensitivity and sometimes immunological assays as well, owing to its sensitivity, specificity, and rapidity in detecting pathogenic microorganisms associated with uveitis. Newer molecular techniques such as PCR followed by sequencing have revealed the involvement of such pathogens in unexplained uveitic entities which were earlier not thought to be involved in ocular inflammation. In spite of a few drawbacks involving false-positive and false-negative results, PCR still holds an important role as an adjunct test for a case of suspected infectious uveitis.

ACKNOWLEDGMENT

The authors would like to thank Molecular Diagnostic Laboratory, Medical Research Foundation, Chennai, Tamil Nadu.

REFERENCES

1. Bispo PJM, Davoudi S, Sahm ML, Ren A, Miller J, Romano J, et al. Rapid detection and identification of uveitis pathogens by qualitative multiplex real-time PCR. Invest Ophthalmol Vis Sci. 2018;59(1):582-9.
2. Mochizuki M, Watanabe T, Yamaguchi K, Yoshimura K, Nakashima S, Shirao M, et al. Uveitis associated with human T-cell lymphotropic virus type I. Am J Ophthalmol. 1992;114(2):123-9.
3. Mochizuki M, Sugita S, Kamoi K, Takase H. A new era of uveitis: impact of polymerase chain reaction in intraocular inflammatory diseases. Jpn J Ophthalmol. 2017;61(1):1-20.
4. Kadri K. 'Polymerase chain reaction (PCR): principle and applications.' Synthetic biology—new interdisciplinary science, Intech Open, 12 Feb. 2020. [online] Available from: https://www.intechopen.com/chapters/67558 [Last accessed September, 2024].

5. Singh J, Niti B, Sinha S, Goswami A. A critical review on PCR, its types and applications. Int J Adv Res Biol Sci. 2014:1(7):65-80.
6. Fallon J, Narayan S, Lin J, Sassoon J, Llop S. The impact of polymerase chain reaction (PCR) on diagnosis and management of infectious uveitis at a tertiary care facility. J Ophthalmic Inflamm Infect. 2022;12(1):1.
7. Knox CM, Cevallos V, Margolis TP, Dean D. Identification of bacterial pathogens in patients with endophthalmitis by 16S ribosomal DNA typing. Am J Ophthalmol. 1999;128(4):511-2.
8. Jaeger EE, Carroll NM, Choudhury S, Dunlop AA, Towler HM, Matheson MM, et al. Rapid detection and identification of Candida, Aspergillus, and Fusarium species in ocular samples using nested PCR. J Clin Microbiol. 2000;38(8):2902-8.
9. Okhravi N, Adamson P, Carroll N, Dunlop A, Matheson MM, Towler HM, et al. PCR-based evidence of bacterial involvement in eyes with suspected intraocular infection. Invest Ophthalmol Vis Sci. 2000;41(11):3474-79.
10. Chiquet C, Cornut PL, Benito Y, Thuret G, Maurin M, Lafontaine PO, et al. Eubacterial PCR for bacterial detection and identification in 100 acute postcataract surgery endophthalmitis. Invest Ophthalmol Vis Sci. 2008;49(5):1971-8.
11. Ogawa M, Sugita S, Shimizu N, Watanabe K, Nakagawa I, Mochizuki M. Broad-range real-time PCR assay for detection of bacterial DNA in ocular samples from infectious endophthalmitis. Jpn J Ophthalmol. 2012;56(5):529-35.
12. Sugita S, Kamoi K, Ogawa M, Watanabe K, Shimizu N, Mochizuki M. Detection of Candida and Aspergillus species DNA using broad-range real-time PCR for fungal endophthalmitis. Graefes Arch Clin Exp Ophthalmol. 2012;250(3):391-8.
13. Sugita S, Ogawa M, Shimizu N, Morio T, Ohguro N, Nakai K, et al. Use of a comprehensive polymerase chain reaction system for diagnosis of ocular infectious diseases. Ophthalmology. 2013;120(9):1761-8.
14. Sugita S, Shimizu N, Watanabe K, Mizukami M, Morio T, Sugamoto Y, et al. Use of multiplex PCR and real-time PCR to detect human herpes virus genome in ocular fluids of patients with uveitis. Br J Ophthalmol. 2008;92(7):928-32.
15. Sugita S, Ogawa M, Inoue S, Shimizu N, Mochizuki M. Diagnosis of ocular toxoplasmosis by two polymerase chain reaction (PCR) examinations: qualitative multiplex and quantitative real-time. Jpn J Ophthalmol. 2011;55(5):495-501.
16. Anand AR, Biswas J. Molecular diagnosis of infectious uveitis: an update. Sci J Med Vis Res Foun. 2019;37(1):7-11.
17. Kharel Sitaula R, Janani MK, Madhavan HN, Biswas J. Outcome of polymerase chain reaction (PCR) analysis in 100 suspected cases of infectious uveitis. J Ophthalmic Inflamm Infect. 2018;8(1):2.
18. Sabhapandit S, Murthy SI, Singh VM, Gaitonde K, Gopal M, Marsonia K, et al. Epidemiology and clinical features of uveitis from urban populations in South India. Ocul Immunol Inflamm. 2017;25(1):S39-45.
19. Borde P, Priyanka, Kumar K, Takkar B, Sharma B. Pattern of uveitis in a tertiary eye care center of Central India: results of a prospective patient database over a period of two years. Indian J Ophthalmol. 2020;68(3):476-81.
20. Verhagen C, Bruinenberg M, Rothova A, Baarsma G, Der LA, Ooyman F, et al. Serologic and polymerase chain reaction analysis of intraocular fluids in the diagnosis of infectious uveitis. Am J Ophthalmol.1996;121(6):650-8.
21. Harper TW, Miller D, Schiffman JC, Davis JL. Polymerase chain reaction analysis of aqueous and vitreous specimens in the diagnosis of posterior segment infectious uveitis. Am J Ophthalmol. 2009;147(1):140-7.

22. Fox GM, Crouse CA, Chuang EL, Pflugfelder SC, Cleary TJ, Nelson SJ, et al. Detection of herpesvirus DNA in vitreous and aqueous specimens by the polymerase chain reaction. Arch Ophthalmol. 1991;109(2):266-71.
23. Tran TH, Rozenberg F, Cassoux N, Rao NA, LeHoang P, Bodaghi B. Polymerase chain reaction analysis of aqueous humour samples in necrotising retinitis. Br J Ophthalmol. 2003;87(1):79-83.
24. Sandhu HS, Hajrasouliha A, Kaplan HJ, Wang W. Diagnostic utility of quantitative polymerase chain reaction versus culture in endophthalmitis and uveitis. Ocul Immunol Inflamm. 2019;27(4):578-82.
25. Mahalakshmi B, Therese KL, Madhavan HN, Biswas J. Diagnostic value of specific local antibody production and nucleic acid amplification technique-nested polymerase chain reaction (NPCR) in clinically suspected ocular toxoplasmosis. Ocul Immunol Inflamm. 2006;14(2):105-12.
26. Sowmya P, Madhavan HN. Diagnostic utility of polymerase chain reaction on intraocular specimens to establish the etiology of infectious endophthalmitis. Eur J Ophthalmol. 2009;19(5):812-7.
27. Arora SK, Gupta V, Gupta A, Bambery P, Kapoor GS, Sehgal S. Diagnostic efficacy of polymerase chain reaction in granulomatous uveitis. Tuber Lung Dis. 1999;79(4):229-33.
28. Sugita S, Takase H, Nakano S. Role of recent PCR tests for infectious ocular diseases: from laboratory-based studies to the clinic. Int J Mol Sci. 2023;24(9):8146.
29. La Distia Nora R, Putera I, Khalisha DF, Septiana I, Sitompul R. The diagnostic value of polymerase chain reaction for ocular tuberculosis diagnosis in relation to antitubercular therapy response: a meta-analysis. Int J Infect Dis. 2021;110:394-402.
30. Drews SJ, Eshaghi AR, Pyskir D, Chedore P, Lombos E, Broukhanski G, et al. The relative test performance characteristics of two commercial assays for the detection of Mycobacterium tuberculosis complex in paraffin-fixed human biopsy specimens. Diagn Pathol. 2008;3:37.
31. Sridhar N. Diagnostic appraisal of simultaneous application of two nested PCRs targeting MPB64 gene and IS6110 region for rapid detection of *M. Tuberculosis* genome in culture proven clinical specimens. Indian J Med Microbiol. 2013;31(4):366-9.
32. Holland GN. Standard diagnostic criteria for the acute retinal necrosis syndrome. Executive Committee of the American Uveitis Society. Am J Ophthalmol. 1994;117(5):663-7.
33. Schoenberger SD, Kim SJ, Thorne JE, Mruthyunjaya P, Yeh S, Bakri SJ, et al. Diagnosis and treatment of acute retinal necrosis. Am J Ophthalmol. 2017;124(3):382-92.
34. Biswas J, Mayr AJ, Martin WJ, Rao NA. Detection of human cytomegalovirus in ocular tissue by polymerase chain reaction and in situ DNA hybridization. Graefes Arch Clin Exp Ophthalmol. 1993;231(2):66-70.
35. Babu K. Clinical profile of isolated viral anterior uveitis in a South Indian patient population. Ocular Immunol Inflamm. 2014;22(5):356-9.
36. Van Gelder RN. CME review: polymerase chain reaction diagnostics for posterior segment disease. Retina. 2003;23(4):445-52.

9 CHAPTER

Management of Hard Cataracts

Raksheeth Nathan Rajagopal, Ramamurthy Dandapani

ABSTRACT

Hard cataracts represent a common surgical challenge for beginner and experienced cataract surgeons. Despite advancements in modern phacoemulsification machines, outcomes in these cases hinge heavily on surgeon skill. Nucleofractis, or nucleus disassembly, is the most technically demanding step and has consequently witnessed the most innovations. Several nucleus chopping and cracking techniques with or without the assistance of specialized instruments have emerged over time. Femtosecond laser-assisted cataract surgery offers greater precision in capsulorhexis creation and can debulk hard nuclei and facilitate easier phacoemulsification. Manual small-incision cataract surgery retains its place in the surgical armamentarium for hard cataracts—especially in an eye with a shallow anterior chamber or corneal endothelial pathology. Ultimately, the surgery and technique are at the operating surgeon's discretion. Further technical and technological advances will aim to make hard cataract management as safe and as predictable as "routine" cataract surgery.

Keywords: Hard cataract, dense cataract, brown cataract, brunescent cataract, black cataract, cataracta nigra, Catarock, total cataract, phacoemulsification, manual small-incision cataract surgery, SICS

INTRODUCTION

The hard cataract, sometimes (infamously) called the "Catarock," is a rather common surgical challenge encountered by cataract surgeons, especially in this part of the world. Although phacoemulsification (phaco) is currently the standard of care, a higher incidence of postoperative complications while operating dense/brunescent cataracts is established.[1-3] While modern phacoemulsification machines are equipped to emulsify even the densest of nuclei, the outcome and incidence of postoperative complications in these cases strongly depend on the competence of the operating surgeon. It is recognized that nucleus disassembly is the step that requires the most skill to perform. Most innovations have thus focused on simplifying this pivotal step. Relatively simple technical modifications in trenching and chopping, the use of specialized instruments (e.g., mi-LOOP), and the emergence of femtosecond laser-assisted cataract surgery (FLACS) have facilitated easier and quicker nucleofractis, thus simplifying the remainder of the surgery.

This chapter will discuss the following concerning hard cataract management:

- A few relevant preoperative and intraoperative considerations
- The different surgical techniques of nucleofractis
- The advantages and disadvantages of FLACS
- The current role of manual small-incision cataract surgery (mSICS).

PREOPERATIVE CONSIDERATIONS

Visual Acuity

Vision can remain excellent even in brunescent cataracts, with the patient retaining 6/6 or 6/9 vision (albeit with poorer contrast sensitivity).[4] Convincing the patient to undergo cataract surgery while at the same time emphasizing the difficult nature of the procedure is challenging.

Slit-lamp Examination

Cornea: The prevalence of peripheral and central corneal degeneration and arcus senilis (and its density) increases with age, contributing to suboptimal intraoperative visualization.[5] Lower corneal endothelial cell density (ECD) is seen with increasing age,[6] and further loss is anticipated with higher intraoperative phaco energy.

Anterior chamber (AC) depth: Shallow AC depth is an established risk factor for higher intraoperative ECD loss.[7,8] It has been suggested that mSICS may be preferable to phacoemulsification for eyes with hard cataracts and an AC depth of ≤2.86 mm.[9] Besides short axial length, a brunescent cataract can itself significantly contribute to lower AC depth.

Pupil: A small pupil is possibly the most commonly encountered surgical challenge and is a known risk factor for intraoperative complications.[10,11] It is recognized that pupil size decreases with increasing age,[12-14] which, in turn, is associated with harder cataracts and other surgical risk factors such as intraoperative floppy iris syndrome (IFIS). **Figure 9.1** depicts a dense brown cataract in an eye with a small pupil.

Anterior lens capsule: Areas of anterior capsular fibrosis should be documented to plan an appropriate capsulorhexis.[15] **Figure 9.2** shows a hypermature brown cataract with central anterior capsular fibrosis.

Cataract and zonules: The presence of phacodonesis is ideally assessed in the undilated state.[16] Whereas all brown or black cataracts have an inherent

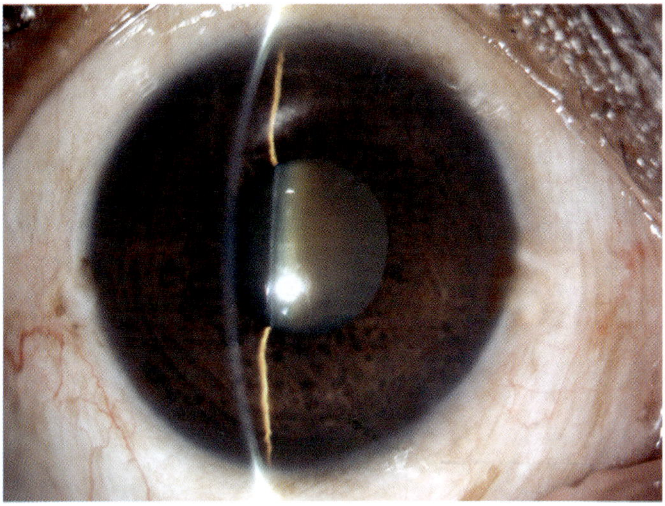

Fig. 9.1: Hard brunescent cataract in an eye with a suboptimally dilated pupil.

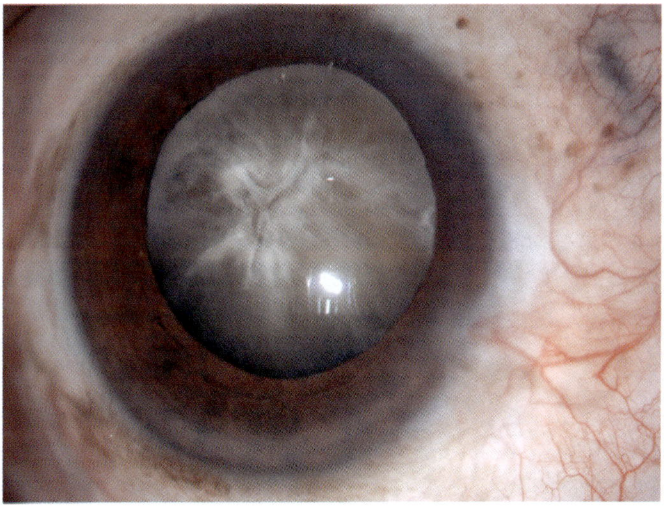

Fig. 9.2: Hypermature brunescent cataract. Note the stellate central area of anterior capsular fibrosis.

hardness, white cataracts may range from hard white (intumescent cortex with a brunescent core; **Figs. 9.3A and B**) to soft/brittle white (bluish-white).[17]

Biometry

The challenges posed by dense cataracts are not restricted to the operating room but begin during preoperative planning. Optical biometry, the current gold standard for intraocular lens (IOL) power calculation, has significant limitations in eyes with dense cataracts.[18] Axial length acquisition failure

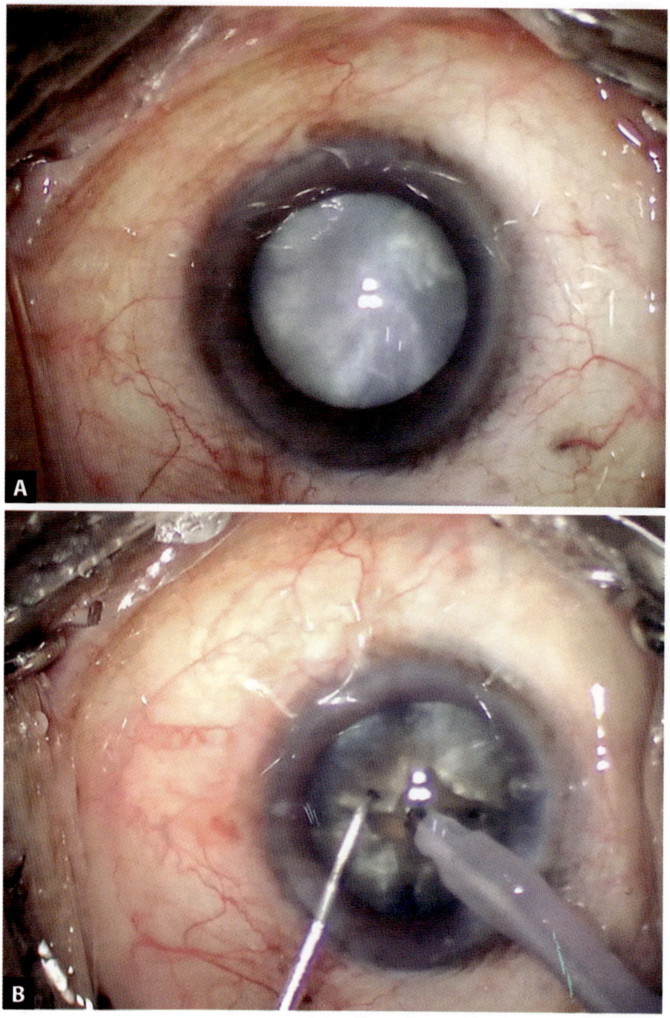

Figs. 9.3A and B: Intumescent white cataract (A), the underlying hard brown nucleus (B) was revealed after the evacuation of the soft white overlying cortex.

rates of up to 30% have been reported in eyes with dense cataracts. Swept source-optical coherence tomography (SS-OCT)-based devices have a clear advantage over partial coherence interferometry-based devices in these eyes.[18,19] In this regard, ultrasound immersion biometry retains a role in everyday surgical practice.

INTRAOPERATIVE CONSIDERATIONS

Incision: An appropriately sized incision (2.8 or 2.4 mm clear corneal incision) with good morphology and adequate tunnel length is recommended. The phaco tip and sleeve must fit snugly into the incision, with minimal fluid

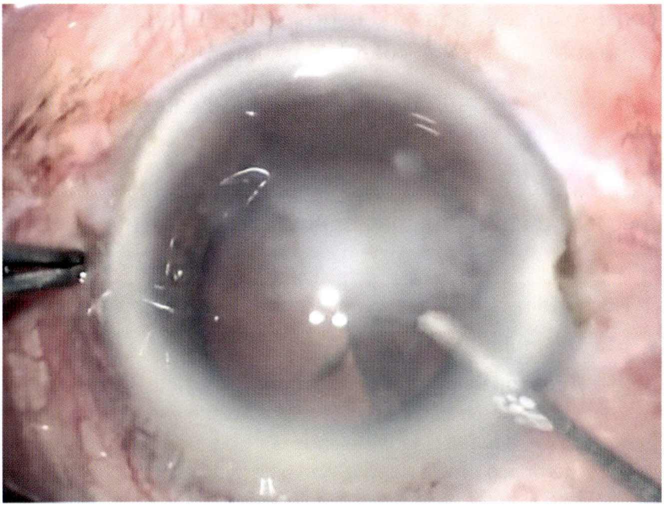

Fig. 9.4: Anterior capsular flap is easily visualized by trypan blue staining, which simplifies CCC creation and visualization, in an eye with dense cataract and significant corneal scarring. (CCC: curvilinear capsulorhexis)

egress, while at the same time avoiding crimping of the sleeve and stretching of the wound, which will predispose to a wound burn, especially in these cases where high phaco energy utilization is anticipated.

Capsulorhexis: It is very useful to stain the anterior lens capsule with trypan blue dye irrespective of the red glow, as this greatly facilitates easier surgery **(Fig. 9.4)**. A continuous curvilinear capsulorhexis (CCC) size of about 5–5.5 mm diameter is recommended in most techniques. A CCC size smaller than 5 mm risks traumatizing the zonules during cracking and chopping maneuvers. A CCC larger than 6 mm may allow free nucleus pieces from within the bag to prolapse into the AC due to fluidics-induced turbulence, risking trauma to the corneal endothelium. Moreover, a well-centered 5–5.5 mm CCC ensures the optical performance of an in-the-bag IOL and reduces the incidence of posterior capsular opacification.[20,21] In the event of a posterior capsular rupture, it allows for a sulcus-placed three-piece IOL to be captured into the anterior capsular rim, allowing for long-term centration and stability.

Hydrodissection: It must be very guarded, as there is minimal potential space between the dense nucleus and capsular bag, with a consequent risk of a sudden rise in intralenticular pressure and posterior capsule blowout. Multiple quadrant hydrodissection or cortical cleaving viscodissection may be required in cataracts with strong corticocapsular adhesions.[15,22]

Nuclear rotation: It must be performed gently, anticipating zonular weakness with hard cataracts. It should, however, be adequate to break any corticocapsular adhesions to ensure a free-floating nucleus, which will greatly aid the subsequent steps of nucleofractis.

Nuclear disassembly: Techniques specific to hard cataracts are summarized in **Table 9.1**.

Phacoemulsification: It becomes easy once proper nucleofractis has been achieved because quadrant management is relatively simple. Hard cataract

TABLE 9.1: Nuclear disassembly techniques for hard cataracts.[15]

Technique	*Description*
Vertical chop	After impaling the phaco tip into the nucleus, the chopper tip is embedded adjacent to the probe. As the vacuum in the phaco probe is maintained, the chopper tip is depressed (keeping the phaco probe steady), and a partial crack is achieved with lateral separation. This maneuver may be repeated multiple times at progressively deeper planes, to realize complete cracking (multilevel chopping).[23] A sharp chopper is required. All instrumentation is performed within the confines of the CCC. Weak zonules may sometimes not withstand the anteroposterior force
Horizontal chop	The phaco tip is impaled into the nucleus in the midperiphery and high vacuum (>500 mm Hg) is maintained, while the chopper tip traverses between the equator and the phaco probe. A sharp or blunt/olive-tipped chopper may be used. The chopper tip must be introduced underneath the distal CCC to reach the equator. The centripetal force generated does not produce zonular stress
Tilt and crack	The primary aim of this technique and its modifications is to facilitate a complete separation of the tenacious posterior plate during the initial chop. This is achieved by prolapsing the distal part of the nucleus outside the capsular bag, providing direct access to the posterior plate while performing a horizontal chop. A large rhexis (≥6 mm) is crucial to avoid zonular damage, which is nevertheless more likely with this technique
Decrease and conquer	The aim is to isolate the epinucleus from the endonucleus and manage each separately. Initially, epinucleus splitting maneuvers are performed, to access the deeper and smaller endonucleus. This technique may not be possible in dense black or brown nuclei where there is no distinction between the epinucleus and endonucleus
Crater and chop/split	The bulk of the hard endonucleus is removed by initial sculpting, to form a central crater. Peripheral chopping can then be performed to obtain wedges of nuclei that can be emulsified in the space created by the crater[24,25]
Drill and crack/chop	The phaco tip is impaled deep into the substance of the nucleus to create a long, thin borehole. Subsequent chopping maneuvers allow the splitting of the endonucleus along with the leathery posterior plate. A prechopper can also be used within the borehole to split the nucleus in the drill and crack technique[26]

emulsification generally requires modifications in all parameters—aspiration flow rate, vacuum, and phaco power. Attention must be paid to phaco fluidics, preventing wound burn and mitigation of postocclusion surge. Phaco power modulations and dynamic parameter adjustments make the surgery safer, more controlled, minimally traumatic, and more efficient. Specific recommendations can be found in this comprehensive review article titled "Phacoemulsification of the rock-hard dense nuclear cataract: Options and Recommendations" from the ASCRS Cataract Clinical Committee.[15]

mi-LOOP

This lens fragmentation device was touted as a game-changer during its introduction and approval by the Food and Drug Administration (FDA) in 2018. It is a pen-like device with a flexible lasso-like Nitinol filament loop of 1.5 mm radius at one end, which can be introduced through a 2.2-mm clear corneal incision and expand up to a 10.5 mm radius. Although trials reported excellent efficacy in achieving complete nucleofractis in dense cataracts and reduced phaco time, these did not translate into superior postoperative day 1 visual acuity or better ECD at 1 month.[27,28] With current phaco machines being equipped to handle nuclei of almost any hardness, the current position of mi-LOOP in the surgeon's toolbox remains under appraisal.

FEMTOSECOND LASER-ASSISTED CATARACT SURGERY

In eyes with hard cataracts with shallow ACs, FLACS (vs. conventional phacoemulsification) in one study was superior with regard to corneal clarity, uncorrected visual acuity, and AC inflammation in the early postoperative period.[29] Other studies comparing FLACS and conventional phacoemulsification did not find meaningful differences between the two groups.[30,31] The superiority of FLACS concerning visual outcomes and endothelial cell loss remains unestablished at the current time. However, the advantages of a precise capsulorhexis and the facilitation of easier nucleus disassembly are more tangible to the operating surgeon. A higher cost, a larger operating room footprint, and an inability to be used in eyes with small pupils and corneal opacities are pertinent disadvantages. **Figures 9.5A and B** depict the FLACS suite view of CCC creation and nucleus fragmentation, and the intraoperative view, respectively.

CURRENT ROLE OF MANUAL SMALL-INCISION CATARACT SURGERY

With the currently available technology, phacoemulsification *can* be performed in any grade of cataract, but certain situations beg the question, "*Should* phacoemulsification be performed in this case?"

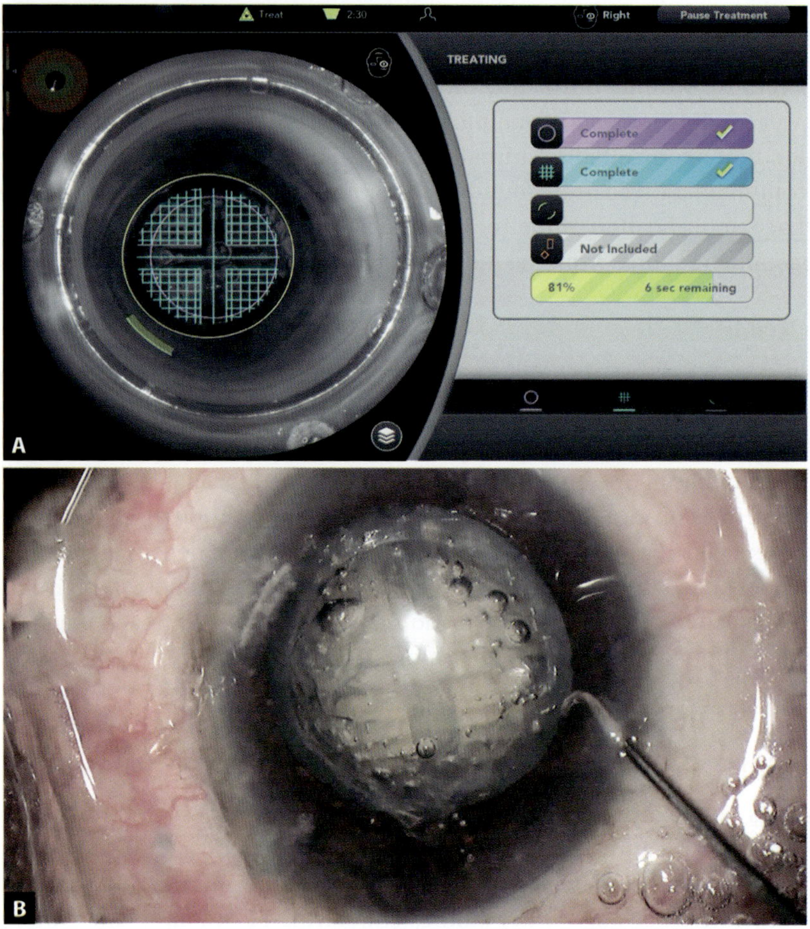

Figs. 9.5A and B: (A) The laser cataract surgery view of femtosecond laser delivery for CCC creation, phacofragmentation, and arcuate incision creation; (B) Intraoperative view of the same case of dense cataract after completion of femtosecond laser delivery. (CCC: curvilinear capsulorhexis)

In these situations, it may be best to step away from the mindset of a "refractive" cataract surgeon and facilitate the fastest, safest, and most minimally traumatic technique. Indeed, this can, on some occasions, be mSICS. For hard cataract eyes with other ocular comorbidities (e.g., small pupil, pseudoexfoliation, diffuse zonular weakness), in resource-poor settings, and for a phaco surgeon in their learning curve, mSICS may be a superior option.[4,32-34]

CONCLUSION

Advances in technology and technique have paved the way for phacoemulsification to emerge as the procedure of choice for even the hardest cataracts while acknowledging that the surgeon's skill has a central role. The importance of careful preoperative examination, planning, and challenges in biometry in these cannot be overemphasized. Relatively recent advances such as the mi-LOOP and FLACS may facilitate easier surgery but require further study to assess if they will improve outcomes. mSICS retains its place in the modern cataract surgeon's armamentarium for specific circumstances. Predictability, precision, and reduced reliance on individual skills should be the goals of future advances.

REFERENCES

1. Dada T, Sharma N, Vajpayee RB, Dada VK. Conversion from phacoemulsification to extracapsular cataract extraction: incidence, risk factors, and visual outcome. J Cataract Refract Surg. 1998;24(11):1521-4.
2. Bourne RRA, Minassian DC, Dart JKG, Rosen P, Kaushal S, Wingate N. Effect of cataract surgery on the corneal endothelium: modern phacoemulsification compared with extracapsular cataract surgery. Ophthalmology. 2004;111(4): 679-85.
3. Muhtaseb M, Kalhoro A, Ionides A. A system for preoperative stratification of cataract patients according to risk of intraoperative complications: a prospective analysis of 1441 cases. Br J Ophthalmol. 2004;88(10):1242-6.
4. Anitha V, Madkaikar A, Ravindran M, Siddique MU. Preferred practice of cataract surgery in brown cataract: a questionnaire-based survey among Indian ophthalmic surgeons. Indian J Ophthalmol. 2022;70(11):3893-7.
5. Ansons AM, Atkinson PL. Corneal mosaic patterns–morphology and epidemiology. Eye (Lond). 1989;3(6):811-5.
6. McCarey BE, Edelhauser HF, Lynn MJ. Review of corneal endothelial specular microscopy for FDA clinical trials of refractive procedures, surgical devices and new intraocular drugs and solutions. Cornea. 2008;27(1):1-16.
7. Storr-Paulsen A, Norregaard JC, Ahmed S, Storr-Paulsen T, Pedersen TH. Endothelial cell damage after cataract surgery: divide-and-conquer versus phaco-chop technique. J Cataract Refract Surg. 2008;34(6):996-1000.
8. Walkow T, Anders N, Klebe S. Endothelial cell loss after phacoemulsification: relation to preoperative and intraoperative parameters. J Cataract Refract Surg. 2000;26(5):727-32.
9. Singh R, Sharma AK, Katiyar V, Kumar G, Gupta SK. Corneal endothelial changes following cataract surgery in hard nuclear cataract: randomized trial comparing phacoemulsification to manual small-incision cataract surgery. Indian J Ophthalmol. 2022;70(11):3904-09.
10. Goverdhan S, Anderson L, Lockwood A, Kirwan J. Risk stratification for posterior capsule rupture and vitreous loss during cataract surgery. Eye. 2010;24(2):389-90.
11. Zare M, Javadi MA, Einollahi B, Baradaran-Rafii AR, Feizi S, Kiavash V. Risk factors for posterior capsule rupture and vitreous loss during phacoemulsification. J Ophthalmic Vis Res. 2009;4(4):208-12.
12. Birren JE, Casperson RC, Botwinick J. Age changes in pupil size. J Gerontol. 1950;5(3):216-21.
13. Guillon M, Dumbleton K, Theodoratos P, Gobbe M, Wooley CB, Moody K. The effects of age, refractive status, and luminance on pupil size. Optom Vis Sci. 2016;93(9):1093-100.

14. Linke SJ, Baviera J, Munzer G, Fricke OH, Richard G, Katz T. Mesopic pupil size in a refractive surgery population (13,959 eyes). Optom Vis Sci. 2012;89(8):1156-64.
15. Foster GJL, Allen QB, Ayres BD, Devgan U, Hoffman RS, Khandelwal SS, et al. Phacoemulsification of the rock-hard dense nuclear cataract: options and recommendations. J Cataract Refract Surg. 2018;44(7):905-16.
16. Recchia FM, Sternberg P. Surgery for ocular trauma: principles and techniques of treatment. Ryan SJ, Sadda SR, Hinton DR, Schachat AP, Sadda SR, Wilkinson CP, et al. (Eds). Retina, 5th edition. London: W.B. Saunders; 2013. pp. 1852-75. [online] Available from: https://www.sciencedirect.com/science/article/pii/B9781455707379001107. [Last accessed September, 2024]
17. Devgan U. White cataracts: they are not all the same! [Internet]. Cataract CoachTM. [Updated March, 2018] Available from https://cataractcoach.com/2018/05/28/not-all-white-cataracts-are-the-same/ [Last accessed September, 2024].
18. González-Godínez S, Saucedo-Urdapilleta R, Mayorquín-Ruiz M, Velasco-Barona C, Moragrega-Adame E, Domínguez-Varela IA, et al. Ocular biometry in dense cataracts: comparison of partial-coherence interferometry, swept-source optical coherence tomography and immersion ultrasound. Indian J Ophthalmol. 2022;70(1):107-11.
19. Tañá-Rivero P, Aguilar-Córcoles S, Tañá-Sanz P, Tañá-Sanz S, Montés-Micó R. Axial length acquisition success rates and agreement of four optical biometers and one ultrasound biometer in eyes with dense cataracts. Eye and Vision. 2023;10(1):35.
20. Ravalico G, Tognetto D, Palomba M, Busatto P, Baccara F. Capsulorhexis size and posterior capsule opacification. J Cataract Refract Surg. 1996;22(1):98-103.
21. Hollick EJ, Spalton DJ, Meacock WR. The effect of capsulorhexis size on posterior capsular opacification: one-year results of a randomized prospective trial. Am J Ophthalmol. 1999;128(3):271-9.
22. Vasavada AR, Raj SM, Praveen MR, Vasavada VA, Vasavada VA. The probable associations for corticocapsular adhesions in patients undergoing cataract surgery: a clinic-based observational study. Indian J Ophthalmol. 2008;56(2):103-8.
23. Vasavada AR, Raj SM. Multilevel chop technique. J Cataract Refract Surg. 2011;37(12):2092-94.
24. Vanathi M, Vajpayee RB, Tandon R, Titiyal JS, Gupta V. Crater-and-chop technique for phacoemulsification of hard cataracts. J Cataract Refract Surg. 2001;27(5):659-61.
25. Aslan BS, Müftüoglu O, Gayretli D. Crater-and-split technique for phacoemulsification: modification of the crater-and-chop technique. J Cataract Refract Surg. 2012;38(9):1526-30.
26. Hwang HS, Kim EC, Kim MS. Drill-and-crack technique for nuclear disassembly of hard nucleus. J Cataract Refract Surg. 2010;36(10):1627-30.
27. Hu EH, Buie T, Jensen RJ, Wu D, Pamnani RD. Comparative study of safety outcomes following nucleus disassembly with and without the miLOOP lens fragmentation device during cataract surgery. Clin Ophthalmol. 2022;16:2391-401.
28. Ianchulev T, Chang DF, Koo E, MacDonald S, Calvo E, Tyson FT, et al. Microinterventional endocapsular nucleus disassembly: novel technique

and results of first-in-human randomised controlled study. Br J Ophthalmol. 2019;103(2):176-80.

29. Vasavada VA, Vasavada S, Vasavada AR, Vasavada V, Srivastava S. Comparative evaluation of femtosecond laser-assisted cataract surgery and conventional phacoemulsification in eyes with a shallow anterior chamber. J Cataract Refract Surg. 2019;45(5):547-52.
30. Kelkar J, Kelkar A, Pandit A, Kelkar S. A prospective comparative study on endothelial cell loss and morphology after femtolaser-assisted cataract surgery and phacoemulsification. Int Ophthalmol. 2020;40(5):1299-305.
31. Ewe SYP, Abell RG, Oakley CL, Lim CHL, Allen PL, McPherson ZE, et al. A comparative cohort study of visual outcomes in femtosecond laser-assisted versus phacoemulsification cataract surgery. Ophthalmology. 2016;123(1):178-82.
32. Ruit S, Tabin G, Chang D, Bajracharya L, Kline DC, Richheimer W, et al. A prospective randomized clinical trial of phacoemulsification vs manual sutureless small-incision extracapsular cataract surgery in Nepal. Am J Ophthalmol. 2007;143(1):32-8.
33. Gajraj M, Mohan A. Safety and efficacy of manual small-incision cataract surgery in patients with brunescent and black cataracts and other ocular comorbidities. Indian J Ophthalmol. 2022;70(11):3898-903.
34. Gogate PM, Kulkarni SR, Krishnaiah S, Deshpande RD, Joshi SA, Palimkar A, et al. Safety and efficacy of phacoemulsification compared with manual small-incision cataract surgery by a randomized controlled clinical trial: six-week results. Ophthalmology. 2005;112(5):869-74.

10 CHAPTER

Management of Retinopathy of Prematurity

Tapas Ranjan Padhi, Akash Belenje, Saurabh Kumar, Inderjeet Kaur, Sameera Nayak, Bhavik Panchal, Subhadra Jalali

ABSTRACT

The global increase in the survival rates of preterm neonates, facilitated by the proliferation of specialized eye care centers, has underscored the necessity for enhanced ocular healthcare for these infants. Preterm neonates are at a heightened risk of developing irreversible blindness within the first few months of life, predominantly due to retinopathy of prematurity (ROP), a vasoproliferative disorder. Addressing this challenge requires a comprehensive approach, incorporating the latest knowledge, standardized protocols, preventive measures, treatment modalities, technological advancements, and international collaboration. This chapter reviews the recent progress in the management of ROP, emphasizing the strategies at the forefront of combating this growing cause of childhood blindness globally.

Keywords: Childhood blindness, newborn eye health, retinopathy of prematurity, neonatal fundus imaging, anti-VEGF injections, laser therapy, prevention and pathophysiology of ROP

INTRODUCTION

Providing care for infants and young children with retinal diseases is profoundly rewarding as these resilient individuals often grow into remarkable adults. These children who strive to live and see despite significant challenges benefit immensely from timely intervention by eye specialists, which can profoundly influence their developmental trajectory and the lives of their families. The global commitment to sustainable development goals further underscores the importance of this care.

Retinopathy of prematurity (ROP) is a potentially blinding ocular disorder that predominantly affects premature infants with low birth weight. Advances in the understanding, diagnosing, and treatment of ROP have markedly enhanced the prognosis of these vulnerable infants. This chapter offers a comprehensive overview of these recent developments highlighting their impact on the management and outcome of ROP.

UPDATED CLASSIFICATION

The International Classification of Retinopathy of Prematurity, 3rd edition (ICROP3, 2021)[1] introduces a revised framework for evaluating and documenting ROP, incorporating significant clarifications of terminology and new definitions to address the globally diverse presentations of this evolving disease. The participants contributing to ICROP3 represent various geographic regions, providing a comprehensive global perspective.

A key update is the reconceptualization of "Plus" and "pre-plus" diseases as a spectrum rather than a binary condition, necessitating closely spaced serial examinations to accurately classify the status. To encompass aggressive disease beyond posterior zones, the term "Aggressive ROP (A-ROP)" is now preferred over aggressive posterior ROP (APROP). A-ROP is characterized by rapidly progressive, flat new vessels with severe plus disease, typically observed in young postmenstrual-age infants without following the traditional staged phases of ROP.

The new classification also introduces the concept of "notch" denoting a focal area of more posterior involvement within a disease zone. Additionally, the terms "regression" (disease involution and resolution) and "reactivation" (recurrence of acute phase characteristics) are defined. Persistent avascular retina (PAR) observed in untreated or spontaneously regressed eyes, or more commonly in injection-treated eyes and rarely in laser-treated eyes, is defined as an area >2 disk diameters or more (>2DD). PAR can also be posterior, especially after antivascular endothelial growth factor (anti-VEGF) injections, and may precede neovascular and tractional disease reactivation or late-onset retinal breaks, lattice degeneration, and rhegmatogenous retinal detachment in later years. More research data on the choroidal supply and retinal development in PAR is awaited.

The ICROP3 update is a critical resource that should be thoroughly understood and integrated into clinical practice from a global perspective.[1,2]

IMPROVED SCREENING AND IMAGING TECHNIQUES

- *Digital imaging:*[3-5] The implementation of mobile, bedside, digital fundus imaging systems, such as the 3Nethra Neo (Forus), Retcam Shuttle, MII Retcam, smartphone-based imaging systems, and video indirect ophthalmoscopes, has significantly enhanced the resolution and accessibility of newborn retinal imaging. Additionally, the recent adaptation of adult outpatient department (OPD) cameras like the Optos ultra-widefield camera and the true color Clarus 700 Zeiss camera has facilitated newborn retinal imaging in OPD settings, eliminating the need for separate equipment for neonatal fundus photography. Utilization of these imaging options is crucial for practitioners managing ROP. Digital imaging in ROP not only aids in documentation and monitoring disease severity but also serves as an educational tool for team members, including parents, neonatal ICU (NICU) staff, and ophthalmology, pediatric, and neonatology subspecialty trainees. Furthermore, it supports meaningful research and facilitates the acquisition of second opinions.

- *Artificial intelligence (AI):*[6,7] To address the interobserver variability in ROP classification and to provide accessible on-site triaging of the babies, AI and machine-learning algorithms integrated with digital imaging platforms are rapidly evolving. These AI platforms are designed to analyze retinal images and accurately determine disease presence and severity, thereby prioritizing the 10–15% of screened infants requiring urgent treatment. Ongoing clinical validation of these systems is expected to standardize their use as "assistants" in the care of ROP shortly. Moreover, AI is employed for not just the diagnosis at screening but also to provide the risk assessment for the treatment versus observation and to help in making better decisions.
- *Other neonatal imaging modalities:* A significant advancement in ROP management is the utilization of optical coherence tomography (OCT). The ICROP3 incorporated OCT imaging.[1] OCT has been used to evaluate abnormal foveal development in preterm infants, detecting pathologies such as macular edema, shallow retinal detachments, and retinoschisis that may affect visual outcomes and necessitate early interventions.[8] Recent studies have employed OCT to identify biomarkers of ischemia and responses to anti-VEGF treatments.[9] Although OCT angiography (OCTA) for neonatal use is not yet widely available, it holds the potential for enhancing our understanding and early intervention strategies for ROP.[10,11] Additional imaging modalities, including B-scan ultrasonography, ultrasound biomicroscopy (UBM), visual electrophysiology, and fundus autofluorescence, contribute to the scientific approach in managing and understanding various stages of ROP as summarized in a recent review.[11]
- *Telemedicine:*[12,13] Telemedicine facilitates remote diagnosis and management by expert ophthalmologists, improving access to care both in underserved populations and in urban areas with limited ROP expertise. The KIDROP model has been well established for over a decade and has been replicated in many regions. With the formal guidelines for teleconsultations provided by the Government of India and the increased acceptance of videoconferencing platforms following the 2020 pandemic, innovative approaches to telemedicine are evolving.[13] This paradigm shift in ROP screening and other neonatal eye disease management is essential for enhancing access, efficiency, and quality of care.[14]
- *National screening guidelines:* Effective dissemination of knowledge and practices to all eligible infants is achievable through the implementation

of National Health Agency guidelines. It is heartening to see multiple countries and regions developing national guidelines tailored to their populations.[2] The government of India's current national guidelines for universal newborn eye screening and ROP screening, available on the Rashtriya Bal Swashthya Shurakshya Karyakram (RBSK)[15] website, provide a framework for establishing ROP programs. While these guidelines outline the mandatory essential components, they also encourage going beyond to optimize program effectiveness.

PHARMACOLOGICAL INTERVENTIONS

Antivascular endothelial growth factor (anti-VEGF) agents, such as bevacizumab, ranibizumab, aflibercept, and their biosimilars, have become prevalent in the treatment of severe ROP. These agents function by inhibiting the abnormal growth of retinal blood vessels. A comparative meta-analysis of various treatment modalities[16] revealed the highest single-treatment success rate for laser therapy at 89%, followed by anti-VEGF drugs with success rates ranging from 87% for bevacizumab to 81% for aflibercept, and 74% for ranibizumab. Specifically, for zone I ROP, bevacizumab demonstrated the highest success rate at 91%, compared to 78% for ranibizumab and 66% for laser therapy.

The recurrence in ROP occurs earlier with ranibizumab compared to bevacizumab. Current evidence indicates that anti-VEGF treatments result in fewer complications and improved structural outcomes, particularly in reducing the incidence of myopia, and have gained approval for use in ROP. However, clinicians should caution parents that high myopia can still occur following any of these treatments.

A significant challenge with anti-VEGF therapy is the need for prolonged and frequent follow-up, due to a small but significant potential of sudden recurrence of neovascularization and rapidly worsening or smoldering retinal detachments which can be overlooked even by ROP experts. Therefore, serial, detailed, evaluations of vascular patterns are crucial for eyes treated with anti-VEGF injections.[17,18] Fundus fluorescein angiography (FFA) has emerged as a vital tool in characterizing eyes post anti-VEGF treatment and guiding subsequent management.[19] Even after laser, some of the vessels may show continued dye leakage on FFA. Despite the limited availability of this imaging modality, innovative low-cost solutions are anticipated to address this challenge. Advances in this field are rapidly evolving.

ADVANCES IN LASER THERAPY

Laser therapy continues to be a cornerstone in the treatment of ROP. Technological advancements in laser systems have enhanced precision and reduced treatment duration, resulting in improved outcomes and fewer side effects. Recent studies have provided new insights into laser posterior to ridge.[20] Combined treatment protocols have been developed for infants with zone I disease who are unable to adhere to close and prolonged follow-up.[21] There is an increased need for laser treatment of PAR, including procedures performed under general anesthesia for older infants.[1,16] Laser therapy has been proven to be highly effective as a standalone treatment for type I ROP.[16] Consequently, proficiency in laser photocoagulation is essential for all clinicians managing ROP.

SURGICAL TECHNIQUES

Modern surgical techniques, particularly microincision vitrectomy surgery (MIVS), have demonstrated the capability to successfully repair complex ROP-related retinal detachment, providing satisfactory anatomical and visual outcomes.[22,23] The choice of the surgical approach varies based on the case specifics. Techniques include scleral buckle using 240- or 42-style silicone bands in infants and other types in older children, lens-sparing vitrectomy, lensectomy combined with vitrectomy, oil or gas tamponade or fibrin-glue-assisted surgery, and scleral imbrication with or without a buckle.[24] Additionally, open-sky vitrectomy and endoscopic vitrectomy are employed, particularly for tractional membranes located behind the clear lens with some cases necessitating a combined surgical approach.

Silicone oil is sparingly used, reserved for complicated rhegmatogenous retinal detachments or iatrogenic retinal breaks with detachment. Complications associated with silicone oil in pediatric patients, similar to those in adults, include intraocular pressure elevation, band-shaped keratopathy, oil emulsification—hyperleon, and cataract formation. However, managing these complications in children is more challenging due to issues such as missed intraocular pressure recordings, contact lens management, rapid onset of strabismus, significant refractive changes due to eye growth, and inability to do precise objective and subjective refractions. In infants, silicone oil is preferably removed 2–3 weeks post surgery and within 6–8 weeks in older children to manage amblyopia and avoid early cataract formation.

Early referral and prompt surgery are crucial, as ROP-related retinal detachments can deteriorate rapidly, often necessitating surgery within 24 hours. When referring to a tertiary center, ensure that the infant has a hemoglobin level of at least 10 g/dL, facilitate blood transfusion to reach the required hemoglobin level, treat any concurrent respiratory infections, and perform laser therapy on the visible attached retina. It is essential for parents to bring all relevant medical records, including antenatal, postnatal, NICU discharge summaries, and previous investigations.

Efforts are made to preserve the lens whenever possible, as removing it, particularly in infants, can significantly worsen visual outcomes. The aphakia often cannot be corrected with intraocular lenses, and hence, a tedious process of heavy aphakic glasses or contact lens usage becomes the pathway to visual rehabilitation. Noncompliance with these leads to severe amblyopia and, ultimately, poor visual outcomes. Herein comes the importance of newborn retinal screening, close follow-up, and early referral of all high-risk babies so that surgery can be done without needing to remove the lens. Compassionate counseling and managing life-threatening situations are additional skills that need to be organized as a multidisciplinary team and become an integral component of ROP care.[25]

UNDERSTANDING THE PATHOPHYSIOLOGY

- *Angiogenesis research:* Advances in understanding the molecular mechanisms of angiogenesis (forming new blood vessels) have shed light on the two phases of ROP: (1) The initial cessation of normal vessel growth and (2) the subsequent abnormal vessel proliferation. This has helped in planning targeted therapy using anti-VEGF injections, especially for more aggressive, atypical, and severe types of ROP.
- *Tear markers and metabolomics and genetics in ROP as a means of recent advancement toward understanding ROP:* ROP has been extensively studied as an oxygen-induced retinopathy in the past while the underlying genetic predisposition and molecular mechanisms in ROP have not been understood very well.[26] A genomic analysis study for preterm born babies revealed a strong role for the genes involved in angiogenesis, growth and development of the fetal retina, transendothelial migration, oxidative stress, inflammation, cholesterol metabolism, and neurodegenerative processes in ROP pathogenesis.[27] We observed strong associations of ROP with increased levels of proteins in the extracellular matrix (ECM) and complement pathways in the vitreous humor samples of ROP patients. It was interesting to note that the levels of matrix metalloprotease (MMP) enzymes (known to induce inflammation and angiogenesis) in tears were significantly higher in severe ROP compared to no-ROP and mild-ROP eyes that underscored its potential use as a biomarker for an early prediction of the condition.[28] Recent advances have been made to measure and quantify the metabolites and protein markers, such as MMP9, in the tear film and vitreous of ROP infants which may be considered as diagnostic and predictive markers of the disease.[29,30]
- *Link between inflammation, oxidative stress, and altered lipid metabolism in ROP pathogenesis:* Prenatal and postnatal inflammation, often triggered by oxygen, sepsis,[31] and metabolic dysregulation, is implicated in ROP pathogenesis. The retina is rich in long-chain polyunsaturated fatty acids (PUFAs), which are prone to frequent lipid peroxidation and structural modifications under oxidative stress. The metabolites of fatty acids (diols) are important structural and signaling molecules in the

vascular endothelial layer and maintain optimal retinal physiology and anatomy. Metabolic dysregulation leads to irregular neovascularization of blood vessels, leading to severe ROP stages.[32] Preliminary data from our laboratory on the metabolic profiling of ROP cases suggested an increased expression of fatty acids with a concurrent increase in severity (abnormal angiogenesis) of the disease. Ongoing studies on the role of altered lipid metabolism with increased inflammation and abnormal angiogenesis are underway. Identification of novel mediators of abnormal lipid metabolism and their genetic regulation can then be tested as new drug targets for checking inflammation and, thus, neovascularization in the retina.

RETINOPATHY OF PREMATURITY AND NEONATAL HEALTH EMBEDDED HEALTHCARE DELIVERY SYSTEMS AND GLOBAL AND NATIONAL PARTNERSHIPS

The eye and neonatal care delivery systems remain a challenge. Partnerships and embedded healthcare delivery systems are still nascent and have started and need to be rapidly upscaled.[33] These have become the primary game-changers in bringing technology and knowledge to the bedside of patients. These will also help parents toward universal acceptance and awareness of the need for early screening and continued follow-up to prevent ROP blindness. Numerous barriers to timely ROP eye care and overall care of newborns result in incurable blindness,[34] even though we have advanced knowledge and technology available. The International Agency for the Prevention of Blindness, the World Health Organization, the Ministry of Health of each country, professional societies of neonatology, pediatrics, obstetricians, nursing counsels, and various subspecialists in ophthalmology, besides NGOs involved in the prevention of blindness and prevention of childhood morbidities (intact survival), need to come together to launch aggressive service delivery models and educational curriculum, thereby reducing the burden of ROP by quality care of neonates.[35] The blinding epidemic is adding more and more blind babies to our population, and the health delivery systems have fallen far behind the need of the ever-increasing survival of premature babies.[36,37]

CONCLUSION

The recent advances in the diagnosis, classification, screening, and treatment approaches for ROP have significantly improved the outcome for premature infants at risk of this condition. The updated classification system, ICROP3, provides a more comprehensive framework for assessing ROP, while improved screening techniques, including digital imaging and artificial intelligence, have enhanced the accuracy and accessibility of early detection. Pharmacological interventions, particularly anti-VEGF therapies, and advancements in laser and surgical techniques have further refined treatment protocols, offering better structural and functional outcomes for affected infants.

Understanding the pathophysiology of ROP has also advanced, highlighting the roles of genetic predisposition, inflammation, and metabolic dysregulation. Continued research in these areas is essential to develop targeted therapies and preventive measures. Telemedicine has emerged as a vital tool in expanding access to expert care, especially in underserved regions.

Overall, the integration of these advancements into clinical practice promises to enhance the quality of care for premature infants worldwide, reducing the incidence of ROP-related blindness and improving the quality of life of affected individuals. Continued innovation and international collaboration will be key to addressing the ongoing challenges in managing this complex disease.[37,38]

ACKNOWLEDGMENT

The authors would like to thank the Hyderabad Eye Research Foundation for the support.

REFERENCES

1. Chiang MF, Quinn GE, Fielder AR, Ostmo SR, Paul, Chan RV, et al. International classification of retinopathy of prematurity, 3rd edition. Ophthalmology. 2021;128(10):51-68.
2. Sabri K, Ells AL, Lee EY, Dutta S, Vinekar A. Retinopathy of prematurity: a global perspective and recent developments. Pediatrics. 2022;150(3):e2021053924.
3. Jayanna S, Padhi TR, Nedhina EK, Agarwal K, Jalali S. Color fundus imaging in retinopathy of prematurity screening: present and future. Indian J Ophthalmol. 2023;71(5):1777-82.
4. Jayanna S, Agarwal K, Doshi V, Reddy RU, Ali H, Dogra A, et al. A retrospective analysis of ultra-widefield photograph (Optos) documentation of retinopathy of prematurity at a tertiary eye care outpatient setup: the Indian Twin Cities ROP Study, report number 11. J AAPOS. 2022;26(2):68.
5. Belenje A, Reddy RU, Agarwal K, Parmeswarappa DC, Jalali S. Non-contact widefield neonatal retinal imaging for retinopathy of prematurity using the Clarus 700 high resolution true colour reflectance imaging. Eye (Lond). 2023;37(9):1904-09.
6. Shah S, Slaney E, VerHage E, Chen J, Dias R, Abdelmalik B, et al. Application of artificial intelligence in the early detection of retinopathy of prematurity: review of the literature. Neonatology. 2023;120(5):558-65.
7. Gilbert C, Malik ANJ, Vinekar A. Artificial intelligence for ROP screening and to assess quality of care: progress and challenges. Pediatrics. 2021;147(3): e2020034314.

8. Vinekar A, Mangalesh S, Jayadev C, Maldonado RS, Bauer N, Toth CA. Retinal imaging of infants on spectral domain optical coherence tomography. Biomed Res Int. 2015:782420.
9. Belenje A, Reddy RU, Parmeswarappa DC, Padhi TR, Subbarao B, Jalali S. Evaluation of optical coherence tomography biomarkers to differentiate favourable and unfavourable responders to intravitreal anti-vascular endothelial growth factor treatment in retinopathy of prematurity. Eye (Lond). 2024;38(6):1097-103.
10. Vinekar A, Chidambara L, Jayadev C, Sivakumar M, Webers CA, Shetty B. Monitoring neovascularization in aggressive posterior retinopathy of prematurity using optical coherence tomography angiography. J AAPOS. 2016;20(3):271-4.
11. Agarwal K, Vinekar A, Chandra P, Padhi TR, Nayak S, Jayanna S, et al. Imaging the pediatric retina: an overview. Indian J Ophthalmol. 2021;69(4):812-23.
12. Vinekar A, Jayadev C, Mangalesh S, Shetty B, Vidyasagar D. Role of tele-medicine in retinopathy of prematurity screening in rural outreach centers in India—a report of 20,214 imaging sessions in the KIDROP program. Semin Fetal Neonatal Med. 2015;20(5):335-45.
13. Padhi TR, Bhunia S, Das, T, Nayak S, Jalan, M, Rath S, et al. Outcome of real-time telescreening for retinopathy of prematurity using videoconferencing in a community setting in Eastern India. Indian J Ophthalmol. 2024;72(5):697-703.
14. Gilbert C, Wormald R, Fielder A, Deorari A, Zepeda-Romero LC, Quinn G, et al. Potential for a paradigm change in the detection of retinopathy of prematurity requiring treatment. Arch Dis Child Fetal Neonatal Ed. 2016;101(1):6-9.
15. Rashtriya Bal Swasthya Karyakram, Ministry of Health and Family Welfare, Government of India. Guidelines for universal eye screening in newborns including retinopathy of prematurity. [online] Available from: http://nhm.gov.in/images/pdf/programmes/ RBSK/ Resource_Documents/ Revised_ROP_Guidelines. [Last accessed September, 2024].
16. Chang E, Josan AS, Purohit R, Patel CK, Xue K. A network meta-analysis of retreatment rates following Bevacizumab, Ranibizumab, Aflibercept, and laser for retinopathy of prematurity. Ophthalmology. 2022;129(12):1389-401.
17. Padhi T, Das, T, Rath S, Pradhan L, Sutar S, Panda KG, et al. Serial evaluation of retinal vascular changes in infants treated with intravitreal bevacizumab for aggressive posterior retinopathy of prematurity in zone I. Eye. 2016;30:392-9.
18. Padhi TR, Bhusal U, Padhy SK, Patel A, Kelgaonker A, Khalsa A, et al. The retinal vascular growth rate in babies with retinopathy of prematurity could indicate treatment need. Indian J Ophthalmol. 2022;70:1270-7.
19. Hans A, Narang S, Sindhu M, Jain S, Chawla D. Fundus fluorescein angiography in retinopathy of prematurity. Eye (Lond). 2022;36(8):1604-9.
20. Regani H, Chandra P, Kumawat D, Chawla R, Agarwal R, Vohra R. Role of additional posterior barrage laser in type 1 zone 2 retinopathy of prematurity: a randomized trial. Indian J Ophthalmol. 2023;71(11):3460-4.
21. Laveti V, Balakrishnan D, Rani PK, Mohamad A, Jalali S. Prospective clinical study of two different treatment regimens of combined laser photocoagulation and intravitreal bevacizumab for retinopathy of prematurity: the Indian Twin Cities ROP Study (ITCROPS) database report number 9. Int Ophthalmol. 2020;40:3539-45.

22. Sen P, Bhende P, Maitra P. Surgical outcomes in aggressive retinopathy of prematurity (AROP)-related retinal detachments. Indian J Ophthalmol. 2023;71(11):3454-9.
23. Sen P, Bhende P, Sharma T, Gopal L, Maitray A, Shah P, Oke Y. Surgical outcomes of microincision vitrectomy surgery in eyes with retinal detachment secondary to retinopathy of prematurity in Indian population. Indian J Ophthalmol. 2019;67(6):889-95.
24. Belenje A, Jalali S. Combined rhegmatogenous and tractional retinal detachment in a child with incontinentia pigmenti managed by scleral imbrication with scleral buckle. BMJ Case Rep. 2023;16(2):253738.
25. Jayanna S, Jalali S, Padhi TR, Agarwal K, Jhingan M, Panchal B, et al. Compassionate and standard operating procedure-based counselling and practice are essential in high-risk infantile anesthesia and managing death in eye surgery. Indian J Ophthalmol. 2022;70(1):266-70.
26. Kaur T, Patnaik S, Kumar S, Kaur I. Molecular mechanisms in the pathogenesis of retinopathy of prematurity (ROP). In: Nema HV, Nema N (Eds). Genetics of Ocular Diseases. Singapore: Springer; 2022.
27. Rathi S, Jalali S, Patnaik S, Shahulhameed S, Musada GR, Balakrishnan D, et al. Abnormal complement activation and inflammation in the pathogenesis of retinopathy of prematurity. Front Immunol. 2017;8:1868.
28. Patnaik S, Rai M, Jalali S, Agarwal K, Badakere A, Puppala L, et al. An interplay of microglia and matrix metalloproteinase MMP9 under hypoxic stress regulates the opticin expression in retina. Sci Rep. 2021;11(1):7444.
29. Ghosh TN, Rotake D, Kumar S, Kaur I, Singh SG. Tear-based MMP-9 detection: a rapid antigen test for ocular inflammatory disorders using vanadium disulfide nanowires assisted chemi-resistive biosensor. Anal Chim Acta. 2023;1263:341281.
30. Kumar S, Joshi MB, Kaur I. Protocol and methods applicable to retinal vascular diseases. Methods Mol Biol. 2023;2625:71-8.
31. Goldstein GP, Leonard SA, Kan P, Koo EB, Lee HC, Carmichael SL. Prenatal and postnatal inflammation-related risk factors for retinopathy of prematurity. J Perinatol. 2019;39(7):964-73.
32. Fu Z, Nilsson AK, Hellstrom A, Smith LEH. Retinopathy of prematurity: metabolic risk factors. Elife. 2022;11:e80550.
33. Jalali S, Azad R. Retinopathy of prematurity: it is time to take swift action. Community Eye Health. 2018;31(101):1-2.
34. Padhi TR, Badhani A, Mahajan S, Savla LP, Sutar S, Jalali S, et al. Barriers to timely presentation for appropriate care of retinopathy of prematurity in Odisha, Eastern India. Indian J Ophthalmol. 2018;67(6):824-7.
35. Kumar P, Chawla D, Thukral A, Deorari A, Shukla R, Gilbert C. Development of a quality improvement package for reducing sight-threatening retinopathy of prematurity. Indian J Ophthalmol. 2020;68(1):115-20.
36. Blencowe H, Lawn JE, Vazquez T, Fielder A, Gilbert C. Preterm-associated visual impairment and estimates of retinopathy of prematurity at regional and global levels for 2010. Pediatr Res. 2013;74(1):35-49.
37. Gilbert CE. Global perspectives of retinopathy of prematurity. Indian J Ophthalmol. 2023;71(11):3431-2.
38. Dammann O, Hartnett ME, Stahl A. Retinopathy of prematurity. Dev Med Child Neurol. 2023;65(5):625-31.

11 CHAPTER

Management of Age-related Macular Degeneration

Kiran Chandra Kedarisetti, Raja Narayanan

ABSTRACT

The main goal of the treatment of age-related macular degeneration (AMD) is to prevent further vision loss. The prevailing treatment over many years for neovascular AMD (nAMD) involves regular intravitreal (IVT) injections of anti-vascular endothelial growth factor (anti-VEGF), imposing a significant strain on patients, caregivers, and physicians alike. Newer molecular agents such as brolucizumab, faricimab, aflibercept, and conbercept aim for longer durability and improvement in visual and anatomic outcomes, with the potential to reduce treatment burden. The standard of care for non-neovascular AMD (nnAMD) has advanced from Age-Related Eye Disease Studies (AREDS) supplementation to newer molecules such as pegcetacoplan, avacincaptad pegol, gene therapy, and stem cell therapy.

Keywords: Neovascular AMD, non-neovascular AMD, anti-VEGF, stem cell therapy, gene therapy

INTRODUCTION

Age-related macular degeneration (AMD) is the leading cause of central visual loss in individuals over the age of 65 years. It is an acquired disease that causes retinal degeneration due to both dry or non-neovascular AMD (nnAMD) and wet or neovascular AMD (nAMD) etiology. The risk of the fellow eye developing choroidal neovascularization (CNV) is 4–12% per year, with increased risk associated with multiple soft drusen, retinal pigment epithelium (RPE) clumping, densely packed drusen, or pigment epithelial detachment (PED). Newer drugs such as brolucizumab, faricimab, conbercept, and aflibercept have shown promising results with less-frequent dosages for the treatment of nAMD. The standard of care for nnAMD is observation and prevention of progression from intermediate to advanced AMD through the Age-Related Eye Disease Studies (AREDS) formulation. Local inflammation, complement activation, genetic variation, oxidative stress, and hypoxia lead to progressive disease with localized areas of RPE cells, photoreceptors (PRs), and choriocapillaris dropouts at the macula.[1]

Complement factor inhibition, gene therapy, and stem cell therapy are novel interventions to tackle geographic atrophy (GA).

BROLUCIZUMAB

Brolucizumab is a single-chain variable fragment (scFV), weighing 26 kilodaltons (kDa), that exhibits a high affinity for vascular endothelial growth factor (VEGF)-A isoforms with the help of an autonomous binding agent.[2] This smaller size enables superior penetration of the retina and choroid compared to alternative anti-VEGF molecules.[3] It exhibits a rapid systemic clearance (5.6 ± 1.5 hours) with a longer ocular duration of action.[4]

The phase 3 multicenter studies HAWK and HARRIER randomized nAMD patients to receive intravitreal (IVT) brolucizumab 3 mg (HAWK only) or 6 mg or aflibercept 2 mg.

Brolucizumab was noninferior to aflibercept in visual function at week 48, and more than 50% of brolucizumab 6 mg-treated eyes were maintained on q12w dosing interval through week 48.[5] Brolucizumab showed a greater decrease in central subfield thickness (CST) (172.8 μm in HAWK and 193.8 μm in HARRIER with brolucizumab vs. 143 μm with aflibercept in both studies) with fewer injections and comparable visual gains. **Figures 11.1A to C** are representative images of a patient with macular neovascularization (MNV) who responded to brolucizumab.[6] Adverse drug effects were observed in 5.8% of eyes treated with brolucizumab.[7] Adverse effects such as intraocular inflammation (IOI) (iritis, uveitis, chorioretinitis, and retinal vasculitis) have led many practitioners to be cautious with its usage.

FARICIMAB

Faricimab is a bispecific antibody designed to bind and neutralize angiopoietin-2 (Ang-2) and VEGF-A.[8] The angiopoietin-TIE2 (Ang-TIE2) signaling pathway maintains vascular stability; however, in nAMD, the elevated levels inhibit angiopoietin-1 (Ang-1) signaling. Such inhibition upregulates VEGF-A, leading to inflammation, vascular leakage, and neovascularization. By targeting both pathways, faricimab has a more durable efficacy.

In the phase 3, noninferiority trials TENAYA and LUCERNE, faricimab every 16 weeks was compared with aflibercept administered every 8 weeks in nAMD patients.[9] At 12 weeks, during the matched-dosing period, the faricimab group showed a greater reduction in CST from baseline compared to the aflibercept group. The CST was comparable during the maintenance period. The 2-year trial introduced a treat-and-extend (T&E)-based personalized treatment interval (PTI) regimen allowing a patient's dosing to be individualized based on disease activity following fixed treatment intervals of the first year.[10] The T&E-based faricimab treatment maintained visual gains through year 2, with most patients achieving

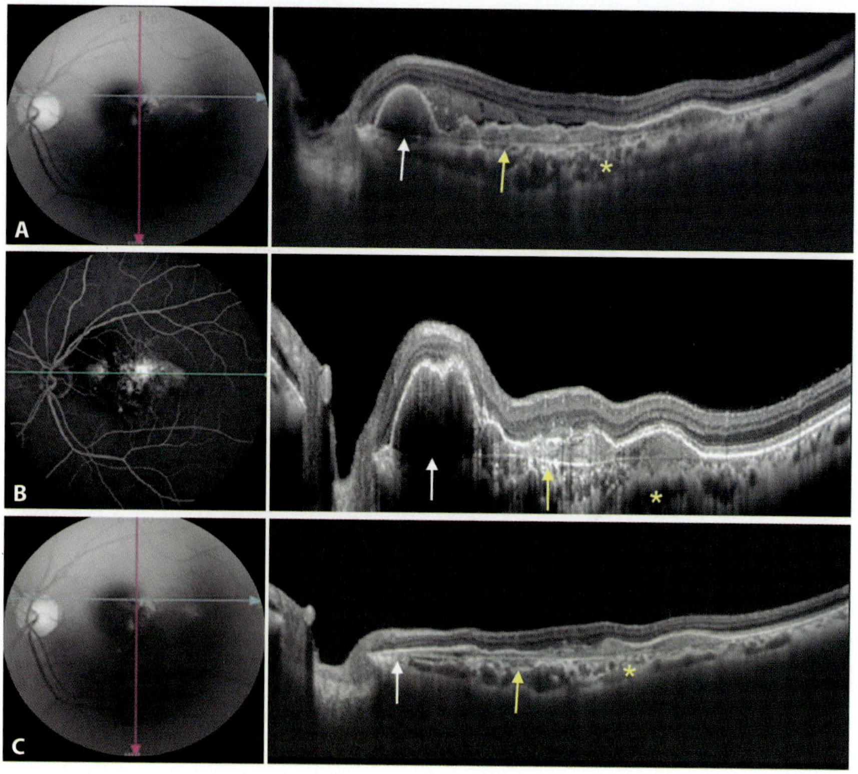

Figs. 11.1A to C: (A) The OCT of the LE shows SHRM, thumb-like PED nasal to fovea, multiple hemorrhagic PEDs, and SRF. Pachyvessels are seen subfoveally; (B) IVT brolucizumab injection was administered. Subsequent OCT at 6 months shows a decrease in SRF and SHRM; (C) The OCT at 1 year following three IVT injections of brolucizumab administered pro re nata shows complete flattening of PED and resolution of SRF. (IVT: intravitreal; LE: left eye; OCT: optical coherence tomography; PED: pigment epithelial detachment; SHRM: subretinal hyperreflective material; SRF: subretinal fluid)
Source: Chandra et al.[6]

extended dosing intervals. The safety profile was comparable in both groups. **Figures 11.2A to C** are representative images of a patient with MNV who showed resolution of intraretinal fluid (IRF) with faricimab.

The phase 2 double-masked trial AVENUE was a superiority trial that assessed the efficacy and safety of different doses and regimens of faricimab versus ranibizumab in patients with nAMD.[11] The AVENUE trial did not show superiority of faricimab over ranibizumab in best-corrected visual acuity (BCVA) at week 36. However, the visual and anatomical gains observed with faricimab suggest it as a viable alternative to monthly anti-VEGF therapy.

CONBERCEPT

Conbercept targets VEGF-A, VEGF-B, VEGF-C, and placental growth factor (PlGF) and was approved for the treatment of nAMD by the China Food and

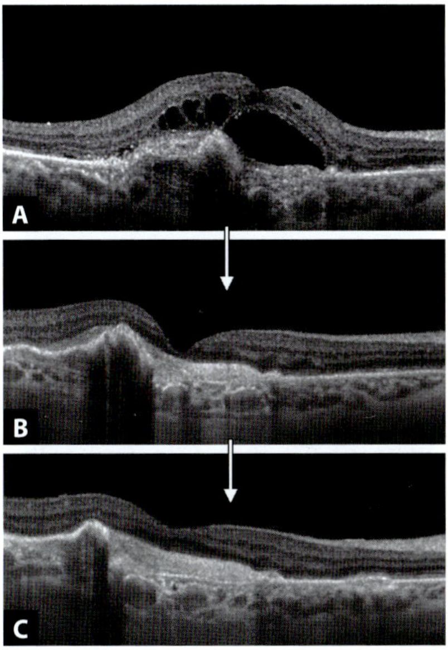

Figs. 11.2A to C: (A) The OCT of the RE shows SHRM, IRF, and SRF; (B) Subsequent OCT at 1 month shows a decrease in SRF and IRF with the persistence of SHRM with a single injection of faricimab; (C) The OCT at 3 months shows complete resolution of SRF. (IRF: intraretinal fluid; OCT: optical coherence tomography; RE: right eye; SHRM: subretinal hyperreflective material; SRF: subretinal fluid)

Drug Administration (FDA) in December 2013.[12] It is a recombinant fusion protein composed of the second immunoglobulin G (IgG) domain of VEGF receptor-1 (VEGFR1) and the third and fourth domains of VEGFR2, fused to the constant region (Fc) of human IgG1.

The PHOENIX trial randomized nAMD patients to receive IVT injections of conbercept (0.5 mg) once monthly for the first 3 months and then once quarterly until month 12 (3 + Q3M).[13] The sham group received first 3-monthly sham injections, followed by 3-monthly injections of conbercept (0.5 mg) and then quarterly administrations until month 12. The BCVA improved at 12 weeks in both groups, with an increase of +9.98 letters in the conbercept group and +8.81 letters in the sham group.

AFLIBERCEPT 8 MG

Aflibercept 8 mg (Bayer) was developed to achieve longer retreatment intervals by using a higher molar concentration of aflibercept. High-dose aflibercept 8 mg (q12w–q16w) was compared with aflibercept 2 mg (q8w) in a randomized controlled phase 3 trial PULSAR.[14] The majority of patients in the aflibercept 8-mg group maintained 12-week or longer dosing (83% in the pooled 8-mg group) and 16-week dosing (77% in the aflibercept 8-mg group every 16 weeks) at week 48. These results indicate that aflibercept 8 mg was effective in controlling the disease during extended intervals in the majority of patients. The pooled aflibercept 8-mg group demonstrated superiority in the absence of intraretinal and subretinal fluid (SRF) in the center subfield at week 16 compared with the aflibercept 2-mg group, while both showed a similar safety profile.

PEGCETACOPLAN

In February 2023, the FDA approved pegcetacoplan (Syfovre), the first-in-class treatment for GA. Pegcetacoplan is a pegylated peptide inhibitor of complement C3, which prevents the activity of C3 convertase, thereby inhibiting the cleavage of C3 into C3a and C3b.[15] This action stops inflammatory responses and opsonization. Additionally, C3b facilitates the enzyme required for C5 cleavage into C5a and C5b, which exacerbates inflammatory reactions and initiates the membrane attack complex, leading to cellular destruction and death. Activation and/or degradation of C3 is associated with increased risks of both exudative and atrophic forms of AMD.[1]

The phase 3 OAKS and DERBY double-masked trials showed a reduction in lesion growth rate in patients treated with pegcetacoplan compared to the sham-administered group at 24 months.[16] Patients were randomly assigned (stratified permuted block randomization) in a 2:2:1:1 ratio to receive 15 mg of pegcetacoplan in 0.1 mL either monthly or every other month, or a sham injection either monthly or every other month.

In the OAKS trial, pegcetacoplan administered monthly and every other month significantly slowed GA lesion growth by 21% and 16%, respectively, compared with the sham group at 12 months.[17] Similarly, in the DERBY trial, pegcetacoplan monthly and every other month injections slowed GA lesion growth by 12% and 11%, respectively, when compared with the sham group at 12 months. At 24 months, pegcetacoplan monthly and every other month injections slowed GA lesion growth by 22% and 18% in the OAKS trial and by 19% and 16% in the DERBY trial, respectively, compared with sham. New-onset nAMD was reported in 11%, 8%, and 2% of patients in the OAKS trial, and in 13%, 6%, and 4% of patients in the DERBY trial receiving pegcetacoplan monthly, pegcetacoplan every other month, and sham, respectively, at 24 months.

AVACINCAPTAD PEGOL

Avacincaptad pegol (ACP), a pegylated RNA aptamer, binds specifically to complement C5 inhibiting its cleavage into C5a and C5b, thus preventing the formation of the membrane attack complex and subsequent cell death, including RPE and PR atrophy. In the phase 3 GATHER trial, comparing

2 mg ACP with sham, there was a 17.3% reduction ($p = 0.0027$) in mean change in GA lesion area compared to the sham arm at 1 year.[18,19] However, there was a higher rate of CNV in patients treated with ACP compared to sham, with rates of 6.7% versus 4.1%. In August 2023, ACP (IZERVAY™) received US-FDA approval.

Intravitreal neuroprotective agents like brimonidine are being studied for nnAMD.[20-22]

GENE THERAPY

Through single-cell sequencing and genome-wide association studies (GWASs), specific genes associated with advanced AMD have been identified. These include *CFH* on chromosome 1 and *ARMS2* and *HTRA1* on chromosome 10.[21] The *CFH* variant is primarily linked to the presence of drusen, while the *ARMS2-HTRA1* variant is correlated with the occurrence of subretinal or sub-RPE hemorrhages. Other genes implicated in AMD pathogenesis include *MMP9, CETP,* and *TIMP3*, which regulate the extracellular matrix, as well as *FGD6, HTRA1,* and *CFH,* which are involved in oxidative stress and inflammation pathways. Current gene therapies primarily target VEGF, VEGFR, PDGF, and PEGF to address AMD progression.

MicroRNAs (miRNAs) evaluated in animal models of AMD exhibit different behavior in human patients, leading to uncertainty regarding their role in the disease.[22]

Retroviruses and lentiviruses have been employed in gene therapy products, such as RetinoStat® (Oxford BioMedica, Oxford, UK, OXB-201) for nAMD (NCT01301443), and in stem cell therapy.[23] However, retroviruses and lentiviruses carry risks, such as potential insertional mutagenesis and germline transmission.

Adeno-associated viruses (AAVs) are commonly used vectors for retinal gene transfer due to advantages, such as extended transgene expression, minimal risk of insertional mutagenesis, slight inflammatory responses, and low chance of germline transmission.[24]

An adenoviral vector containing the pigment epithelium-derived factor (*PEDF*) gene, an endogenous antiangiogenic factor, with deficient replication (achieved by the deletion of E1, E3, and E4), was found to reduce the incidence of MNV in a phase 1 trial.[25,26]

An AAV2-derived vector, ixoberogene soroparvovec (AAV.7m8-aflibercept), named ADVM-22, was administered via IVT injection in nAMD aflibercept responder patients. The OPTIC phase 1 multicenter randomized trial showed that vision and CST remained stable throughout 2 years, with annual anti-VEGF injections reduced by 80% (10 mean annual anti-VEGF injections to 1.9) in 2×10^{11} vg/eye and 98% (9.8 mean annual anti-VEGF injections to 0.2) in 6×10^{11} vg/eye cohorts.[27] IOI responding to topical corticosteroids was observed in 60% of the patients with no systemic or long-term ocular adverse effects at the end of 2 years. In patients with diabetic macular edema (DME) (INFINITY trial), a suspected unexpected serious adverse reaction (SUSAR) hypotony not responding to steroids was seen at 16–32 weeks after the administration of 6×10^{11} vg/eye high-dose ADVM.[28] This led to halting treatment in DME patients; however, no similar SUSAR was observed in nAMD patients.

A gene encoding the monoclonal portion of an anti-VEGF antibody structurally similar to ranibizumab, called RGX-314, administered via subretinal injection, was tested in a phase 1/2a trial (ATMOSPHERE).[29] The rescue treatment consisted of IVT anti-VEGF in the case of vision loss of five or more ETDRS letters; persistent, increased, or new intra-/SRF on optical coherence tomography (OCT); or the appearance of new macular hemorrhage. The open-label, multiple-cohort, multicenter, phase 1/2a dose-escalation study conducted at eight sites in the USA involved participants aged 50–89 years with nAMD who had previously undergone anti-VEGF injections.[30] The study comprised five cohorts receiving different doses of *RGX-314* via subretinal delivery. *RGX-314* administration was generally well tolerated, with no clinically recognized immune responses observed. Most participants showed stable or improved BCVA and central retinal thickness, requiring few or no supplemental anti-VEGF-A injections.

The phase 2 AAVIATE trial aims to assess the suprachoroidal route of *RGX-314* in patients with nAMD.[31]

PHOTOBIOMODULATION

The LIGHTSITE III study evaluated multiwavelength photobiomodulation (PBM) treatment using the LumiThera Valeda® Light Delivery System in dry AMD.[32] The LumiThera technology utilizes near-infrared light (590, 660, and 850 nm) exposure in multiple cycles to selected tissues. The light is absorbed by mitochondrial cytochrome C in the RPE and improves cellular respiration by increasing adenosine triphosphate (ATP) production, reducing free radical production, and decreasing oxidative stress. 55% of PBM-treated eyes showed ≥5 letter gain (mean 9.7 ± 3.7), 26.4% showed ≥10 letter gain (mean 12.8 ± 2.7), and 5.5% showed ≥15 letter gain with a good compliance among patients. The treated patients had a reduction in drusen volume, reduced risk of progression to GA, and an improvement in visual acuity.

STEM CELL THERAPY

Stem cell transplantation holds promise for regenerating the RPE cells and impaired PRs. The ongoing phase 1/2a study is evaluating the safety and tolerability of OpRegen, comprising RPE cells derived from human embryonic stem cells (ClinicalTrials.gov Identifier: NCT02286089).[33]

TABLE 11.1: Comparison of anti-VEGF drugs.

Drugs	*Structure*	*Molecular weight (kDa)*	*Mechanism of action*	*Binding affinity to VEGF-A165 (pm)*	*Clinical dose for nAMD (mg/0.5 mL)*	*Equivalent number of molecules per injection*	*FDA approval*	*Half-life in vitreous (days)*
Bevacizumab	Monoclonal IgG antibody	149	All isoforms of VEGF-A	58	1.25 mg	0.4	Not approved	6.7
Ranibizumab	Monoclonal IgG antibody fragment (Fab)	48	All isoforms of VEGF-A	21.8	0.5 mg	0.5	2006 MARINA and ANCHOR	7.2
Aflibercept	*Fusion protein:* Domain 2 of VEGFR-1 and domain 3 of VEGFR-2 fused with IgG1 Fc15	115	All isoforms of VEGF-A, VEGF-B, and PlGF15	0.172	2 mg	1	2011 VEIW1 and VEIW2	9.1
Conbercept	*Fusion protein:* Domain 2 of VEGFR-1 and domains 3 and 4 of VEGFR-2 fused with IgG1	143	All isoforms of VEGF-A, VEGF-B, VEGF-C, and PlGF	0.5	0.5 mg	0.2	In China in 2013 PHOENIX	4.2 days in rabbits
Brolucizumab	scFV, with an autonomous binding agent	26	High affinity to VEGF-A	1.3	6 mg	11	2019 HAWK and HARRIER	4.3–5.1
Faricimab	Bispecific antibody with Fab arm, anti-Ang-2 arm, and modified Fc region	149	Binds to VEGF-A and Ang-2	22,000	6 mg	1.9–2.3	2022 TENAYA and LUCERNE	7.5

(Ang-2: angiopoietin 2; FDA: Food and Drug Administration; IgG: immunoglobulin G; kDa: kilodaltons; nAMD: neovascular AMD; PlGF: placental growth factor; scFV: single-chain variable fragment; VEGF-A: vascular endothelial growth factor-A; VEGFR: vascular endothelial growth factor receptor)

TABLE 11.2: Different treatment modalities for AMD.

Treatment modality	*Trial name*	*Drug tested*	*Treatment arms*	*Results*
Complement system	DERBY and OAKS[15]	Pegcetacoplan	24-month, multicenter, randomized, double-masked, sham-controlled, phase 3 studies, patients with GA. Randomly assigned (2:2:1:1) to IVT 15 mg per 0.1 mL pegcetacoplan monthly or every other month, or sham monthly or every other month using stratified permuted block randomization	At 24 months, pegcetacoplan monthly and every other month slowed GA lesion growth by 22% and 18% in OAKS, and by 19% and 16% in DERBY, respectively, compared with sham. New-onset nAMD was reported in 11%, 8%, and 2% patients in OAKS and in 13%, 6%, and 4% patients in DERBY receiving pegcetacoplan monthly, every other month, and sham, respectively, at 24 months
	GATHER[18]	ACP	Randomized patients into 2 mg and 4 mg ACP with sham groups	The phase 3 trial showed 17.3% ($p = 0.0027$) reduction in mean change in GA lesion area compared to the sham arm at 1 year. There was a higher rate of CNV in patients treated with ACP compared to sham, 6.7% versus 4.1%
Neuroprotective agents	BEACON[20]	Brimonidine IVT implant	Patients were randomized to receive either 400 µg or sham, 3-monthly	There was a significant decrease in GA growth in the treated arm of 0.36 mm^2 ($p = 0.047$) and 0.52 mm^2 ($p = 0.017$) at months 24 and 30, respectively

Contd...

Contd...

Treatment modality	***Trial name***	***Drug tested***	***Treatment arms***	***Results***
Ocular gene therapy	OPTIC trial[28]	Ixoberogene soroparvovec, ADVM-22	Phase 1 multicenter randomized trial	Vision and CST remained stable throughout 2 years with annualized anti-VEGF injections reduced by 80% in 2×10^{11} vg/eye and 98% in 6×10^{11} vg/eye cohorts
	ATMOSPHERE trial[31]	*RGX-314*	Open-label, multiple-cohort, multicenter, phase 1/2a, dose-escalation study conducted at eight sites in the USA; participants with nAMD who have been previously treated with anti-VEGF injections were classified into five cohorts (with five different doses of *RGX-314*)	• Well tolerated with no clinically recognized immune responses. Asymptomatic pigmentary changes seen • Stable or improved BCVA and CST with few or no supplemental anti- VEGF-A injections in most participants
Stem cell therapy	(Phase 1/2): NCT0228608[37,38]	OpRegen	Open-label, single-arm, multicenter, dose-escalation trial evaluating a single administration of OpRegen delivered subretinally in patients with bilateral GA secondary to dry-form ARMD. Twenty-four patients were enrolled into four cohorts based on BCVA	• Well tolerated • 18% ERM formation, 12% RD • Imaging findings suggested presence of transplanted cells in the subretinal space

(ACP: avacincaptad pegol; AMD: age-related macular degeneration; BCVA: best-corrected visual acuity; CNV: choroidal neovascularization; CST: central subfield thickness; ERM: epiretinal membrane; GA: geographic atrophy; IVT: intravitreal; nAMD: neovascular AMD; RD: retinal detachment)

Twenty-four subjects were enrolled and divided into four cohorts. Positive safety indicators were observed, with no instances of inflammatory or immune responses reported. Additionally, patients demonstrated improved visual functions.[34]

The human-induced pluripotent stem cells (hiPSCs)-derived Eyecyte-RPE™, developed by Eyestem, aim to replace damaged or lost RPE cells and potentially enable tissue regeneration in the diseased retina.[35] Preclinical safety and efficacy studies with Eyecyte-RPE™ have demonstrated significant beneficial effects on the degenerating retina in animals, with no significant safety concerns. The phase 1/2a trial to evaluate the safety and efficacy of Eyecyte-RPE™ is currently underway.

ARTIFICIAL INTELLIGENCE

Machine-learning models to predict at baseline and treatment outcomes in patients with nAMD receiving anti-VEGF treatment like faricimab are being studied.[36] These models can help answer questions as to how many injections will be required, the prognosis, and so forth.

CONCLUSION

Drugs such as brolucizumab, faricimab, conbercept, and aflibercept 8 mg demonstrated stable BCVA with improvement in CST with less frequent dosages for the treatment of nAMD **(Table 11.1)**. Complement factor inhibition, gene therapy, and stem cell therapy are novel interventions to tackle GA **(Table 11.2)**.

ACKNOWLEDGMENT

The authors acknowledge the Rights Reprints and Licensing team at the *Indian Journal of Ophthalmology Case Reports*.

REFERENCES

1. Khan H, Aziz AA, Sulahria H, Sulahria H, Ahmed A, Choudhry N, et al. Emerging treatment options for geographic atrophy (GA) secondary to age-related macular degeneration. Clin Ophthalmol. 2023;17:321-7.
2. Nguyen QD, Das A, Do DV, Dugel PU, Gomes A, Holz FG, et al. Brolucizumab: evolution through preclinical and clinical studies and the implications for the management of neovascular age-related macular degeneration. Ophthalmology. 2020;127(7):963-76.
3. Tadayoni R, Sararols L, Weissgerber G, Verma R, Clemens A, Holz F. Brolucizumab: a newly developed anti-VEGF molecule for the treatment of neovascular age-related macular degeneration. Ophthalmologica. 2021;244:93-101.
4. Gaudreault J, Gunde T, Floyd HS, Ellis J, Tietz J, Binggeli D, et al. Preclinical pharmacology and safety of ESBA1008, a single-chain antibody fragment, investigated as potential treatment for age related macular degeneration. Invest Ophthalmol Vis Sci. 2012;53(14):3025.

5. Dugel PU, Koh A, Ogura Y, Jaffe GJ, Schmidt-Erfurth U, Brown DM, et al. HAWK and HARRIER study investigators. HAWK and HARRIER: phase 3, multicenter, randomized, double-masked trials of brolucizumab for neovascular age-related macular degeneration. Ophthalmology. 2020;127(1):72-84.
6. Chandra KK, Reddy NG, Narayanan R. Indocyanine green angiographic documentation of regression of polypoidal lesions after brolucizumab injection in polypoidal choroidal vasculopathy. Indian J Ophthalmol. 2023;3(3):764-6.
7. Pakravan P, Shaheen A, Chau V, Lai J, Patel V, Yannuzi N. Adverse events following intravitreal brolucizumab for exudative age-related macular degeneration. Invest Ophthalmol Vis Sci. 2022;63(7):1342.
8. Khanani AM, Patel SS, Ferrone PJ, Osborne A, Sahni J, Grzeschik S, et al. Efficacy of every four monthly and quarterly dosing of faricimab vs ranibizumab in neovascular age-related macular degeneration: the STAIRWAY phase 2 randomized clinical trial. JAMA Ophthalmol. 2020;138(9):964-72.
9. Heier JS, Khanani AM, Quezada CR, Basu K, Ferrone PJ, Brittain C, et al; TENAYA and LUCERNE Investigators. Efficacy, durability, and safety of intravitreal faricimab up to every 16 weeks for neovascular age-related macular degeneration (TENAYA and LUCERNE): two randomised, double-masked, phase 3, non-inferiority trials. Lancet. 2022;399(10326):729-40.
10. Khanani AM, Kotecha A, Chang A, Chen SJ, Chen Y, Guymer R, et al; TENAYA and LUCERNE Investigators. TENAYA and LUCERNE: two-year results from the phase 3 neovascular age-related macular degeneration trials of faricimab with treat-and-extend dosing in year 2. Ophthalmology. 2024;S0161-6420(24):00134-9.
11. Sahni J, Dugel PU, Patel SS, Chittum ME, Berger B, Del Valle Rubido M, et al. Safety and efficacy of different doses and regimens of faricimab vs ranibizumab in neovascular age-related macular degeneration: the AVENUE phase 2 randomized clinical trial. JAMA Ophthalmol. 2020;138(9):955-63.
12. Wang F, Bai Y, Yu W, Han N, Huang L, Zhao M, et al. Anti-angiogenic effect of KH902 on retinal neovascularization. Graefes Arch Clin Exp Ophthalmol. 2013;251(9):2131-9.
13. Liu K, Song Y, Xu G, Ye J, Wu Z, Liu X, et al; PHOENIX study group. Conbercept for treatment of neovascular age-related macular degeneration: results of the randomized phase PHOENIX study. Am J Ophthalmol. 2019;197:156-67.
14. Lanzetta P, Korobelnik JF, Heier JS, Leal S, Holz FG, Clark WL, et al; PULSAR Investigators. Intravitreal aflibercept 8 mg in neovascular age-related macular degeneration (PULSAR): 48-week results from a randomised, double-masked, non-inferiority, phase 3 trial. Lancet. 2024;403(10432):1141-52.
15. Liao DS, Grossi FV, El Mehdi D, Gerber MR, Brown DM, Heier JS, et al. Complement C3 inhibitor pegcetacoplan for geographic atrophy secondary to age-related macular degeneration: a randomized phase 2 trial. Ophthalmology. 2020;127(2):186-95.
16. Heier JS, Lad EM, Holz FG, Rosenfeld PJ, Guymer RH, Boyer D, et al; OAKS and DERBY study investigators. Pegcetacoplan for the treatment of geographic atrophy secondary to age-related macular degeneration (OAKS and DERBY): two multicentre, randomised, double-masked, sham-controlled, phase 3 trials. Lancet. 2023;402(10411):1434-48.
17. Goldberg R, HeieR JS, Wykoff CC, Staurenghi G, Singh RP, Steinle N, et al. Efficacy of intravitreal pegcetacoplan in patients with geographic atrophy (GA):

12-month results from the phase 3 OAKS and DERBY studies. Invest Ophthalmol Vis Sci. 2022;63(7):1500.

18. IVERIC bio. A phase 3 safety and efficacy study of intravitreal administration of Zimura (complement C5 inhibitor). ClinicalTrials.gov identifier:[online] Available from https://classic.clinicaltrials.gov/ct2/show/NCT04435366 [Last accessed September, 2024].
19. Khanani AM, Patel SS, Staurenghi G, Tadayoni R, Danzig CJ, Eichenbaum DA, et al; GATHER2 trial investigators. Efficacy and safety of avacincaptad pegol in patients with geographic atrophy (GATHER2): 12-month results from a randomised, double-masked, phase 3 trial. Lancet. 2023;402(10411):1449-58.
20. Doozandeh A, Yazdani S. Neuroprotection in glaucoma. J Ophthal Vis Res. 2016;11:209-20.
21. Kuppermann BD, Patel SS, Boyer DS, Augustin AJ, Freeman WR, Kerr KJ, et al; Brimo DDS Gen 1 Study Group. Phase 2 study of the safety and efficacy of brimonidine drug delivery system (brimo dds) generation 1 in patients with geographic atrophy secondary to age- related macular degeneration. Retina. 2021;41(1):144-55.
22. Freeman WR, Bandello F, Souied EH, Guymer RH, Garg S, Chen FK, et al. Lopez phase 2b study of brimonidine DDS: potential novel treatment for geography Vic atrophy. Invest Ophthalmol Vis Sci. 2019;60(9):971.
23. Williams BL, Seager NA, Gardiner JD, Pappas CM, Cronin MC, Amat di San Filippo C, et al. Chromosome 10q26-driven age-related macular degeneration is associated with reduced levels of HTRA1 in human retinal pigment epithelium. Proc Natl Acad Sci USA. 2021;118(30):e2103617118.
24. Cruz MA, Groman SL, Jimenez-Martınez MC. MicroRNAs as potential biomarkers and therapeutic targets in age-related macular degeneration. Front Ophthalmol. 2023;3:1023782.
25. Lauer AK, Campochiaro PA, Sohn EH, Kelleher M, Harrop R, Loader J, et al. Phase I safety and tolerability results for RetinoStat®, a lentiviral vector expressing endostatin and angiostatin, in patients with advanced neovascular age-related macular degeneration. Investig Ophthalmol Vis Sci. 2016;57(12).
26. Day TP, Byrne LC, Schaffer DV, Flannery JG. Advances in AAV vector development for gene therapy in the retina. Adv Exp Med Biol. 2014;801:687-93.
27. Bennett J, Wilson J, Sun D, Forbes B, Maguire A. Adenovirus vector-mediated in vivo gene transfer into adult murine retina. Invest Ophthalmol Vis Sci. 1994;35:2535-42.
28. Parks RJ, Chen L, Anton M, Sankar U, Rudnicki MA, Graham FL. A helper-dependent adenovirus vector system: removal of helper virus by Cre-mediated excision of the viral packaging signal. Proc Natl Acad Sci USA. 1996;93: 13565-70.
29. Khanani AM, Boyer DS, Wykoff CC, Regillo CD, Busbee BG, Pieramici D, et al. Safety and efficacy of ixoberogene soroparvovec in neovascular age-related macular degeneration in the United States (OPTIC): a prospective, two-year, multicentre phase 1 study. EClinical Med. 2023;67:102394.
30. Adverum Biotechnologies. Intravitreal gene therapy for DME(INFINITY); Adverum Biotechnologies, Inc. ClinicalTrials.gov ID NCT04418427; ADVM-022. [online] Available from https://classic.clinicaltrials.gov/ct2/show/NCT04418427 [Last accessed September, 2024].

31. AbbVie. Pivotal 1 study of *RGX-314* gene therapy in participants with nAMD (ATMOSPHERE). ClinicalTrials.gov ID NCT04704921. Available from https://classic.clinicaltrials.gov/ct2/show/NCT0470492 [Last accessed September, 2024].
32. Campochiaro PA, Avery R, Brown DM, Heier JS, Ho AC, Huddleston SM, et al. Gene therapy for neovascular age-related macular degeneration by subretinal delivery of RGX-314: a phase 1/2a dose-escalation study. Lancet. 2024; 403(10436):1563-73.
33. Khanani AM. Suprachoroidal delivery of *RGX-314* gene therapy for neovascular AMD: the phase II AAVIATE™ study. Invest Ophthalmol Vis Sci. 2022;63(7):1497.
34. Munk MR, Gonzalez V, Boyer DS, Rosen RB, Xavier S, Hu A, et al. LIGHTSITE III 24-month analysis: evaluation of multiwavelength photobiomodulation in dry age-related macular degeneration using the LumiThera Valeda light delivery system. Invest Ophthalmol Vis Sci. 2023;64(8):5059.
35. Eyestem Research. Safety and efficacy study of Eyecyte-RPE™ in patients with geographic atrophy secondary to dry age-related macular degeneration. clinicalTrials.gov identifier: NCT06394232. [online] Available from https://classic.clinicaltrials.gov/ct2/show/NCT0639423 [Last accessed September, 2024].
36. Kikuchi Y, Kawczynski MG, Anegondi N, Neubert A, Dai J, Ferrara D, et al. Machine learning to predict faricimab treatment outcome in neovascular age-related macular degeneration. Ophthalmol Sci. 2023;4(2):100385.
37. Hoffmann-La Roche. Safety and efficacy study of OpRegen for treatment of advanced dry-form age-related macular degeneration. clinicalTrials.gov identifier: NCT02286089. [online] Available from https://classic.clinicaltrials.gov/ct2/show/NCT02286089 [Last accessed September, 2024].
38. Ho AC, Banin E, Barak A, Boyer DS, Ehrlicj R, Jouni T, et al. Safety and efficacy of a phase 1/2a clinical trial of transplanted allogeneic retinal pigmented epithelium (RPE, OpRegen) cells in advanced dry age-related macular degeneration (AMD). Invest Ophthalmol Vis Sci. 2022;63(7):1862.

12 CHAPTER

Diagnosis and Management of Diabetic Macular Edema

Samya Singh, Shilpi Arya, Sandeep Saxena

ABSTRACT

Worldwide, approximately 93 million people suffer from diabetic retinopathy (DR), of which 21 million have treatable diabetic macular edema (DME). Elevated blood sugar levels cause a disruption in the blood–retinal barrier, which leads to DME. Ellipsoid zone (EZ) disruption happens when the external limiting membrane (ELM) loses its barrier function. Since vascular endothelial growth factor (VEGF) is essential to the pathophysiology of DME, anti-VEGFs are the recommended course of treatment. Research has demonstrated a relationship between enhanced optical coherence tomography (OCT) biomarkers and better visual results. Anti-VEGF treatments and OCT-based measures show promise in treating DME and improving our knowledge of this blinding illness.

Keywords: Diabetic retinopathy, diabetic macular edema, ellipsoid zone, external limiting membrane, retinal pigment epithelium, spectral domain-optical coherence tomography, disorganization of retinal inner layers

INTRODUCTION

Globally, diabetic retinopathy (DR) impacts approximately 93 million individuals, with around 21 million among them experiencing treatable forms of diabetic macular edema (DME) **(Fig. 12.1)**.[1] Within the realm of DR, DME exhibits a prevalence ranging from 11 to 15%,[1-3] standing as the primary contributor to vision impairment.[4] Among those affected, roughly 20% of patients with Type 1 diabetes mellitus (DM) and 14–25% of those with Type 2 DM are influenced by DME.[5]

Persistently elevated blood sugar sets off a series of chemical changes that ultimately result in the blood–retinal barrier being compromised, which opens the door to DME. Vascular endothelial growth factor (VEGF) is a key player in the pathophysiology of DME. Anti-VEGFs have consequently become the gold standard for treating DME **(Figs. 12.2A and B)**. Spectral-domain optical coherence tomography (SD-OCT) is a powerful tool that allows for the accurate distinction and detailed viewing of retinal layers. Making use of it, a range of OCT-based biomarkers have been used to predict the course of treatment for patients with DME receiving intravitreal anti-VEGFs.

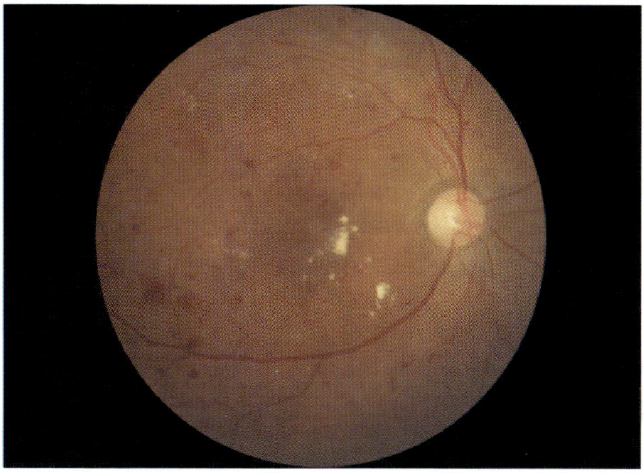

Fig. 12.1: Fundus image showing nonproliferative diabetic retinopathy changes with diabetic macular edema.

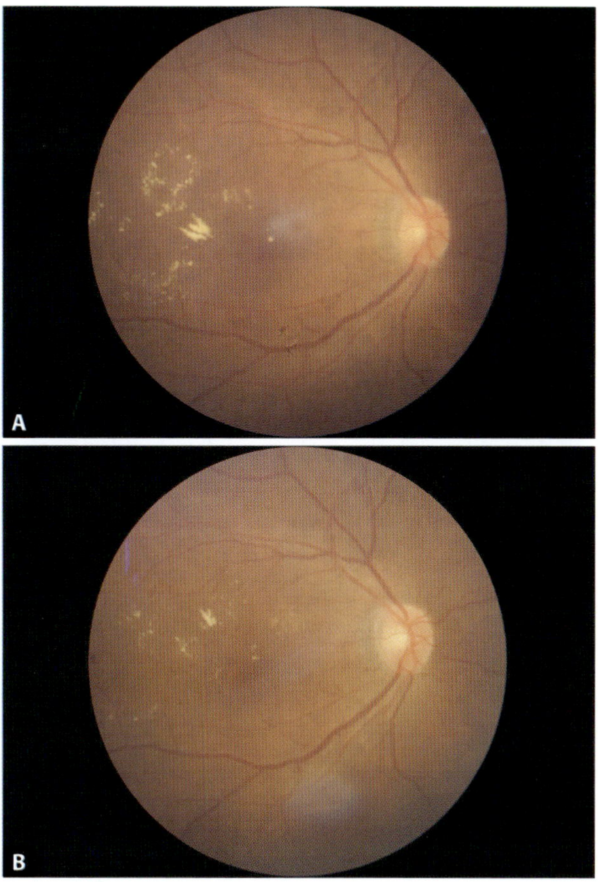

Figs. 12.2A and B: (A) Fundus image showing diabetic macular edema; (B) Fundus image showing resolving diabetic macular edema post anti-VEGF injection. (VEGF: vascular endothelial growth factor)

SPECTRAL DOMAIN-OPTICAL COHERENCE TOMOGRAPHY: ROLE IN THE ASSESSMENT OF RETINAL MORPHOLOGY

Optical coherence tomography is a noninvasive imaging method that provides cross-sectional, topographical, and three-dimensional retinal imaging, providing an in vivo view of retinal histology. Ten distinct layers make up the human retina, which are generally divided into inner and outer retinal layers. Three hyper-reflective bands are prominently identified in the outer retinal region by SD-OCT, and they are important because of their crucial involvement in retinal function.

The International Nomenclature for OCT (IN-OCT) Panel developed a nomenclature to describe the different hypo- and hyper-reflective layers seen on SD-OCT in order to promote the characterization of these layers.[6] This nomenclature demarcates specific zones **(Table 12.1)**.

Spaide et al. conducted a retrospective analysis of scientific literature and publications concerning the histology of the outer retina. Their study concluded that the SD-OCT bands linked to the external limiting membrane (ELM), positioned as the innermost band, and the retinal pigment epithelium (RPE), positioned as the outermost band, were indeed accurately designated. However, they found that the second band, often associated with the division between the inner and outer segments of photoreceptors, in reality, corresponds to the ellipsoid part of the inner segments. The third band was identified as corresponding to the enveloping of the cone's outer segments by the apical processes of the RPE, forming a structure known as the *contact cylinder*.[7]

It is possible to identify ultrastructural alterations in the retina during the early stages of the disease by using biomarkers derived from SD-OCT. The grading of these biomarkers can be correlated with the severity of DME and is an important factor in determining treatment approaches.

Reliable estimations for DME screening can be obtained by applying SD-OCT-based measures, such as cube average thickness (CAT) and macular central subfield thickness (CST).[8] Numerous investigations have demonstrated the relationship between visual acuity in DME and retinal thickness determined by OCT.[8-11]

As substitute indicators for determining the disease severity, CST and CAT are useful. Using these imaging biomarkers for targeted DME screening in a population is a useful indicator of disease progression across various grades of retinopathy, especially in cases where it is not evident clinically.[12] Notably, elevated CST and CAT values are associated with a higher probability of ellipsoid zone (EZ) disruption, indicating that these parameters function as bio-imaging markers for EZ disruption in DME.[13] In cases with center-involving-DME (CI-DME), disarray within the foveal retinal inner layers and

TABLE 12.1: International nomenclature for optical coherence tomography (IN-OCT).

Layer number	*OCT description*	*Nomenclature by consensus*
1	Hyper-reflective	Posterior cortical vitreous
2	Hyporeflective	Preretinal space
3	Hyper-reflective	Nerve fiber layer
4	Hyporeflective	GCL
5	Hyper-reflective	IPL
6	Hyporeflective	INL
7	Hyper-reflective	OPL
8	Hyporeflective	*Inner half:* Henle's nerve fiber layer; *outer half:* ONL
9	Hyper-reflective	ELM
10	Hyporeflective	Myoid zone of photoreceptors
11	Hyper-reflective	EZ of photoreceptors
12	Hyporeflective	Outer segments of photoreceptors
13	Hyper-reflective	Cone interdigitation with RPE
14	Hyper-reflective band	RPE/Bruch's membrane complex. On occasion, this can be separated into more than one band
15	A thin layer of moderate reflectivity in the inner choroid	Choriocapillaris
16	A thick layer of round- or oval-shaped hyper-reflective profiles with hyper-reflective cores in the mid-choroid	Sattler's layer
17	A thick layer of oval-shaped hyper-reflective profiles with hyper-reflective cores in the outer choroid	Haller's layer
18	Zone at the outer choroid with a marked change in texture, in which large circular or ovoid profiles abut a homogenous region of variable reflectivity	Choroidal–Scleral juncture

(ELM: external limiting membrane; EZ: ellipsoid zone; GCL: ganglion cell layer; INL: inner nuclear layer; IPL: inner plexiform layer; OCT: optical coherence tomography; ONL: outer nuclear layer; OPL: outer plexiform layer; RPE: retinal pigment epithelium)

disruption of the photoreceptors' ELM are crucial SD-OCT-based imaging markers for predicting visual outcomes.

Parallelism: A Novel Parameter

A novel parameter, called "parallelism," has been proposed for assessing retinal layer integrity using SD-OCT. Utilizing skeletonization, this technique examines the orientation of segmented lines, or "parallelism," inside OCT pictures. This measure is used to categorize the condition of the photoreceptor layer at the fovea, which includes the continuity of the ELM, the inner segment of the EZ, and the existence of hyper-reflective foci in the outer retinal layers. When comparing the parallelism of eyes with DME to normal eyes, a significant difference is observed. It also shows a favorable relationship with visual acuity. Comparing eyes with an intact EZ or ELM to eyes with a disrupted or nonexistent EZ or ELM, the former exhibits much higher visual acuity and stronger parallelism. This innovative "parallelism" parameter emerges as a potential biomarker, holding promise for predicting visual outcomes in cases of DME.[14]

BASIC CONSIDERATIONS FOR INNER AND OUTER RETINAL LAYERS

The inner layers of retina include a ganglion cell layer–inner plexiform layer (GCL–IPL) complex, an inner nuclear layer (INL), and an outer plexiform layer (OPL).

The outer layers of retina include ELM, EZ, and RPE:

- ELM is the innermost hyper-reflective band, composed of junctional complexes connecting Muller cells and photoreceptors.[15] This band is generally thinner and less pronounced compared to the surrounding bands. Functionally, the ELM acts as a boundary, separating the layers of rods and cones from the outer nuclear layer (ONL) above while simultaneously providing a barrier against macromolecules.
- EZ, the next discernible band, represents the demarcation between the inner and outer segments of the photoreceptors, closely corresponding to the ellipsoid segment within the inner segments.[16] Photoreceptors are made up of an inner segment that carries out essential metabolic functions including protein synthesis and energy production and an outer segment that is in charge of absorbing light and converting it into electrical impulses.
- RPE is the outermost band, which has a high reflectivity and contains Bruch's membrane, the RPE, and potentially the choriocapillaris to RPE is the outermost band, which has a high reflectivity.[17,18] The RPE, which is the pigmented cell layer located just outside the neurosensory retina, is essential for maintaining the retinal visual cells. It remains firmly attached to both the surrounding retinal vision cells and the underlying choroid. The RPE is made up of a single layer of hexagon-shaped cells that are densely packed with pigment granules. It performs a number of vital tasks, including immune response control, phagocytosis, light absorption, epithelial transport, and spatial ion buffering.

The behavior of the ELM and EZ was explored through OCT examination in brown Norwegian rats. It has been shown that the EZ and ELM disappeared following euthanasia. The origin of these structures is linked to the biological activities of the photoreceptor cells.[19]

INNER RETINAL LAYERS IN DIABETIC MACULAR EDEMA

Vascular lesions and apparent thickening of the sensory retina are frequent in the clinical setting of DME. Histological studies have shown that cystoid spaces are mostly found in the OPL and INL, which may be partially responsible for the macular thickening that has been seen.[20-22] The intricate mechanism of DME is further revealed by electron microscopy, which also reveals the intracytoplasmic swelling of Müller cells and the accumulation of extracellular fluid. OCT imaging reveals a variety of foveal morphologies associated with DME, including sponge-like diffuse retinal swelling, serous retinal detachment (SRD), and cystoid macular edema (CME).[23] Within the retinal layers, each of these unique lesions has been described. For instance, cystoid spaces predominantly manifest in the INL and OPL, while SRD involves the pooling of extracellular fluid between the outer segments and the RPE.[24,25] Sponge-like retinal swelling localized at the fovea is observed in the OPL.

Another factor that leads to macular thickening in DME is vitreomacular traction.[26,27] Notably, as seen in cases of idiopathic epiretinal membrane (ERM), pathological alterations in the vitreomacular interface frequently occur at the same time as sponge-like retinal swelling.[28] The thickening of the retinal parenchyma within the OPL at the fovea is a result of anomalies in the vitreomacular interface. As in the case of idiopathic macular holes, OCT occasionally reveals cystoid spaces in addition to vitreoretinal abnormalities. It has also been observed that anomalies affecting the vitreomacular interface may also cause SRD in DME.[29,30]

The inability to discriminate between the GCL–IPL complex, the INL, and the OPL, which are the limits of the inner retinal layers, is referred to as *disorganization of retinal inner layers (DRIL)*. DRIL is not considered to be present if intraretinal cysts develop in the OPL and cause an overall thickness of the retina while maintaining discernible inner retinal layers. If the loss of retinal layer boundaries is not present, the absence of the typical foveal contour does not alone suggest DRIL. Interestingly, foveal DRIL, or DRIL affecting at least 50% of the central 1-mm wide zone focused on the fovea, is linked to worse visual acuity. This is still the case when edema resolution does not improve vision or, in the opposite situation, when edema is present but vision is still good.[31]

Additional histology research is necessary to clarify the precise processes by which DRIL affects vision. The disruption-induced incapacity to distinguish retinal layer boundaries appears to indicate a structural break in the visual transmission system. It has been hypothesized that this disruption happens when bipolar axons break because edema causes them to exceed their elasticity limit.[10] In essence, DRIL refers to the disorder or death of bipolar, amacrine, or horizontal cells found in the inner layers of the retina. It is an indication of a disruption in the pathways that carry visual information from photoreceptors to ganglion cells.

OUTER LAYERS OF RETINA IN DIABETIC MACULAR EDEMA

The complex pathophysiology of DR encompasses multiple molecular pathways that are impacted by metabolic disruptions. Persistent hyperglycemia causes protein glycosylation, which results in the production of advanced glycation end products (AGEs). These AGEs affect the metabolism of calcium and vitamin D, the retinal microvasculature, VEGF, intercellular adhesion molecule-1 (ICAM-1), nitrosative and oxidative stress, and more.

Proangiogenic factors are released when endothelial dysfunction is triggered by the activation of AGEs and their receptors. This cascade damages the retinal vascular components by inducing pericyte death, vascular inflammation, and angiogenesis.[32,33] This ultimately results in fluid leakage and buildup, which is known as *DME*. Furthermore, in RPE cells and retinal pericytes, AGEs increase VEGF expression.[34] Interaction between photoreceptors and the RPE is essential for a healthy retina. It is acknowledged that preserving the ELM is necessary to preserve the integrity of the EZ.[35] Notably, DME and the disruption of EZ and ELM are related.[36,37]

Based on animal models, the ELM is made up of the glial Müller cells' outer processes that link them to inner photoreceptor segments.[38] Tight connections between glial Müller cells and photoreceptors are seen in the ELM, and occludin has been found to be an essential element. Glial Müller cells at the ELM level enlarge and lose their occludin content in patients with DME. Therefore, ELM junctions may be specifically targeted for treatment as distinct regulatory sites. Vascular permeability can be increased and tight junctions can be disrupted by VEGF. Murakami et al. have highlighted the importance of occludin in controlling endothelial barrier characteristics.[39]

The EZ serves as a clinical indicator of photoreceptor integrity. It is mostly made up of mitochondria in a biological sense, which allow photoreceptors to use more energy.[40] Mitochondrial impairment in the foveal photoreceptors is a common feature of DME. The anatomical lack of EZ or decreased reflectivity is associated with the absence of subfoveal EZ on SD-OCT.

Research showcasing early-stage retinal degeneration in experimental diabetes has brought attention to RPE morphological alterations.[41] In the diabetic retina, oxidative stress plays a role in the oxidation of glycated proteins and lipid peroxidation (LPO).[42] It has been demonstrated that nitrosative and oxidative stresses are related to alterations in the retinal photoreceptor

EZ and RPE topography.[43] Research conducted through experiments has demonstrated that the interaction between RPE and endothelial cells leads to a VEGF-mediated loss of RPE barrier function. The progression of DR depends critically on the balance between VEGF and the antiangiogenic factor pigment epithelium-derived factor (PEDF), which is released by RPE.[44] The VEGF that is released by the RPE is essential for preserving the choriocapillaris and outer retina's structural integrity.

The production of ICAM-1 is triggered by retinal VEGF, and this results in leukostasis and the disruption of the blood–retinal barrier.[45] The relationship between VEGF and ICAM-1 and the disruption of the ELM and EZ were illustrated by Jain et al.[35] AGEs cause oxidative stress, which, in turn, causes thrombogenic and inflammatory responses. Under diabetic conditions, mitochondrial superoxide generation affects the formation and accumulation of AGEs.[46] Sharma et al. discovered a connection between the disturbance of ELM and EZ and nitric oxide (NO) and oxidative stress in DR.[43] ELM and EZ dysfunction in DME is linked to elevated serum antimyeloperoxidase antibody levels.[47] Diabetes-related metabolic disturbances lead to a weakened nutritional state. ELM and EZ dysfunction is linked to vitamin D deficiency.[48] Furthermore, vitamin D is essential for maintaining calcium homeostasis. Retinal photoreceptor apoptosis is triggered by elevated serum ionized calcium levels, which, in turn, causes the breakdown of ELM and EZ in DR.[49]

EFFECT OF OUTER LAYERS OF RETINA ON VISUAL FUNCTION IN DIABETIC MACULAR EDEMA

The ELM and EZ integrity is essential for the maintenance of normal vision. Many cross-sectional or longitudinal studies have shown the clinical importance of both layers in DME. The length of the disrupted or absent EZ has been associated with visual impairment.[50] DME is known to be associated with the disruption of ELM and EZ, which, in turn, affects vision. An increase in VEGF and ICAM-1 levels correlates with increased macular thickness (CST), sequential disruption of ELM and EZ, and an increase in the severity of DME.[35] EZ disruption is found to be significantly associated with the severity of retinopathy. RPE, which forms the outer retinal barrier, in turn, maintains the nutrition and normal physiology of photoreceptors and inner retinal layers. The RPE alterations (RPE-A) have been reported to be associated with the severity of DME and a decrease in visual acuity.[51]

Blood flow to adjacent retinal capillaries is increased due to retinal ischemia, increasing vessel wall shear stress.[52] Capillary closure and alterations in the rheological properties of blood also result in increased shear stress. Locking of the vessel occurs due to increased glycation and thickening of the basement membrane.[53] Also in the presence of a dilated vasculature, the systemic blood pressure is more easily transmitted to the microcirculation, resulting in increased capillary pressure. As a result, shear stress in the vessel wall increases as the vessel diameter is unable to change, leading to mechanical injury to the vascular endothelium. This circumferential stress resulting in mechanical damage to the endothelium is directly proportional to the perfusion pressure and radius of the vessel wall and inversely proportional to the thickness of the vessel wall.[54] Hence, circumferential stress damage occurs more on vessels with larger diameters, resulting in further dilatation of the vessel. The tension resisting the circumferential stress in the vessel wall has an inverse relationship with the radius of the vessel; as a result, tension to counteract circumferential stress is not attained in a dilated vessel, and, therefore, there is a tendency toward dilatation with consequent hyperperfusion.

Additionally, several other factors resulting in hyperperfusion are abnormal autoregulation of the retinal circulation, increased conductance as an autoregulatory response to retinal ischemia, endothelin-1 resistance, inhibition of calcium influx channel in smooth muscle cells, and increased activity of NO synthase.[55,56] As these changes occur in retinal vasculature, the resistive index (RI) increases.

Retinal pigment epithelium is essential for the maintenance and survival of the overlying photoreceptor cells and thereby sustains the structural and functional integrity of EZ. It is also involved in the regulation of the integrity of the choroidal capillaries.[57,58] RPE is necessary for the maintenance of photoreceptor excitability by stabilizing ion composition in the subretinal space,[59] phagocytosis of shed photoreceptor outer segments,[57] and rebuilding light-sensitive outer segments from the base of the photoreceptors. Moreover, the structural integrity of choriocapillaris endothelium and photoreceptors is maintained by a variety of growth factors secreted by RPE. These growth factors function in both endothelial cell differentiation and photoreceptor differentiation.[60,61] Thus, RPE is essential for visual function and the development of retinal structures. Failure of any one of these functions can lead to degeneration of the retina, loss of visual function, and blindness. RPE cells are dependent on the choroid for their metabolic needs. Khatri et al.[62] showed that the RI of the ophthalmic artery (OA) and central retinal artery (CRA) increases the severity of DR. As a result, the choroidal blood supply is hampered due to a lack of autoregulation. Thus, an increase in the RI of OA also impairs the blood supply of RPE, resulting in structural changes expressed as topographical alterations in RPE on SD-OCT. Alterations in RPE correlate with EZ disruption. Our earlier studies have shown a negative correlation between grades of EZ disruption and visual acuity.[50]

Inner and outer retinal layer grading systems in DME:

DRIL has been graded as follows:[63]

- *Grade 0:* DRIL absent
- *Grade 1:* DRIL present

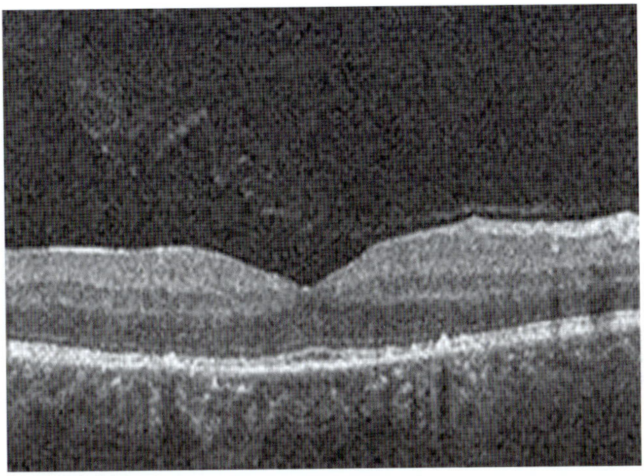

Fig. 12.3: SD-OCT image. Grade 0: External limiting membrane and ellipsoid zone are intact. (SD-OCT: spectral-domain optical coherence tomography)

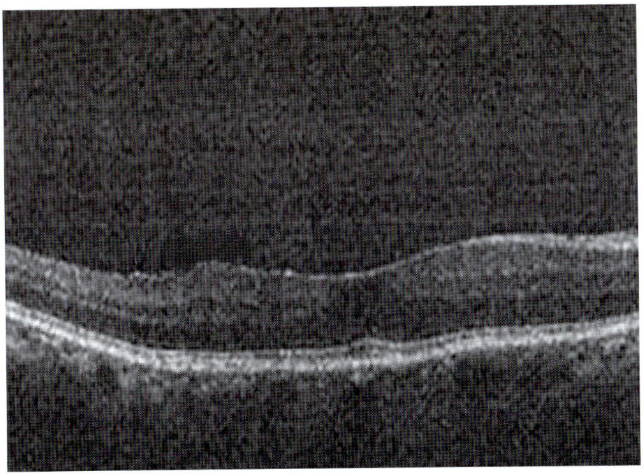

Fig. 12.4: SD-OCT image. Grade 1: Subfoveal disruption of the external limiting membrane with an intact ellipsoid zone. (SD-OCT: spectral-domain optical coherence tomography)

The severity of DR, EZ disruption, and retinal nerve fiber layer (RNFL) thinning can be correlated with the presence of DRIL.

The disruption of ELM and EZ has been graded as per our published classification:

- *Grade 0:* ELM and EZ not disrupted
- *Grade 1:* ELM disrupted, EZ intact
- *Grade 2:* ELM and EZ both disrupted

This grading system is user-friendly for physicians, has good repeatability, and aids in illness prognosis.

Ellipsoid zone disruption **(Figs. 12.3 to 12.5)** has been graded as follows:[64]

- *Grade 0:* Intact EZ

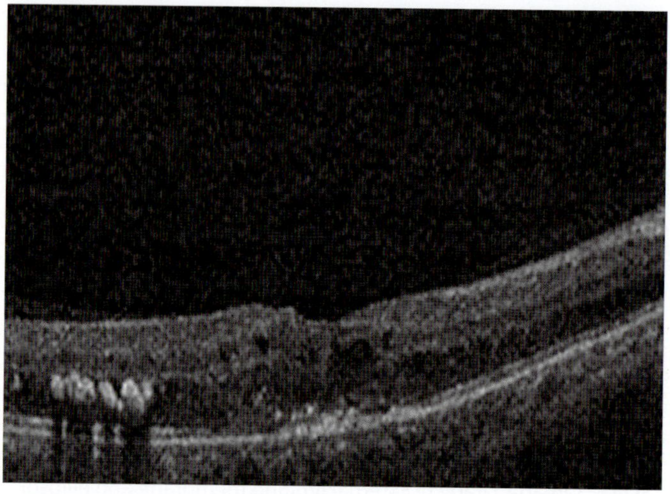

Fig. 12.5: SD-OCT image. Grade 2: Subfoveal disruption of the external limiting membrane and the ellipsoid zone. There are associated cystic changes and hard exudates suggested by the hyper-reflective foci. The foveal contour is lost. (SD-OCT: spectral-domain optical coherence tomography)

- *Grade 1:* Subfoveal focal disruption
- *Grade 2:* Global disruption of EZ involving the macular cube

The grades of RPE-A are assessed using single-layer RPE (SL-RPE) map as follows:

- *Grade 0:* No alterations
- *Grade 1:* Two-quadrant alteration
- *Grade 2:* More than two-quadrant alteration

EFFECT OF ANTIVASCULAR ENDOTHELIAL GROWTH FACTOR THERAPY ON INNER AND OUTER RETINAL LAYERS IN DIABETIC MACULAR EDEMA

The mainstay of care for DME is anti-VEGF therapy. The cornerstone of DME management is now these agents. Aptamers like pegaptanib, VEGF-specific antibodies like bevacizumab, VEGF-specific antibody fragments like ranibizumab, and fusion proteins like aflibercept and conbercept, which are a fusion of VEGF receptor with an immunoglobulin Fc fragment, are among the variety of anti-VEGF medications available. While antibodies and fusion proteins attach to all VEGF-A isoforms, the fusion proteins additionally bind VEGF-B and placental growth factor. Given their higher affinity for VEGF, fusion proteins hold the potential for reduced injection frequency in DME treatment.[65,66] Bevacizumab, approved by the Food and Drug Administration (FDA) for advanced solid cancers, is commonly employed off-label for DME due to its cost-effectiveness when compared to FDA-approved ocular anti-VEGF drugs.[67] Ziv-aflibercept, a systemically formulated aflibercept with higher osmolarity, is an alternative.[68] The first anti-VEGF drug for DME, pegaptanib, selectively blocked the 165-isoform of VEGF but yielded superior outcomes with agents that target all VEGF isoforms.[69] The efficacy of ranibizumab and aflibercept was established through randomized controlled trials in 2010 and 2014, respectively.[70,71] A comparative study involving these drugs in CI-DME with good visual acuity showed no disparity in efficacy after 1 or 2 years of follow-up. However, for patients with poor visual acuity, aflibercept outperformed ranibizumab and bevacizumab after 1 year while maintaining superiority over bevacizumab at the 2-year mark.[72]

As previously discussed, ELM junctions hold unique potential as treatment targets.[38] Murakami et al. demonstrated VEGF treatment-induced phosphorylation, ubiquitination, and fragmentation of tight junction protein occludin in primary bovine retinal endothelial cells, implying its role in barrier regulation and therapeutic potential.[39]

Our prior SD-OCT-based study highlights an association between increased VEGF levels and the severity of DME, coupled with sequential disruptions of ELM and EZ. This underscores the importance of an intact ELM for an intact EZ in DME.[35,37] De et al. shed light on ELM and EZ restoration following anti-VEGF therapy, with the barrier effect of ELM being restored first, followed by EZ restoration.[73] Hence, our research group has established ELM as a novel structural retinal barrier besides the already-known blood–retinal barriers.

Intervention induced an improvement in SD-OCT biomarkers, such as DRIL, ELM, and EZ **(Figs. 12.6A to C)**. The relevance of DRIL as a predictor of visual acuity in DME has been suggested.[74] There is a direct relationship between the amelioration of DRIL and visual acuity improvement. The correlation of DRIL with EZ disruption indicates its potential involvement in interrupting the transmission pathway between ganglion cells and photoreceptors, ultimately decreasing the vision.[75] Anti-VEGF therapy ameliorates DRIL, thereby re-establishing synaptic connections, promoting impulse transmission from photoreceptors, and enhancing visual acuity. A similar pattern emerged regarding ELM and EZ disruption in DME. The extent of EZ disruption correlates with vision in DME. ELM and EZ integrity are positive predictors for visual outcomes, with EZ integrity having the strongest impact.[76,77] Our prior work has established ELM as the primary structural retinal barrier.[78]

Intravitreal anti-VEGF administration correlates with decreased CST and improved vision.[79,80] Foveal photoreceptor restoration after intravitreal ranibizumab administration in DME has been demonstrated.[40] Notably, reductions in CST and CAT were significant post-anti-VEGF treatment.[72,81] A connection has been established between the magnitude of CST reduction in various treatment regimens and improved visual outcomes.[70]

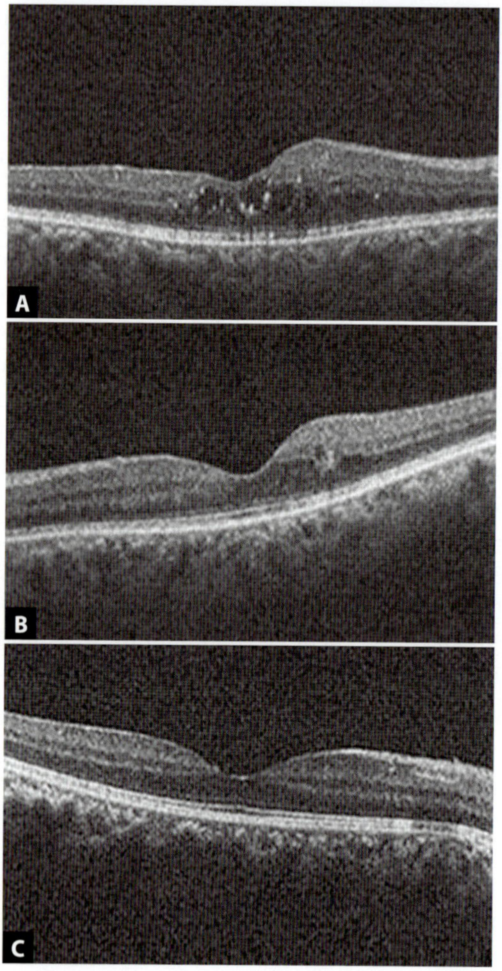

Figs. 12.6A to C: (A) SD-OCT image (pretreatment) shows global disruption of the ellipsoid zone within the macular cube. DRIL can be seen along with cystic changes and hard exudates; (B) SD-OCT image (1 month after ranibizumab injection) shows focal subfoveal disruption of the ellipsoid zone. Associated hard exudates can be seen temporally; (C) SD-OCT image (3 months after ranibizumab injection): DRIL resolved and the external limiting membrane and ellipsoid zone restored. Few hard exudates can be seen temporally. (DRIL: disorganization of retinal inner layers; SD-OCT: spectral-domain optical coherence tomography)

Hareedy et al. noted that photoreceptor integrity enhancement occurs after the second and third ranibizumab doses, correlating with improved visual acuity and color vision. Best-corrected visual acuity improvement aligns with EZ recovery after the second and third injections. Restoration of foveal photoreceptor microstructure following anti-VEGF therapy is linked with visual improvement.[82] Larger foveal photoreceptor microstructure defects correlate with lower vision. Chatziralli et al. also observed substantial EZ photoreceptor restoration in patients with DME after intravitreal ranibizumab treatment over 12 months.[83]

Intravitreal anti-VEGF therapy exhibits an association with improved RPE-A grades and consequently improved vision.[84] Functional RPE with intact tight junctions is crucial for regulated fluid removal from the subretinal space.[85] RPE-secreted growth factors maintain structural integrity for choriocapillaris, endothelium, and photoreceptors, vital for endothelial and photoreceptor differentiation.[61] RPE plays a pivotal role in maintaining photoreceptor excitability by stabilizing ion composition.[59] It also facilitates outer segment shedding through phagocytosis and rebuilding light-sensitive outer segments.[86] Additionally, RPE functions as a major VEGF secretor. Increased VEGF levels result in RPE proliferation, implying that elevated VEGF in DR coincides with increased RPE-A.[87] Anti-VEGF therapy reduces RPE-A grades, ultimately influencing CST and logMAR visual acuity reduction.

By comparing three intravitreal anti-VEGF medicines, the Diabetic Retinopathy Clinical Research Network (DRCR.net) Protocol T conducted a ground-breaking study on the management of DME. In this study, the safety and effectiveness of aflibercept, bevacizumab, and ranibizumab were compared. With a primary goal of change in visual acuity at 1 year, 0.05 mL of 2 mg aflibercept, 1.25 mg bevacizumab, or 0.3 mg ranibizumab was administered to masked individuals. Follow-up was scheduled for 2 years and recalled at 5 years. Based on the results of the OCT and vision tests, a modified pro re nata protocol served as the treatment plan. Participants received monthly injections for the first 6 months unless their OCT central thickness was better than the qualifying level and their visual acuity was 20/20 or above. The mean visual acuity decreased over 2 and 5 years, despite the mean retinal thickness being similar.[88]

The following anti-VEGFs are commercially available:

- *Ranibizumab* (Lucentis, Genentech, Inc., CA, USA) is a Fab fragment of the humanized monoclonal antibody (48 kDa) with affinity to all isoforms of VEGF.
- *Aflibercept* (Eylea, Regeneron Pharmaceuticals, NY, USA), which was approved by the FDA in 2011, is a soluble fusion protein that has an extracellular VEGF-binding domain derived from the VEGF receptors 1 and 2 and acts by blocking the biological effect of VEGF. It has an increased affinity for VEGF-A, VEGF-B, and placental growth factors 1 and 2. It also has a much higher VEGF-binding affinity than ranibizumab, which can last up to 10–12 weeks, double the period of bevacizumab and ranibizumab.
- *Brolucizumab* (Beovu, Novartis, Basel, Switzerland) is a single-chain variable fragment, which is a fusion protein of the variable regions of

the heavy and light chain regions of immunoglobulins. The single-chain fragment variable is the smallest functional unit of an antibody, the Fv region. The small fragments can penetrate tissue more rapidly and evenly. Because it lacks the Fc region, brolucizumab has a molecular weight of 26 kDa, allowing for a higher molar dosing. Brolucizumab binds VEGF-A in a 2:1 ratio and has been shown to have a higher binding affinity to VEGF-A isoforms than bevacizumab or ranibizumab.[89]

- *Faricimab* (Vabysmo™, Genentech, San Francisco, CA) is a combined-mechanism medication with simultaneous and independent binding on both VEGF-A and angiopoietin-2 (Ang-2). It has been approved for the treatment of DME by the FDA, USA, in 2022.

IMPORTANT BIOMOLECULAR BIOMARKERS AFFECTING THE INNER AND OUTER RETINAL LAYERS

As a fat-soluble vitamin, vitamin D has several functions in DME, including anti-inflammatory, antioxidant, and antiangiogenic effects.[90,91] The retinal GCL, IPL, INL, OPL, ONL, and photoreceptor layers are among the retinal layers that contain vitamin D receptors (VDRs).[92] The expression of micro RNA (mRNA) and protein for every component involved in the synthesis and metabolism of vitamin D3 is particularly evident in the mature ARPE-19. There is a strong correlation between reduced serum vitamin D levels and the severity of DME.[93,94] Serum vitamin D levels are found to be significantly correlated with measures, such as CST, CAT, DRIL, grades of EZ disruption, and RPE-A. Furthermore, there is a positive correlation between reduced serum vitamin D levels and visual acuity.[48]

Increased macular CST, progressive disruption of the ELM and EZ, and greater severity of DME are all correlated with elevated VEGF and ICAM-1 levels.[35]

According to Mishra et al., there is a correlation between elevated N(ε)-(carboxymethyl)lysine (CML) levels and more severe DR, DME, and structural changes such as ELM and EZ disruption in the macula, which may have predictive significance for visual outcomes.[95]

Increased plasma NO levels have been linked to increased DR severity, as shown by Sharma et al. Their research demonstrated that in vivo structural alterations seen in the EZ and RPE correspond with elevated plasma levels of NO and LPO, as well as decreased levels of glutathione (GSH).[43]

In DME, serum urea and creatinine levels serve as stand-in indicators for the disruption of retinal photoreceptor ELM and EZ.[37]

Furthermore, an escalation in the RI of OA and CRA corresponds with the severity of DR, grades of RPE-A, and disruptions in the EZ.[62]

ROLE OF OPTICAL COHERENCE TOMOGRAPHY-ANGIOGRAPHY

Advancements in OCT-angiography (OCT-A) technology have significantly deepened our comprehension of retinal vasculature in DME. The extent of recovery in the ELM and EZ has shown a robust correlation with the initial state of the deep capillary plexus vascular density (DCP VD) and the foveal avascular zone (FAZ) in the baseline. Those who positively respond to anti-VEGF treatment exhibit stronger baseline integrity of the DCP and notably greater photoreceptor recovery. The degree of DCP preservation during the initial resolution of DME is closely associated with the sustained recuperation of photoreceptor integrity and eventual visual outcomes among patients whose DME has been resolved.[96]

ARTIFICIAL INTELLIGENCE AND DIABETIC RETINOPATHY: THE FUTURE

Artificial intelligence (AI) rooted in deep learning (DL) has garnered substantial global attention in recent times. Its potential is gradually extending to the realm of healthcare, including ophthalmology. In this field, DL techniques have been successfully applied to interpret fundus photographs, OCT, and visual fields. These applications have demonstrated robust capabilities in classifying conditions such as DR, retinopathy of prematurity, glaucoma-like disk appearance, macular edema, and age-related macular degeneration. DL's incorporation into ocular imaging holds the promise of synergizing with telemedicine, offering a viable strategy to screen, diagnose, and monitor prevalent eye diseases among patients in primary care and community settings.

Singh et al.[97] developed a tool that can assist in screening for DRIL in both research and clinical decision-making settings. Creating a DL algorithm to detect DRIL in DME opens up distinctive possibilities. DRIL's link to poorer visual prognosis underscores the significance of identifying it in patients, potentially within OCT screening initiatives. This approach could aid in pinpointing individuals who would gain from early intervention and referral to specialized retinal care. Additionally, incorporating DRIL identification into the baseline assessment during clinical trials holds importance, serving to categorize patients according to their prognosis. Given that manually grading DRIL is laborious and time-intensive, automation has the potential to facilitate extensive investigations into the connections between DRIL development and treatment response through large-scale studies.

CONCLUSION

With SD-OCT, we have an unparalleled chance to investigate the complex in vivo histology of retinal layers and explore the morphological changes that take place in each layer in DME. DME causes complex structural changes, including DRIL, disruption of EZ and ELM, and changes in the RPE, all of which add up to a visual impairment. The administration of anti-VEGF contributes to the restoration of damaged layers, which subsequently enhances visual acuity. The trajectory of AI is undeniably transformative for humanity, and its involvement in addressing DME is already well established.

REFERENCES

1. Yau JW, Rogers SL, Kawasaki R, Lamoureux EL, Kowalski JW, Bek T, et al. Global prevalence and major risk factors of diabetic retinopathy. Diabetes Care. 2012;3:152-60.
2. Xie XW, Xu L, Wang YX, Jonas JB. Prevalence and associated factors of diabetic retinopathy. The Beijing eye study. Graefes Arch Clin Exp Ophthalmol. 2008;246:1519-26.
3. Wong TY, Klein R, Islam FM, Cotch MF, Folsom AR, Klein BE, et al. Diabetic retinopathy in a multi-ethnic cohort in the United States. Am J Ophthalmol. 2006;141:446-55.
4. Lee R, Wong TY, Sabanayagam C. Epidemiology of diabetic retinopathy, diabetic macular edema and related vision loss. Eye Vis (Lond). 2015;2:17.
5. Klein R, Knudtson MD, Lee KE, Gangnon R, Klein BE. The Wisconsin Epidemiologic Study of Diabetic Retinopathy XXIII: the twenty-five-year incidence of macular edema in persons with type 1 diabetes. Ophthalmology. 2009;116:497-503.
6. Staurenghi G, Sadda S, Chakravarthy U, Spaide RF. International Nomenclature for Optical Coherence Tomography (IN•OCT) Panel. Proposed lexicon for anatomic landmarks in normal posterior segment spectral-domain optical coherence tomography: the IN•OCT consensus. Ophthalmology. 2014;121:1572-8.
7. Spaide RF, Curcio CA. Anatomical correlates to the bands seen in the outer retina by optical coherence tomography: literature review and model. Retina. 2011;31:1609-19.
8. Ruia S, Saxena S, Prasad S, Sharma SR, Akduman L, Khanna VK. Correlation of biomarkers thiobarbituric acid reactive substance, nitric oxide and central subfield and cube average thickness in diabetic retinopathy: a cross-sectional study. Int J Retina Vitreous. 2016;2:8.
9. Browning DJ, Glassman AR, Aiello LP, Beck RW, Brown DM, Fong DS, et al. Diabetic Retinopathy Clinical Research Network. Relationship between optical coherence tomography-measured central retinal thickness and visual acuity in diabetic macular edema. Ophthalmology. 2007;114:525-36.
10. Pelosini L, Hull CC, Boyce JF, McHugh D, Stanford MR, Marshall J. Optical coherence tomography may be used to predict visual acuity in patients with macular edema. Invest Ophthalmol Vis Sci. 2011;52:2741-8.
11. Alkuraya H, Kangave D, El-Asrar AM. The correlation between optical coherence tomographic features and severity of retinopathy, macular thickness, and visual acuity in diabetic macular edema. Int Ophthalmol. 2005;26:93-9.
12. Phadikar P, Saxena S, Ruia S, Lai TY, Meyer CH, Eliott D. The potential of spectral domain optical coherence tomography imaging based retinal biomarkers. Int J Retina Vitreous. 2017;3:1.

13. Ahuja S, Saxena S, Meyer CH, Gilhotra JS, Akduman L. Central subfield thickness and cube average thickness as bioimaging biomarkers for ellipsoid zone disruption in diabetic retinopathy. Int J Retina Vitreous. 2018;4:41.
14. Uji A, Murakami T, Unoki N, Ogino K, Horii T, Yoshitake S, et al. Parallelism for quantitative image analysis of photoreceptor-retinal pigment epithelium complex alterations in diabetic macular edema Parallelism in DME. Invest Ophthalmol Vis Sci. 2014;55(5):3361-7.
15. Drexler W, Sattmann H, Hermann B, Ko TH, Stur M, Unterhuber A, et al. Enhanced visualization of macular pathology with the use of ultrahigh-resolution optical coherence tomography. Arch Ophthalmol. 2003;121(5):695-706.
16. Srinivasan VJ, Ko TH, Wojtkowski M, Carvalho M, Clermont A, Bursell SE, et al. Noninvasive volumetric imaging and morphometry of the rodent retina with high-speed, ultrahigh-resolution optical coherence tomography. Invest Ophthalmol Vis Sci. 2006;47(12):5522-8.
17. Puche N, Querques G, Benhamou N, Tick S, Mimoun G, Martinelli D, et al. High-resolution spectral domain optical coherence tomography features in adult onset foveomacular vitelliform dystrophy. Br J Ophthalmol. 2010;94(9):1190-6.
18. Gloesmann M, Hermann B, Schubert C, Sattmann H, Ahnelt PK, Drexler W. Histologic correlation of pig retina radial stratification with ultrahigh-resolution optical coherence tomography. Invest Ophthalmol Vis Sci. 2003;44(4):1696-703.
19. Yamauchi Y, Yagi H, Usui Y, Kimura K, Agawa T, Tsukahara R, et al. Biological activity is the likely origin of the intersection between the photoreceptor inner and outer segments of the rat retina as determined by optical coherence tomography. Clin Ophthalmol. 2011;5:1649-53.
20. Fine BS, Brucker AJ. Macular edema and cystoid macular edema. Am J Ophthalmol. 1981;92(4):466-81.
21. Tso MOM. Pathology of cystoid macular edema. Ophthalmology. 1982;89:902-15.
22. Yanoff M, Fine BS, Brucker AJ, Eagle RC Jr. Pathology of human cystoid macular edema. Surv Ophthalmol. 1984;28(Supp l):505-11.
23. Otani T, Kishi S, Maruyama Y. Patterns of diabetic macular edema with optical coherence tomography. Am J Ophthalmol.1999;127(6):688-93.
24. Otani T, Kishi S. Correlation between optical coherence tomography and fluorescein angiography findings in diabetic macular edema. Ophthalmology. 2007;114(1):104-7.
25. Bolz M, Ritter M, Schneider M, Simader C, Scholda C, Schmidt-Erfurth U. A systematic correlation of angiography and high-resolution optical coherence tomography in diabetic macular edema. Ophthalmology. 2009;116(1):66-72.
26. Gandorfer A, Rohleder M, Grosselfinger S, Haritoglou C, Ulbig M, Kampik A. Epiretinal pathology of diffuse diabetic macular edema associated with vitreomacular traction. Am J Ophthalmol. 2005;139(4):638-52.
27. Gaucher D, Tadayoni R, Erginay A, Haouchine B, Gaudric A, Massin P. Optical coherence tomography assessment of the vitreoretinal relationship in diabetic macular edema. Am J Ophthalmol. 2005;139(5):807-13.
28. Ophir A, Martinez MR. Epiretinal membranes and incomplete posterior vitreous detachment in diabetic macular edema, detected by spectral-domain optical coherence tomography. Invest Ophthalmol Vis Sci. 2011;52(9):6414-20.
29. Kaiser PK, Riemann CD, Sears JE, Lewis H. Macular traction detachment and diabetic macular edema associated with posterior hyaloidal traction. Am J Ophthalmol. 2001;131(1):44-9.

30. Takahashi A, Nagaoka T, Ishiko S, Kameyama D, Yoshida A. Foveal anatomic changes in a progressing stage 1 macular hole documented by spectral-domain optical coherence tomography. Ophthalmology. 2010;117(4):806-10.
31. Sun JK, Lin MM, Lammer J, Prager S, Sarangi R, Silva PS, et al. Disorganization of the retinal inner layers as a predictor of visual acuity in eyes with center-involved diabetic macular edema. JAMA Ophthalmol. 2014;132(11):1309-16.
32. Kollias AN, Ulbig MW. Diabetic retinopathy: early diagnosis and effective treatment. Dtsch Arztebl Int. 2010;107(5):75-83.
33. Xu J, Chen LJ, Yu J, Wang HJ, Zhang F, Liu Q, et al. Involvement of advanced glycation end products in the pathogenesis of diabetic retinopathy. Cell Physiol Biochem. 2018;48(2):705-17.
34. Yamagishi S, Amano S, Inagaki Y, Okamoto T, Koga K, Sasaki N, et al. Advanced glycation end products-induced apoptosis and overexpression of vascular endothelial growth factor in bovine retinal pericytes. Biochem Biophys Res Commun. 2002;290(3):973-8.
35. Jain A, Saxena S, Khanna VK, Shukla RK, Meyer CH. Status of serum VEGF and ICAM-1 and its association with external limiting membrane and inner segment-outer segment junction disruption in type 2 diabetes mellitus. Mol Vis. 2013;19:1760-8.
36. Sharma SR, Saxena S, Mishra N,Akduman L, Meyer CH. The association of grades of photoreceptor inner segment-ellipsoid band disruption with severity of retinopathy in type 2 diabetes mellitus. J Case Rep Stud. 2014;2:502-8.
37. Saxena S, Ruia S, Prasad S, Jain A, Mishra N, Natu SM, et al. Increased serum levels of urea and creatinine are surrogate markers for disruption of retinal photoreceptor external limiting membrane and inner segment ellipsoid zone in type 2 diabetes mellitus. Retina. 2017;37(2):344-9.
38. Omri S, Omri B, Savoldelli M, Jonet L, Thillaye-Goldenberg B, Thuret G,et al. The outer limiting membrane (OLM) revisited: clinical implications. Clin Ophthalmol. 2010;4:183-95.
39. Murukami T, Felinski EA, Antonetti DA. Occludin phosphorylation and ubiquitination regulate tight junction trafficking and vascular endothelial growth factor (VEGF)-induced permeability. J Biol Chem. 2009;284(31):21036-46.
40. Mori Y, Suzuma K, Uji A, Ishihara K, Yoshitake S, Fujimoto M, et al. Restoration of foveal photoreceptors after intravitreal ranibizumab injections for diabetic macular edema. Sci Rep. 2016;6(39161):3-5.
41. Decanini A, Karunadharma PR, Nordgaard CL, Feng X, Olsen TW, Ferrington DA. Human retinal pigment epithelium proteome changes in early diabetes. Diabetologia. 2008;51(6):1051-61.
42. Van Reyk DM, Gillies MC, Davies MJ. The retina: oxidative stress and diabetes. Redox Rep. 2003;8:187-92.
43. Sharma S, Saxena S, Srivastav K, Shukla RK, Mishra N, Meyer CH, et al. Nitric oxide and oxidative stress is associated with severity of diabetic retinopathy and retinal structural alterations. Clin Exp Ophthalmol. 2015;43(5):429-36.
44. Hartnett ME, Lappas A, Darland D, McColm JR, Lovejoy S, D'Amore PA. Retinal pigment epithelium and endothelial cell interaction causes retinal pigment epithelial barrier dysfunction via a soluble VEGF-dependent mechanism. Exp Eye Res. 2003;77(5):593-9.

45. Vlassara H, Cai W, Crandall J, Goldberg T, Oberstein R, Dardaine V, et al. Inflammatory mediators are induced by dietary glycotoxins, a major risk factor for diabetic angiopathy. Proc Natl Acad Sci U S A. 2002;99(24):15596-601.
46. Yamagishi S, Maeda S, Matsui T, Ueda S, Fukami K, Okuda S. Role of advanced glycation end products (AGEs) and oxidative stress in vascular complications in diabetes. Biochim Biophys Acta. 2012;1820(5):663-71.
47. Sinha S, Saxena S, Prasad S, Mahdi AA, Bhasker SK, Das S, et al. Association of serum levels of anti-myeloperoxidase antibody with retinal photoreceptor ellipsoid zone disruption in diabetic retinopathy. J Diabetes Complications. 2017;31(5):864-8.
48. Nadri G, Saxena S, Kaur A, Ahmad K, Garg P, Mahdi AA, et al. Correlation between vitamin D serum levels and severity of diabetic retinopathy in patients with type 2 diabetes mellitus. JEMDSA. 2021;26:82-8.
49. Ankita, Stefanickova J, Saxena S, Nim DK, Ahmad K, Mahdi AA, et al. Hyperglycemia potentiates the effect of ionic calcium in photoreceptor ellipsoid zone disruption in diabetic retinopathy. Int Ophthalmol. 2019;39(10): 2237-43.
50. Maheshwary AS, Oster SF, Yuson RM, Cheng L, Mojana F, Freeman WR. The association between percent disruption of the photoreceptor inner segment-outer segment junction and visual acuity in diabetic macular edema. Am J Ophthalmol. 2010;150(1):63-7.
51. Mishra N, Saxena S, Ruia S, Prasad S, Singh V, Khanna V, et al. Increased levels of N(ε)-Carboxy methyl lysine (N(ε)-CML) are associated with topographic alterations in retinal pigment epithelium: a preliminary study. J Diabetes Complications. 2016;30(5):868-72.
52. Fry DL. Certain histological and chemical responses of the vascular interface to acutely induced mechanical stress in the aorta of the dog. Circ Res. 1969;24(1):93-108.
53. Tooke JE. Microvascular hemodynamics in diabetes mellitus. Clin Sci. 1986;70(2):119-25.
54. Burton AC. Relation of structure to function of the tissues of the walls of blood vessels. Physiol Rev. 1954;34(4):619-42.
55. Grunwald JE, DuPont J, Riva CE. Retinal hemodynamics in patients with early diabetes mellitus. Br J Ophthalmol. 1996;80(4):327-31.
56. Grunwald JE, Riva CE, Martin DB, Quint AR, Epstein PA. Effect of an insulin-induced decrease in blood glucose on the human diabetic retinal circulation. Ophthalmology. 1987;94(12):1614-20.
57. Bok D. The retinal pigment epithelium: a versatile partner in vision. J Cell Sci Suppl. 1993;17:189-95.
58. Boulton M, Dayhaw-Barker P. The role of the retinal pigment epithelium: topographical variation and ageing changes. Eye. 2001;15:384-9.
59. Dornonville de la Cour M. Ion transport in the retinal pigment epithelium: a study with double barrelled ion-selective microelectrodes. Acta Ophthalmol Suppl. 1993;209:1-32.
60. Jablonski MM, Tombran-Tink J, Mrazek DA, Iannaccone A. Pigment epithelium-derived factor supports normal development of photoreceptor neurons and opsin expression after retinal pigment epithelium removal. J Neurosci. 2000;20(19):7149-57.

61. King GL, Suzuma K. Pigment-epithelium-derived factor: a key coordinator of retinal neuronal and vascular functions. N Engl J Med. 2000;342(5):349-51.
62. Khatri M, Saxena S, Kaur A, Bhasker SK, Kumar M, Meyer CH. Resistive index of ophthalmic artery correlates with retinal pigment epithelial alterations on spectral domain optical coherence tomography in diabetic retinopathy. Int J Retina Vitreous. 2018;4:12.
63. Nadri G, Saxena S, Stefanickova J, Ziak P, Benacka J, Gilhotra JS, et al. Disorganization of retinal inner layers correlates with ellipsoid zone disruption and retinal nerve fiber layer thinning in diabetic retinopathy. J Diabetes Complications. 2019;33(8):550-3.
64. Andrade GC, Dias JR, Maia A, Farah ME, Meyer CH, Rodrigues EB, et al. Intravitreal injections of ziv-aflibercept for diabetic macular edema: a pilot study. Retina. 2016;36(9):1640-5.
65. de Oliveira Dias JR, Badaró E, Novais EA, Colicchio D, Chiarantin GM, Matioli MM, et al. Preclinical investigations of intravitreal ziv-aflibercept. Ophthalmic Surg Lasers Imaging Retina. 2014;45(6):577-84.
66. Wells JA, Glassman AR, Ayala AR, Jampol LM, Aiello LP, Antoszyk AN, et al. Aflibercept, bevacizumab, or ranibizumab for diabetic macular edema. N Engl J Med. 2015;372(13):1193-203.
67. de Andrade GC, de Oliveira Dias JR, Maia A, Farah ME, Meyer CH, Rodrigues EB, et al. Intravitreal ziv-aflibercept for diabetic macular edema: 48-week outcomes. Ophthalmic Surg Lasers Imaging Retina. 2018;49(4):245-50.
68. Cunningham ET Jr, Adamis AP, Altaweel M, Aiello LP, Bressler NM, D'Amico DJ. A phase II randomized double-masked trial of pegaptanib, an anti-vascular endothelial growth factor aptamer, for diabetic macular edema. Ophthalmology. 2005;112(10):1747-57.
69. Rajendram R, Fraser-Bell S, Kaines A, Michaelides M, Hamilton RD, Esposti SD, et al. A 2-year prospective randomized controlled trial of intravitreal bevacizumab or laser therapy (BOLT) in the management of diabetic macular edema: 24-month data: Report 3. Arch Ophthalmol. 2012;130(8):972-9.
70. Nguyen QD, Brown DM, Marcus DM, Boyer DS, Patel S, Feiner L, et al. RISE and RIDE Research Group. Ranibizumab for diabetic macular edema: results from 2 phase III randomized trials: RISE and RIDE. Ophthalmology. 2012;119(4):789-801.
71. Brown DM, Schmidt-Erfurth U, Do DV, Holz FG, Boyer DS, Midena E, et al. Intravitreal aflibercept for diabetic macular edema: 100-week results from the VISTA and VIVID studies. Ophthalmology. 2015;122(10):2044-52.
72. Wells JA, Glassman AR, Ayala AR, Jampol LM, Bressler NM, Bressler SB, et al. Aflibercept, bevacizumab, or ranibizumab for diabetic macular edema: Two-year results from a comparative effectiveness randomized clinical trial. Ophthalmology. 2016;123(6):1351-9.
73. De S, Saxena S, Kaur A, Mahdi AA, Misra A, Singh M, et al. Sequential restoration of external limiting membrane and ellipsoid zone after intravitreal anti-VEGF therapy in diabetic macular edema. Eye (Lond). 2021;35(5):1490-5.
74. Soliman AZ, Radwan SH, Prager SG, Kewak H, Silva PS, Aiello GP, et al. Spectral-domain optical coherence tomography parameters associated with visual acuity in patients with resolved center-involved diabetic macular edema. Invest Ophthalmol Vis Sci. 2012;53(14):1338.

75. Saxena S, Srivastav K, Cheung CM, Ng JY, Lai TY. Photoreceptor inner segment ellipsoid band integrity on spectral domain optical coherence tomography. Clin Ophthalmol. 2014;8:2507-22.
76. Uji A, Murakami T, Nishijima K, Akagi T, Horii T, Arakawa N, et al. Association between hyper reflective foci in the outer retina, status of photoreceptor layer, and visual acuity in diabetic macular edema. Am J Ophthalmol. 2012;153(4):710-7.
77. Kang HM, Chung EJ, Kim YM, Koh HJ. Spectral-domain optical coherence tomography (SD-OCT) patterns and response to intravitreal bevacizumab therapy in macular edema associated with branch retinal vein occlusion. Graefes Arch Clin Exp Ophthalmol. 2013;251(2):501-8.
78. Saxena S, Meyer CH, Akduman L. External limiting membrane and ellipsoid zone structural integrity in diabetic macular edema. Eur J Ophthalmol. 2022;32(1):15-6.
79. Rosenfeld PJ, Fung AE, Puliafito CA. Optical coherence tomography findings after an intravitreal injection of bevacizumab (Avastin®) for macular edema from central retinal vein occlusion. Ophthalmic Surg Lasers Imaging. 2005;36(4):336-9.
80. Kriechbaum K, Michels S, Prager F, Georgopoulos M, Funk M, Geitzenauer W, et al. Intravitreal Avastin for macular edema secondary to retinal vein occlusion: a prospective study. Br J Ophthalmol. 2008;92(4):518-22.
81. Comyn O, Sivaprasad S, Peto T, Neveu MM, Holder GE, Xing W, et al. A randomized trial to assess functional and structural effects of ranibizumab versus laser in diabetic macular edema (the LUCIDATE study). Am J Ophthalmol. 2014;157(5):960-70.
82. Hareedy NH, Gaafar AA, El-Dayem HK, El-Shinawy RF. The relation between inner segment/outer segment junction and visual acuity before and after ranibizumab in diabetic macular edema. J Egypt Ophthalmol Soc. 2018;111:102-7.
83. Chatziralli I, Theodossiadis G, Dimitriou E, Kazantzis D, Theodossiadis P. Association between the patterns of diabetic macular edema and photoreceptors' response after intravitreal ranibizumab treatment: a spectral-domain optical coherence tomography study. Int Ophthalmol. 2020;40(10):2441-8.
84. Saxena S, Singh M, Chaubey A, Mohan A, De S, Kaur A, et al. Anti-VEGF therapy leads to an improvement in grade of retinal pigment epithelium alterations on single layer retinal pigment epithelium map in diabetic macular edema. Eur J Ophthalmol. 2023;33(3):1412-7.
85. Marmor MF. Mechanisms of fluid accumulation in retinal edema. Doc Ophthalmol. 1999;97(3-4):239-49.
86. Strauss O, Stumpff F, Mergler S, Wienrich M, Wiederholt M. The Royal College of Surgeons rat: an animal model for inherited retinal degeneration with a still unknown genetic defect. Acta Anat (Basel). 1998;162(2-3):101-11.
87. Ablonczy Z, Crosson CE. VEGF modulation of retinal pigment epithelium resistance. Experiment Eye Res. 2007;85(6):762-71.
88. Glassman AR, Wells JA 3rd, Josic K, Maguire MG, Antoszyk AN, Baker C, et al. Five-year outcomes after initial aflibercept, bevacizumab, or ranibizumab treatment for diabetic macular edema (Protocol T Extension Study). Ophthalmology. 2020;127(9):1201-10.
89. Tadayoni R, Sararols L, Weissgerber G, Verma R, Clemens A, Holz FG. Brolucizumab: a newly developed anti-VEGF molecule for the treatment

of neovascular age-related macular degeneration. Ophthalmologica. 2021;244(2):93-101.

90. Palomer X, González-Clemente JM, Blanco-Vaca F, Mauricio D. Role of vitamin D in the pathogenesis of type 2 diabetes mellitus. Diabetes Obes Metab. 2008;10(3):185-97.
91. Albert DM, Scheef EA, Wang S, Mehraein F, Darjatmoko SR, Sorenson CM, et al. Calcitriol is a potent inhibitor of retinal neovascularization. Invest Ophthalmol Vis Sci. 2007;48(5):2327-34.
92. Craig TA, Sommer S, Sussman CR, Craig TA, Sommer S, Sussman CR, et al. Expression and regulation of the vitamin D receptor in the zebrafish, Danio rerio. J Bone Miner Res. 2008;23(9):1486-96.
93. Luo BA, Gao F, Qin LL. The association between vitamin D deficiency and diabetic retinopathy in type 2 diabetes: a meta-analysis of observational studies. Nutrients. 2017;9(3):307.
94. Zhang J, Upala S, Sanguankeo A. Relationship between vitamin D deficiency and diabetic retinopathy: a meta-analysis. Can J Ophthalmol. 2017;52(1):219-24.
95. Mishra N, Saxena S, Shukla RK, Singh V, Meyer CH, Kruzliak P, et al. Association of serum N(ε)-Carboxy methyl lysine with severity of diabetic retinopathy. J Diabetes Complications. 2016;30(3):511-7.
96. Moon BG, Um T, Lee J, Yoon YH. Correlation between deep capillary plexus perfusion and long-term photoreceptor recovery after diabetic macular edema treatment. Ophthalmol Retina. 2018;2(3):235-43.
97. Singh R, Singuri S, Batoki J, Lin K, Luo S, Hatipoglu D, et al. Deep learning algorithm detects presence of disorganization of retinal inner layers (DRIL)-an early imaging biomarker in diabetic retinopathy. Transl Vis Sci Technol. 2023;12(7):6.

13 CHAPTER

Pachychoroid: The Disease Spectrum

Anand Rajendran, Aditya Maitray, Ritesh Chainani, Debolina Deb

ABSTRACT

With the advent of advanced imaging modalities, especially optical coherence tomography (OCT), our ability to study the choroid and its role in influencing retinal pathology has been significantly enhanced over the last decade. One of the key outcomes of this has been the recognition of "pachychoroid" or thickened choroid as an entity underlying and unifying several subretinal conditions that are causal to a range of macular exudative and hemorrhagic pathologies. The clinical features common to the pachychoroid conditions are decreased fundus tessellation (reduced choroidal vascular markings), increased choroidal thickness, presence of pachyvessels (dilated Haller layer vessels), choriocapillaris thinning, and choroidal hyperpermeability. The pachychoroid disease spectrum (PDS) currently encompasses six distinct clinical entities—pachychoroid pigment epitheliopathy (PPE), central serous chorioretinopathy (CSCR), pachychoroid neovasculopathy (PNV), polypoidal choroidal vasculopathy (PCV), peripapillary pachychoroid syndrome (PPS), and focal choroidal excavation (FCE).

Keywords: Pachychoroid, OCT, ICGA, central serous chorioretinopathy, polypoidal choroidal vasculopathy, neovascularization

INTRODUCTION

Advances in optical coherence tomography (OCT) such as enhanced depth imaging (EDI) with spectral-domain OCT (SD-OCT) and swept-source OCT (SS-OCT) have enabled us to image and study the subretinal structures, especially the choroid with greater clarity. Several macular pathologies are now understood to have their pathophysiological basis in the choroid. This has, consequently, led to a better understanding of these pathologies and their therapy. Choroidal thickness and vascularity are more accurately assessed now and have been well demonstrated as being relevant to retinal pathology. The term "pachychoroid" (pachy means thick) was first coined by Warrow et al. to characterize an atypical and persistent increase in choroidal thickness, typically associated with dilated Haller layer vessels ("pachyvessels").[1] They described the retinal pigment epithelial changes terming them "pachychoroid pigment epitheliopathy" (PPE) in patients with thickened choroid devoid of subretinal fluid (SRF), which resembled that seen in the fellow eyes of patients with central serous chorioretinopathy (CSCR). Subsequently, multiple conditions associated with a thickened choroid with pachyvessels have been brought under the umbrella term of "pachychoroid disease spectrum" (PDS).

With the advent of EDI and SS-OCT imaging, greater information regarding choroid is becoming available. Yamashita et al. used three different SD-OCT machines and reported high intraclass coefficient and intraraster correlation coefficient in the assessment of choroidal thickness.[2] However, on comparing SD-OCT and SS-OCT, Matsuo et al. showed that choroidal thickness between these machines was not comparable and the choroid is measured thicker in SS-OCT.[3]

The thickness of the choroid thus far has been estimated, via automated software or manually, in the perpendicular drawn from the external edge of the hyper-reflective retinal pigment epithelium (RPE) to the internal edge of the sclera (choroid–sclera junction). Such measurements are seen to be highly reproducible.[4] Copete et al. demonstrated that SS-OCT identified the choroidoscleral junction better and showed more reproducible results as compared to SD-OCT.[5]

Choroidal thickness is affected by age (6 μm decrease for every decade), refraction value, axial length (thinner in myopes), gender (thinner in females), circadian rhythm (statistically significant variations in subjects with thick choroids compared to subjects with thin choroids, especially in the mornings), and several other factors.[6,7] The mean subfoveal choroid thickness (SFCT) reported in healthy subjects varies in different studies, ranging from 191 ± 74.2 to 354 ± 111 μm.[4-11]

The choroid is thickest in the subfoveal area, with the nasal zone being thinner than the temporal.[8,9] A study described pachychoroid as choroidal thickness of over 395 μm.[10] Recent articles have suggested >300 μm as pathological choroidal thickness. Also, pachychoroid may include eyes with a relatively normal choroidal thickness but with pachyvessels, which are the predominant drivers of the pathology (as can be seen in PDS involving high myopes), or eyes with normal SFCT but having extrafoveal foci of greater choroidal thickness (defined as thickness >50 μm of the SFCT).[12]

Choroidal thickness and vascularity have been demonstrated to have a critical role in the pathophysiology of several diseases, such as age-related macular degeneration (AMD), CSCR, Vogt–Koyanagi–Harada (VKH) disease, and pathologic myopia. Evidence of isolated pachychoroid in all generations of subjects with CSCR has suggested that pachychoroid could be a dominant inherited condition.[10] Choroidal vascular hyperpermeability, another important feature in PDS, is best illustrated by indocyanine green angiography (ICGA).[13]

Pachyvessel morphology: Wide-field ICGA studies have shown a possible role of anomalous intervortex vein anastomosis as one of the factors driving the choroidal vascular hyperpermeability in PDS.[14] Choroidal veins invariably disappear close to the macula on ICGA. In pachychoroid eyes, dilated choroidal veins may come in close proximity to the macula, often passing by it.[13,15]

The features common to all pachychoroid phenotypes are as follows:[13,15]

- Reduced fundus tessellation on clinical examination or white light photography
- Relatively increased choroidal thickness, which may be focal or diffuse
- Pathological dilation of outer choroidal (Haller) vessels, referred to as "pachyvessels"
- Attenuation/compression of choriocapillaris and Sattler layers overlying pachyvessels
- Choroidal vascular hyperpermeability

The pachychoroid disease is understood to constitute a spectrum of six different pathologies. These pathologies are considered to be the stages of the disease itself as the increased severity in the preceding group leads the patient to the succeeding group of disease. The spectrum comprises the following six disease groups:

1. PPE
2. CSCR
3. Pachychoroid neovasculopathy (PNV)
4. Polypoidal choroidal vasculopathy (PCV)
5. Peripapillary pachychoroid syndrome (PPS)
6. Focal choroidal excavation (FCE)

PACHYCHOROID PIGMENT EPITHELIOPATHY

First described by Warrow et al., PPE is considered a "forme-fruste" variant of CSCR as it shares the features of CSCR without the presence of any SRF or any history suggestive of prior collection of SRF.[1] It is often found in the other eye of patients presenting with acute unilateral CSCR. Pigment epithelial detachments (PEDs) may then occur in areas of choroidal hyperpermeability, increasing the risk of local RPE disruption, eventually resulting in the leakage of serous fluid into the subretinal space with subsequent macular detachment.

The characteristic findings of PPE are as follows:

- The presence of the pachychoroid phenotype with increased choroidal thickness and dilated larger choroidal vessels as seen on SD-OCT/SS-OCT
- Reddish orange hue of the fundus with decreased tessellation (reduced choroidal vascular markings) on fundoscopic evaluation

- Absence of SRF and absent history/evidence of SRF
- Nonspecific drusenoid RPE changes/pigmentary abnormalities and/or small PEDs visible on fundus evaluation/OCT/fundus autofluorescence (AF) directly overlying the focal areas and thickened choroid/dilated choroidal vessels

Pachychoroid pigment epitheliopathy is, therefore, commonly mixed up with other diseases, such as AMD, pigment epitheliitis, and pattern dystrophy. Diagnosis of the disease may help in monitoring the patient and avoiding unnecessary testing and intervention.

The pachyvessels can compress the overlying choriocapillaris and lie close to the vicinity of the RPE–Bruch membrane complex, signaling that they may be mechanically inciting pigment epitheliopathy. OCT also highlights sub-RPE drusen-like deposits and focal RPE hyperplasia represented by several scattered small elevations of the RPE. Occasionally, small serous PEDs may be found. SS-OCT and EDI-OCT have also additionally shown increased choroidal thickening, pachyvessels within the Haller layer, thinning of the Sattler layer and choriocapillaris and outer nuclear layer thinning.[1]

Choroidal hyperpermeability, seen as diffuse leakage and hyperfluorescence in mid and late phases on ICGA, underlies these areas of RPE disturbances. Foci of both hyper-AF and hypo-AF may be revealed on fundus AF imaging of these areas of retinal pigment epitheliopathy. Retinal pigment epithelial hyperplasia is shown up on OCT scans through hyperautofluorescent foci. PPE is never associated with signs of previous SRF, such as tear-drop tracts, zonal areas of hyperautofluorescence, or focal areas of speckled hyperautofluorescence.[1]

CENTRAL SEROUS CHORIORETINOPATHY

Central serous chorioretinopathy is an idiopathic noninflammatory condition characterized by serous detachment of the neurosensory retina and alterations of RPE, with or without serous retinal PEDs.

It is now known to be associated with choroidal vascular hyperpermeability and dilated large choroidal vessels, which is proposed to cause alterations/decompensation of the overlying RPE and effusion under the retina.[15,16] The predisposing factors for CSCR are type A personality, hypertension, smoking, corticosteroid use in any form/Cushing syndrome, pregnancy, hysteria and hypochondria, systemic lupus erythematosus, and psychopharmacological medication.[1]

Fundus fluorescein angiography (FFA) typically shows the ink-blot or smoke-stack pattern of focal leaks in acute CSCR. ICGA shows choroidal vascular hyperpermeability in areas where fluorescein angiogram (FA) shows leakage at the level of the RPE. ICGA also typically shows dilated choroidal vessels at the posterior pole that are oriented diagonally and are noted to communicate with the vortex ampulla **(Fig. 13.1A)**.

Optical coherence tomography frequently demonstrates SRF, subretinal precipitates/shaggy photoreceptors underlying the detached retina, with or without subretinal fibrin, irregular RPE, and serous PEDs, alongside a thickened choroid with dilated Haller layer vessels, better appreciated on EDI-OCT and SS-OCT **(Fig. 13.1B)**. Fundus AF may reveal focal areas of speckled hyper-AF, denoting the chronic presence of fluid. Gravitational descending tear-drop tracts with a mottled AF can also be noted in several cases. Chronic CSCR can also have zonal areas of hyper-AF or hypo-AF reflecting the widespread RPE dysfunction. OCT-angiography (OCTA) is likely to demonstrate pachyvessels in the Haller layer.[17,18]

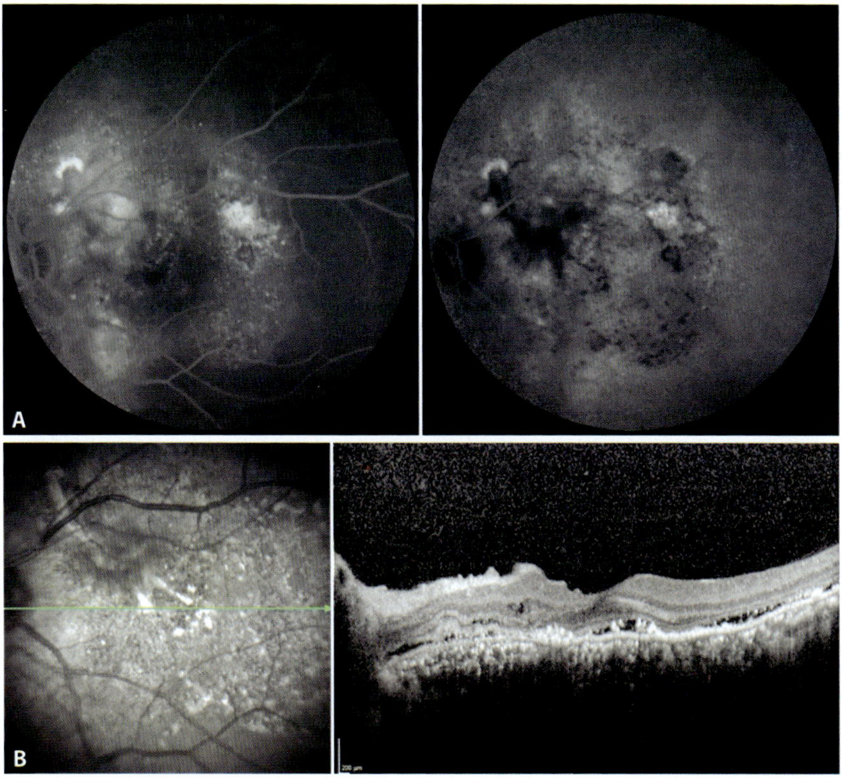

Figs. 13.1A and B: (A) FFA and ICGA images of a case of chronic CSCR showing the intense hyperfluorescence from leaking areas on FFA with corresponding choroidal hyperpermeable areas showing up as areas of hypercyanescence on ICGA. A tear-drop tract is also evident; (B) OCT shows chronic CSCR with diffuse shallow subretinal fluid with extensive subretinal precipitates and fibrin alongside the thickened choroid. (CSCR: central serous chorioretinopathy; FFA: fundus fluorescein angiography; ICGA: indocyanine green angiography; OCT: optical coherence tomography)

Acute CSCR generally is self-limited in majority of cases. However, persistent SRF/multiple recurrences of CSCR can lead to diffuse widespread RPE decompensation seen in chronic CSCR, also referred to as *diffuse retinal pigment epitheliopathy (DRPE)*. It is generally seen in older age groups, typically sixth to seventh decades, and can be associated with secondary choroidal neovascularization (CNV).[19] It is not established yet whether a continuum exists between acute simple CSCR and the chronic variant. FFA in chronic CSCR typically shows ill-defined leakage/mottling due to progressive pathologic changes in the RPE.

PACHYCHOROID NEOVASCULOPATHY

Freund et al. described the development of a type 1 CNV as a late complication of chronic CSCR and PPE.[18] In susceptible individuals, a hyperpermeable, congested, and chronically exuding pachychoroid with dilated Haller layer vessels may compress the overlying vessels in the Sattler layer and choriocapillaris and lead to long-term degenerative effects on the RPE, Bruch's membrane, and choriocapillaris. This, in turn, may induce, subsequently, neovascularization beneath the RPE. A relative absence of drusen, with reduced choroidal vascular markings in the affected area, a younger age at the onset of neovascularization, and a thick choroid with pachyvessels distinguish PNV from AMD and other degenerative conditions that lead to type 1 neovascularization.[13,18,19] Occasionally, the neovascular tissue of PNV in some eyes may evolve into PCV. Also, the contralateral eyes of subjects with PNV may show changes consistent with PPE or resolved CSCR, further reinforcing the idea that PPE, CSCR, PNV, and PCV may all lie on the PDS. OCT highlights its prime features: The presence of a wide shallow irregular elevation of the RPE signifying the type 1 CNV proliferation between RPE and Bruch's membrane, classically described as the "double-layer sign." It is associated with choroidal thickening and dilated choroidal vessels **(Fig. 13.2B)** below the RPE irregularity.[13,18] The double-layer sign can also be seen in choroidal neovascular membrane (CNVM) secondary to chronic CSCR and in PCV. OCTA highlights the complex, tangled vein network under these irregular shallow PEDs. FFA shows an ill-defined area of hyperfluorescence and/or late leakage of indeterminate origin corresponding to the area of irregular RPE elevation seen on OCT. In these cases, ICGA often reveals both patchy areas of choroidal hyperpermeability in the mid phases and a discrete plaque of late hyperfluorescence **(Fig. 13.2A)**, reflective of the type 1 neovascular tissue.[17]

POLYPOIDAL CHOROIDAL VASCULOPATHY

Yannuzzi et al. asserted that PCV constituted 7.8% of the exudative AMD cases, while studies from Asia place that incidence in the range

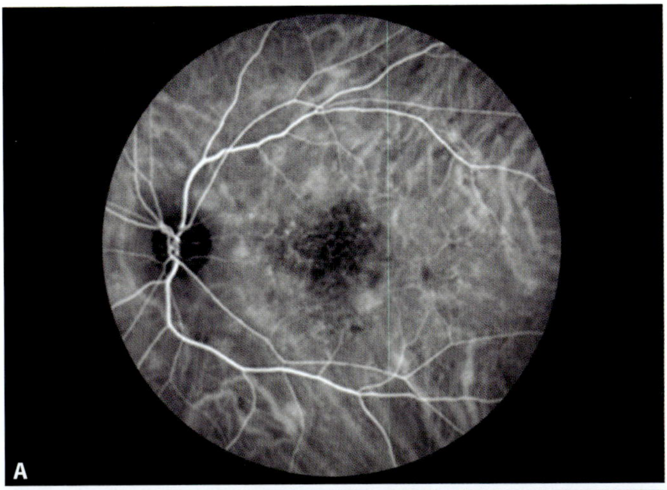

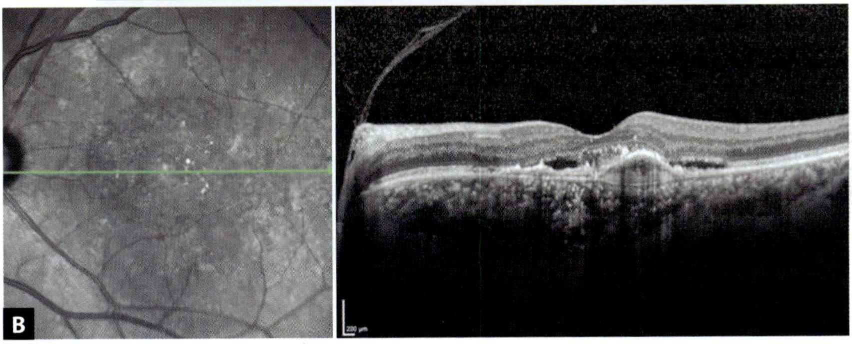

Figs. 13.2A and B: (A) PNV with areas of distinctive choroidal hyperpermeability seen as hypercyanescent zones on indocyanine green angiography; (B) OCT image of the PNV case with elevated retinal pigment epithelium resembling a type 1 choroidal neovascular membrane. A thickened choroid is also noted. (OCT: optical coherence tomography; PNV: pachychoroid neovasculopathy)

of 25–50%.[20-22] The hallmark of PCV is the proliferation of an abnormal branching vascular network (BVN) from choroidal capillaries under the RPE with terminal aneurysmal dilations in the form of polyps.[20] These choroidal vascular polyps, the pathognomonic lesions, are clearly diagnosed by ICGA. ICGA helps identify these polyps as early focal areas of intense hyperfluorescence that may reveal either late leakage or "wash-out" features depending on their degree of activity **(Fig. 13.3A)**. These polypoidal structures cause leakage or hemorrhage beneath the RPE and neurosensory retina. The spectrum of clinical lesions ranges from the presence of orangish nodular lesions to serosanguinous PEDs, subretinal exudates and neurosensory detachments to bullous retinal detachments, and breakthrough vitreous hemorrhages with associated subretinal hemorrhage.[23] The OCT features of PCV cause it to be likened to a form of type 1 neovascularization,

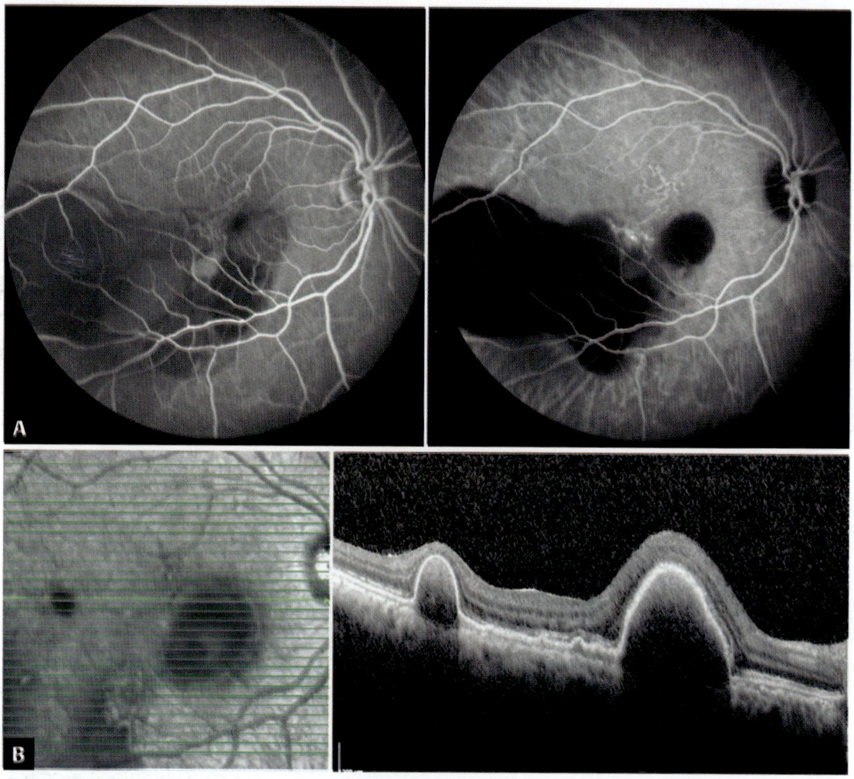

Figs. 13.3A and B: (A) A case of PCV with massive subretinal hemorrhage seen as blocked fluorescence on FFA and ICGA. The ICGA additionally shows the branching vascular network terminating in the classic polyps seen as the hypercyanescent bulbs; (B) The tall-peaked, thumb-shaped PEDs typical of PCV are noted on OCT with a thickened choroid. (FFA: fundus fluorescein angiography; ICGA: indocyanine green angiography; OCT: optical coherence tomography; PCV: polypoidal choroidal vasculopathy; PEDs: pigment epithelial detachments)

and it remains a close differential to neovascular AMD.[24] It has been reported that long-standing PNV, essentially type 1 CNV secondary to CSCR or PPE, can develop polypoidal features at it margins and converts to PCV.[18,19]

Hemorrhages and lipid exudation occur through these polyps. The scrutiny of the OCT morphology of the choroids of several patients diagnosed with PCV shows characteristics consistent with those of the pachychoroid phenotype (**Figs. 13.3A and B**): Choroids thicker than what are usual for AMD, minimal or absent drusen, dilated Haller layer vessels with inner choroidal thinning, and shallow irregular PEDs.[1,13,21] The OCT evidence of sharp-peaked PEDs/thumb-like PEDs, notched PEDs, and the presence of a hyporeflective lumen surrounded by a hyper-reflective ring attached to the undersurface of RPE within a PED are all characteristic of PCV and denote polyps.

The previously used terminology, aneurysmal type 1 neovascularization, is again being considered as a better term to define PCV. The recent advent of SS-OCT and EDI-OCT has confirmed that BVN and aneurysmal dilation are present between the basal lamina of the RPE layer and the inner collagenous layer of Bruch's membrane (seen as the classic double-layer sign), with more evidence that mechanisms that underlie aneurysm formation differ from those which promote neovascularization in AMD.[25]

Indocyanine green angiography remains the gold standard for diagnosing PCV.[26] However, recent studies have recommended that using multimodal imaging, a combination of three features on SD-OCT, namely sharp-peaked PED (identified as PED with a sharp vertical inclination of >70° and a height:base ratio >1), a sub-RPE ring-like structure, and complex RPE elevation on en face OCT along with the presence of an orange nodule on clinical fundus photograph, PCV can be diagnosed and differentiated from neovascular AMD with high accuracy in most scenarios.[27,28] OCTA has been shown superior to ICGA in the detection of BVN but has a poorer polypoidal lesion detection rate possibly due to their variable flow and partially obstructed lumen. Its utility/sensitivity is also limited by difficulty in segmentation and imaging due to hemorrhages, exudates, and irregular PEDs.[26,27]

PERIPAPILLARY PACHYCHOROID SYNDROME

Peripapillary pachychoroid syndrome is a recently described entity by Phasukkijwatana et al. as a PDS variant characterized by isolated peripapillary choroidal thickening (thicker nasal vs. temporal macular choroids), associated with nasal macular intraretinal fluid (IRF) and/or SRF and occasional disk edema **(Figs. 13.4A to D)**. Associated findings include

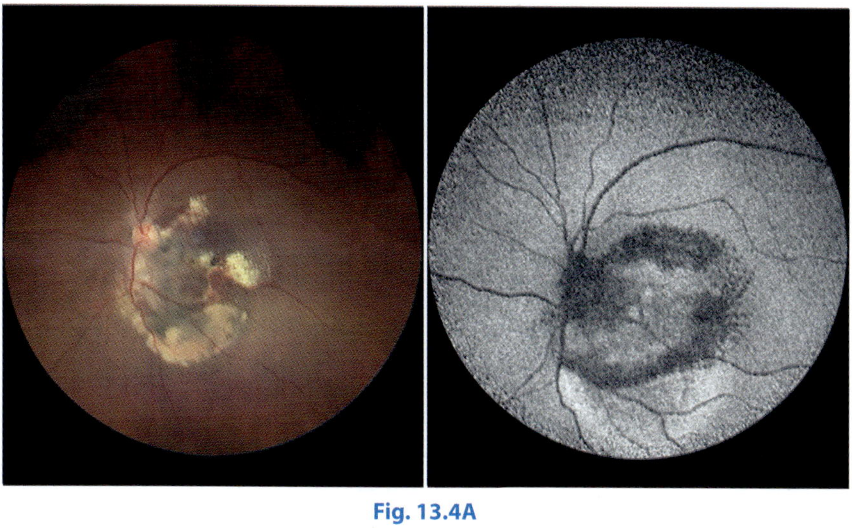

Fig. 13.4A

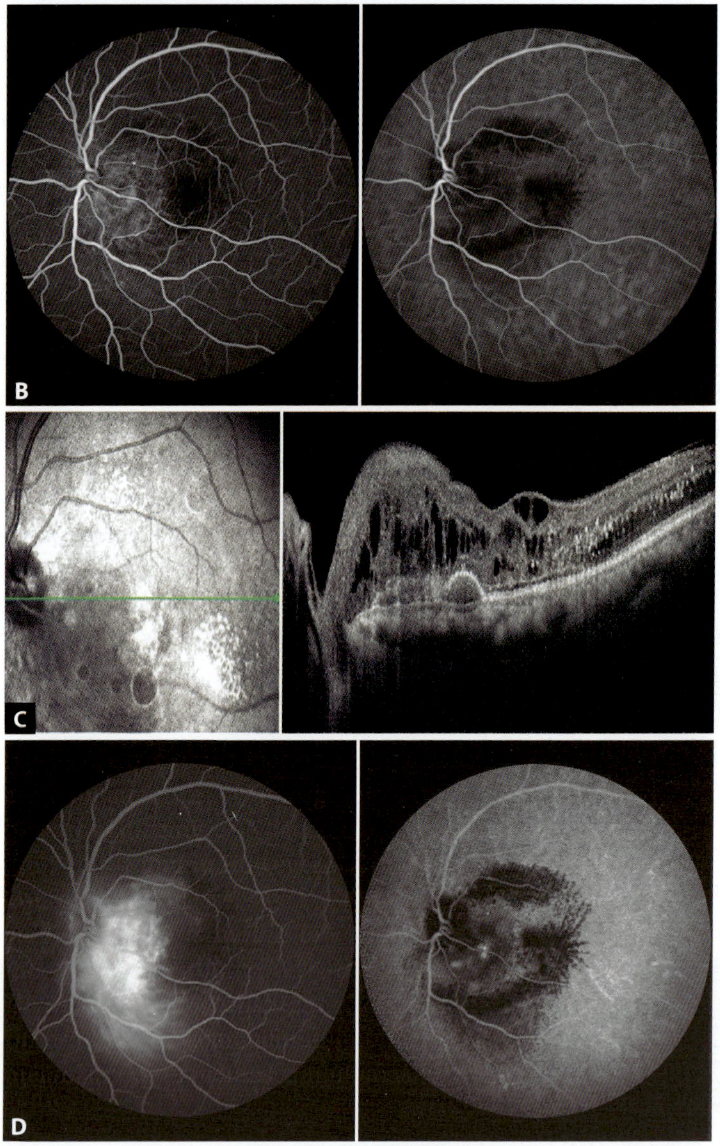

Figs. 13.4B to D

Figs. 13.4A to D: (A) Color fundus photograph and fundus autofluorescence of the left eye of a patient with peripapillary pachychoroid syndrome demonstrating subretinal hemorrhage and exudates extending from the optic nerve head to the macula; (B) Early-phase FFA and ICGA showing window defects of early hyperfluorescence in the peripapillary area; (C) OCT of the left eye showing IRF and SRF in the papillomacular bundle, with increased choroidal thickness nasal to fovea; (D) Late-phase FFA and ICGA showing hypercyanescence nasal to fovea, indicating thickened and leaking choroidal vessels, suggestive of choroidal hyperpermeability. (FFA: fundus fluorescein angiography; ICGA: indocyanine green angiography; IRF: intraretinal fluid; OCT: optical coherence tomography; SRF: subretinal fluid) peripapillary serous PEDs, choroidal hyperpermeability (as seen on ICGA), and pachyvessels (seen on OCT and ICGA), suggesting that this is a pachychoroid-driven entity. Fundus AF and fluorescein angiography typically illustrate peripapillary pigmentary mottling without focal leakage. It is commonly associated with hyperopia and choroidal folds.[29]

FOCAL CHOROIDAL EXCAVATION

The hallmark characteristics of FCE are localized area(s) of choroidal excavation without features of posterior staphyloma or scleral ectasia in patients who usually lack evidence of a disease known to result in choroidal attenuation. It is most commonly seen in the fourth to fifth decade with no gender predilection. Most cases are seen in moderate myopes. OCT shows two types of FCE: The "conforming type" where the photoreceptor tips are directly in contact with the RPE and the "nonconforming" type where they are detached from the RPE **(Figs. 13.5A to C)**. Eyes with FCE have been

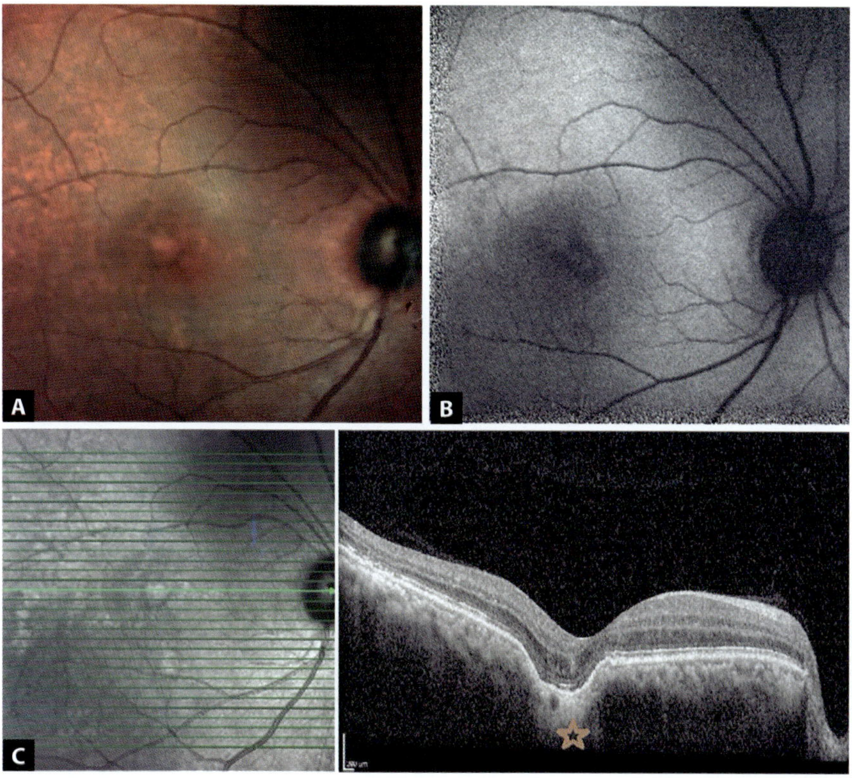

Figs. 13.5A to C: (A) Multicolor image of the right eye fundus showing subtle RPE alterations; (B) Irregular hypoautofluorescence corresponding to the same area on fundus autofluorescence; (C) OCT of the right eye showing focal choroidal excavation with pachychoroidal vessels nasal to it. (OCT: optical coherence tomography; RPE: retinal pigment epithelium)

shown to have pachychoroid features, including greater SFCT and choroidal vascular hyperpermeability in ICGA.[30]

Lim et al. reported FCE in eyes with PCV, CSCR, and CNV (both type 1 and type 2).[31] Most FCEs remain stable or show minimal change with time. Some cases may rarely develop neovascularization.[32]

With advances in multimodal imaging techniques, there has been a progressive improvement in our ability to image and study the choroid and its thickness and vascularity. As a result, the spectrum of the pachychoroid phenotype is expanding. Further research on this topic is mandated to enhance our knowledge regarding the pachychoroid pathology and its many clinical ramifications in the posterior segment.

PERIPHERAL LEPTOCHOROID

In contrast to pachychoroid conditions, the entity of peripheral leptochoroid has been described by Francis et al., which includes eyes with significantly thinner peripheral (extramacular) choroid **(Fig. 13.6)** and relatively normal or preserved choroidal thickness in the macular area.[33] These cases show a geographic hyperpigmented appearing macular fundus with a relatively hypopigmented adjacent fundus, with the hyperpigmentation and hypopigmentation actually corresponding to the normal and decreased choroidal thickness areas, respectively. The condition does not appear to

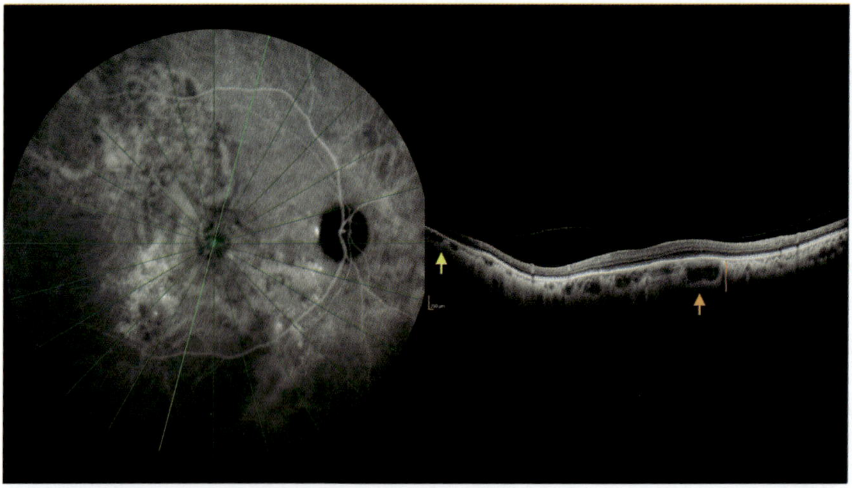

Fig. 13.6: Radial scan OCT of the right eye of a patient with peripheral leptochoroid. The OCT shows increased choroidal thickness centrally (represented by the orange arrow and orange line) and peripheral reduced choroidal thickness (represented by the yellow arrow). The central thickened choroid typically corresponds to the hyperpigmented area of the fundus, whereas the peripheral leptochoroid corresponds to the hypopigmented area of the fundus. (OCT: optical coherence tomography)

impact visual acuity [best-corrected visual acuity (BCVA) 20/40 or better in all reported eyes], and there is no correlation between the leptochoroid findings with iris pigmentation, ethnicity, and refractive error when compared to controls; however, it appears to be more common in older females. It has been postulated that there may be reduced choroidal circulation in the areas of peripheral leptochoroid, leading to an increased risk of chorioretinal atrophy in these areas.[33]

USE OF ARTIFICIAL INTELLIGENCE IN PACHYCHOROID

Since the diagnosis of many retinal pathologies depends largely on imaging, artificial intelligence (AI) technologies, especially machine learning and deep learning, have been actively applied in many areas of retina-associated diseases, including diabetic retinopathy and AMD.[34,35]

These techniques analyze vast amounts of imaging data to identify subtle patterns that may not be easily noticeable by human examiners. These AI systems can aid in the early diagnosis of retinal diseases, improving the accuracy and efficiency of screening processes. Recently, reports have emerged about the use of AI in the diagnosis of pachychoroid conditions with good accuracy. Lee et al. have reported the use of deep convolutional neural network (DCNN) models trained on OCT en face images to distinguish pachychoroid from nonpachychoroid with 90% accuracy.[36]

An AI model has also been reported to yield good accuracy (89%) in the classification of pachychoroid diseases including CSCR and PCV using wide-field ICGA images.[37] This automated classification of pachychoroid may be useful for tailored treatment of individual patients with exudative maculopathy, differentiating it from typical AMD, since they differ in terms of their typical clinical course and response to treatment.

CONCLUSION

The study of choroidal morphology and thickness profile, with the aid of advanced OCT and angiographic imaging capability, has led to the recognition of the PDS and the associated clinical entities. The role of choroid in the pathophysiologic mechanisms of a variety of macular diseases has given us the opportunity to hone our diagnostic ability in terms of detecting them early as well as enhance our therapeutic strategies. It is envisaged that continued research on the choroid and its influence on retinal diseases will further uncover such etiological relationships and help refine our management paradigms.

REFERENCES

1. Warrow DJ, Hoang QV, Freund KB. Pachychoroid pigment epitheliopathy. Retina. 2013;33(8):1659-72.

2. Yamashita T, Yamashita T, Shirasawa M, Arimura N, Terasaki H, Sakamoto T. Repeatability and reproducibility of subfoveal choroidal thickness in normal eyes of Japanese using different SD-OCT devices. Invest Ophthalmol Vis Sci. 2012;53(3):1102-7.
3. Matsuo Y, Sakamoto T, Yamashita T, Tomita M, Shirasawa M, Terasaki H. Comparisons of choroidal thickness of normal eyes obtained by two different spectral-domain OCT instruments and one swept-source OCT instrument. Invest Ophthalmol Vis Sci. 2013;54(12):7630-6.
4. Rahman W, Chen FK, Yeoh J, Patel P, Tufail A, Da Cruz L. Repeatability of manual subfoveal choroidal thickness measurements in healthy subjects using the technique of enhanced depth imaging optical coherence tomography. Invest Ophthalmol Vis Sci. 2011;52(5):2267-71.
5. Copete S, Flores-Moreno I, Montero JA, Duker JS, Ruiz-Moreno JM. Direct comparison of spectral-domain and swept-source OCT in the measurement of choroidal thickness in normal eyes. Br J Ophthalmol. 2014;98(3):334-3.
6. Margolis R, Spaide RF. A pilot study of enhanced depth imaging optical coherence tomography of the choroid in normal eyes. Am J Ophthalmol. 2009; 147(5):811-5.
7. Ikuno Y, Kawaguchi K, Nouchi T, Yasuno Y. Choroidal thickness in healthy Japanese subjects. Invest Ophthalmol Vis Sci. 2010;51(4):2173-6.
8. Wei WB, Xu L, Jonas JB, Shao L, Du KF, Wang S, et al. Subfoveal choroidal thickness: the Beijing Eye Study. Ophthalmology. 2013;120(1):175-80.
9. Bidaut-Garnier M, Schwartz C, Puyraveau M, Montard M, Delbosc B, Saleh M. Choroidal thickness measurement in children using optical coherence tomography. Retina. 2014;34(4):768-74.
10. Lehmann M, Bousquet E, Beydoun T, Behar-Cohen F. Pachychoroid: an inherited condition? Retina. 2015;35(1):10-6.
11. Chhablani JK, Deshpande R, Sachdeva V, Vidya S, Rao PS, Panigati A, et al. Choroidal thickness profile in healthy Indian children. Indian J Ophthalmol. 2015;63(6):474-7.
12. Dansingani KK, Balaratnasingam C, Naysan J, Freund KB. En face imaging of pachychoroid spectrum disorders with swept-source optical coherence tomography. Retina. 2016;36(3):499-516.
13. Gallego-Pinazo R, Dolz-Marco R, Gomez-Ulla F, Mrejen S, Freund KB. Pachychoroid diseases of the macula. Med Hypothesis Discov Innov Ophthalmol. 2014;3(4):111-5.
14. Sharma A, Parachuri N, Kumar N, Bandello F, Kuppermann BD, Loewenstein A, et al. Vortex vein anastomosis and pachychoroid—an evolving understanding. Eye. 2021;35(6):1545-7.
15. Akkaya S. Spectrum of pachychoroid diseases. Int Ophthalmol. 2018;38(5): 2239-46.
16. Spaide RF, Goldbaum M, Wong DW, Tang KC, Iida T. Serous detachment of the retina. Retina. 2003;23(6):820-46.
17. Imamura Y, Fujiwara T, Margolis R, Spaide RF. Enhanced depth imaging optical coherence tomography of the choroid in central serous chorioretinopathy. Retina. 2009;29(10):1469-73.
18. Pang CE, Freund KB. Pachychoroid neovasculopathy. Retina. 2015;35(1):1-9.

19. Fung AT, Yannuzzi LA, Freund KB. Type 1 (sub-retinal pigment epithelial) neovascularization in central serous chorioretinopathy masquerading as neovascular age-related macular degeneration. Retina. 2012;32(9):1829-37.
20. Yannuzzi LA, Wong DW, Sforzolini BS. Polypoidal choroidal vasculopathy and neovascularised age-related macular degeneration. Arch Ophthalmol. 1999;117(11):1503-10.
21. Maruko I, Iida T, Saito M, Nagayama D, Saito K. Clinical characteristics of exudative age-related macular degeneration in Japanese patients. Am J Ophthalmol. 2007;144(1):15-22.
22. Kwok AK, Lai TY, Chan CW, Neoh EL, Lam DS. Polypoidal choroidal vasculopathy in Chinese patients. Br J Ophthalmol. 2002;86(8):892-7.
23. Imamura Y, Engelbert M, Iida T, Freund KB, Yannuzzi LA. Polypoidal choroidal vasculopathy: a review. Surv Ophthalmol. 2010;55(6):501-15.
24. Squirrel DM, Bacon JF, Brand CS. To investigate the prevalence of polypoidal choroidal vasculopathy in presumed age-related peripapillary subretinal neovascular membranes. Clin and Exp Ophthalmol. 2009;37(4):367-82.
25. Dansingani KK, Gal-Or O, Sadda SR, Yannuzzi LA, Freund KB. Understanding aneurysmal type 1 neovascularization (polypoidal choroidal vasculopathy): a lesson in the taxonomy of 'expanded spectra' - a review. Clin Exp Ophthalmol. 2018;46(2):189-200.
26. Koh A, Lee WK, Chen LJ, Chen SJ, Hashad Y, Kim H, et al. EVEREST study. Efficacy and safety of verteporfin photodynamic therapy in combination with ranibizumab or alone versus ranibizumab monotherapy in patients with symptomatic macular polypoidal choroidal vasculopathy. Retina. 2012;32(8):1453-64.
27. Cheung CMG, Lai TYY, Teo K, Ruamviboonsuk P, Chen SJ, Kim JE, et al. Polypoidal choroidal vasculopathy: consensus nomenclature and non-indocyanine green angiograph diagnostic criteria from the Asia-Pacific ocular imaging society PCV workgroup. Ophthalmology. 2021;128(3):443-52.
28. Sheth JU, Narayanan R, Anantharaman G, Bhende M, Agarwal A, Chawla S, et al. Updated guidelines for the management of polypoidal choroidal vasculopathy: recommendations from the Indian Polypoidal Choroidal Vasculopathy Panel and the Vitreoretinal Society of India. Indian J Ophthalmol. 2022;70(8): 3102-11.
29. Phasukkijwatana N, Freund KB, Dolz-Marco R, Al-Sheikh M, Keane PA, Egan CA, et al. Peripapillary pachychoroid syndrome. Retina. 2018;38(9):1652-67.
30. Margolis R, Mukkamala SK, Jampol LM, Spaide RF, Ober MD, Sorenson JA, et al. The Expanded spectrum of focal choroidal excavation. Arch Ophthalmol. 2011;129(10):1320-5.
31. Lim FP, Wong CW, Loh BK, Chan CM, Yeo I, Lee SY, et al. Prevalence and clinical correlates of focal choroidal excavation in eyes with age-related macular degeneration, polypoidal choroidal vasculopathy and central serous chorioretinopathy. Br J Ophthalmol. 2016;100(7):918-23.
32. Chung H, Byeon SH, Freund KB. Focal choroidal excavation and its association with pachychoroid spectrum disorders: a review of the literature and multimodal imaging findings. Retina. 2017;37(2):199-221.
33. Francis JH, Habib LA, Abramson DH. Peripheral leptochoroid: clinical and anatomical findings. Br J Ophthalmol. 2018;102(1):120-5.

34. Burlina PM, Joshi N, Pekala M, Pacheco KD, Freund DE, Bressler NM. Automated grading of age-related macular degeneration from color fundus images using deep convolutional neural networks. JAMA Ophthalmol. 2017;135(11):1170-6.
35. Gargeya R, Leng T. Automated identification of diabetic retinopathy using deep learning. Ophthalmology. 2017;124(7):962-9.
36. Lee K, Ra H, Lee JH, Baek J, Lee WK. Classification of pachychoroid on optical coherence tomographic en face images using deep convolutional neural networks. Transl Vis Sci Technol. 2021;10(7):28.
37. Kim IK, Lee K, Park JH, Baek J, Lee WK. Classification of pachychoroid disease on ultrawide-field indocyanine green angiography using auto-machine learning platform. Br J Ophthalmol. 2021;105(6):856-61.

14 CHAPTER

Integrated Intraoperative Optical Coherence Tomography During Posterior Segment Surgeries

Lingam Gopal, Chetan Rao, Su Xinyi

ABSTRACT

Optical coherence tomography (OCT) is a technology that enables the evaluation of retinal anatomy at a high resolution and has become a standard of care in the management of vitreoretinal disorders. With advances in technology, OCT has been integrated with operating microscopes for intraoperative use. In the posterior segment, intraoperative OCT (iOCT) has been explored for its utility in various surgeries, including surgery for macular disorders, retinal detachment, and diabetic retinopathy. While stop-and-scan technique is the commonly adopted technique wherein OCT is used for the evaluation and modification of surgical steps, its real-time use while performing surgery is being exploited. For real-time use of iOCT, the major obstacle appears to be the shadow caused by the metallic instruments. Attempts are being made to address this problem by manufacturing OCT-compatible instruments for intraoperative use. The future should see the integration of OCT with operating microscopes as a standard feature, and its routine use should see wider applications and potential enhancement of surgical competence.

Keywords: Optical coherence tomography, vitrectomy, epiretinal membrane, operating microscope

INTRODUCTION

Optical coherence tomography (OCT) has taken the vitreoretinal world by storm after its humble introduction in 1991 by Huang et al.[1] The near-histopathological rendition of the layers of the tissue under consideration has enabled a better understanding of many diseases and description of new entities and has provided a crucial guide for monitoring and treating several diseases. However, in most instances, static pictures or videos are reviewed and coupled with clinical information from which the decisions are reached. The instrumentation was designed for office use and mounted on a tabletop.

One important deficiency, thus, was the inability to perform OCT in the supine position. Surgeons have also envisaged the possibility of using OCT during surgery as an aid to tissue visualization. In the field of retina, most of the applications involving OCT have remained in the evaluation of the posterior pole (perimacular area) of the eye. However, diseases beyond the macula can potentially be understood better if wide-angle OCT is made possible. This chapter deals with the journey toward fulfilling this goal and the present-day experience of utilization of OCT for intraoperative use.

GENESIS OF INTRAOPERATIVE OPTICAL COHERENCE TOMOGRAPHY

Optical coherence tomography is based on the principles of Michelson's interferometry. The initial time-domain-based OCTs have been replaced by spectral domain and swept-source technology, which has improved the speed of image acquisition. As alluded to above, the need for adopting the technology for intraoperative use was felt strongly and, hence, a series of adaptations were tried. Initially, supine-position OCT was done by positioning the patient under general anesthesia on one side but using the routine OCT machine. Handheld probes were subsequently developed that permitted OCT in the supine position with substantial ease (Bioptigen). The handheld probes gave greater flexibility but also brought in the difficulty of properly orientating the image vis-à-vis the fundus. Portable OCT scan heads were mounted on the operating microscope to permit the use of the X-Y system of microscope as well as to have a fixed orientation of the image. These adjustments enabled the use of OCT in the operating room but needed the surgeon to stop surgery while performing the OCT.

The next major development was integration of the OCT into the operating microscope and having the display visible to the surgeon by injecting the image either into the optics of the oculars of the microscope (heads-up display) or on an external monitor. Thus, true real-time imaging was made possible. The control for the activation of the OCT was mostly incorporated in the foot switch of the operating microscope. While these technological developments have taken place, the use of intraoperative OCT (iOCT) is still currently not routine, and surgeons are still exploiting its potential to improve surgical maneuvers and, thereby, the outcome of surgeries.

STOP AND SCAN VERSUS REAL-TIME INTRAOPERATIVE USE

Stop and scan is perhaps the commonly used method of iOCT wherein the surgeon stops operating, scans the area of interest, reviews the scans, and proceeds with surgery. While it does not guide the surgeon while operating, it helps them in taking decisions and corrective actions. The quality of scan is also likely to be better since the scan can be optimized and is free of shadowing caused by the intraocular instruments.

In contrast, real-time scanning can guide the step of surgery while it is in progress. However, the shadowing caused by the metallic instruments is a major issue that reduces the value of real-time scanning in vitreous surgery.

COMMONLY AVAILABLE SYSTEMS

The Zeiss Rescan 700 was built on the Lumera microscope platform and Zeiss OCT. The controls are on the operating microscope foot switch, and the image is injected into the optics of the oculars of the microscope and is parfocal to the surgeon's view. Leica microscope has a similar integrated OCT (Enfocus) using the Bioptigen OCT. The Haag-Streit system uses the OPMed T OCT system.

INTRAOPERATIVE HANDHELD OPTICAL COHERENCE TOMOGRAPHY FOR PEDIATRIC RETINAL DISORDERS[2]

Nguyen et al. have developed an OCT that could be used in supine position on children and provides a field of view of 55° and 105°. The authors have shown better detection of peripheral retinal detachments of stage 4a of retinopathy of prematurity (ROP) than was possible by indirect ophthalmoscopy. The authors used OCT to follow-up patients after surgery for rhegmatogenous retinal detachment to document the resolution of subretinal fluid. There is also potential to use wide-field OCT in eyes with retinoblastoma to locate and monitor the tumors with treatment and to evaluate the vascularity of the tumor using OCT angiography. The authors have also found its use in evaluating eyes with hereditary retinal dystrophies—to chart the extent of photoreceptor damage—as well as in evaluating the vitreoretinal relationship. Eyes with retinoschisis are especially good candidates for evaluation with OCT. Not only is the schisis identified clearly but any shallow outer layer detachment due to outer layer breaks can also be clearly defined. **Figure 14.1** depicts the value of iOCT in clearly delineating the schisis and excluding shallow retinal detachment in an eye after surgery for stage 4 ROP.

ISSUES THAT CAN POTENTIALLY BE IMPROVED

- *Image quality and speed of acquisition:* Only with high-speed image acquisition, it is possible to observe tissue–instrument interaction during the surgery. Real-time volumetric scanning, approaching video rates, is possible with an increase in the speed of scanning.[3]
- *Automated tracking:* Current systems need the assistant or surgeon to direct the area of scanning to the point of interest. The future should see some degree of automation where the system detects the operating field and directs the scan to the area of interest.
- *Image processing and enhancement in software:* The display to the surgeon can be improved with better image processing.

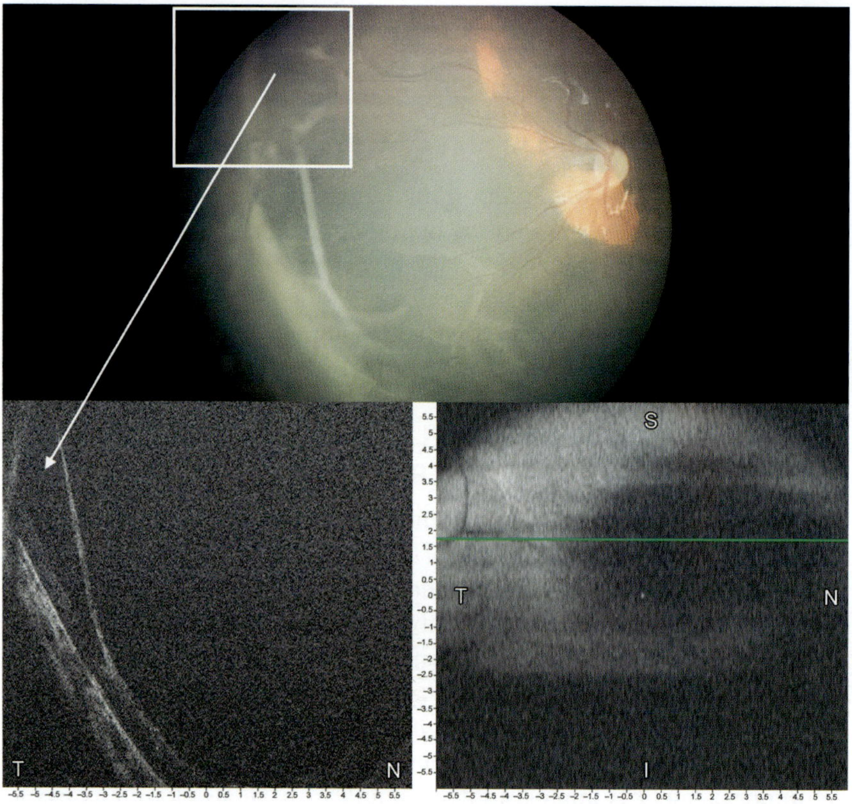

Fig. 14.1: OCT of posterior pole of an eye with ROP stage 4 following scleral buckling. Observe the retinoschisis on OCT that could potentially be confused with shallow retinal detachment. (OCT: optical coherence tomography; ROP: retinopathy of prematurity)

- *Intraocular instruments with OCT sensors:* Microsurgical instruments can incorporate OCT within them and can continuously monitor the area of interest during surgery.[4] Cereda et al. have developed an OCT-based distance sensor that was used along with robotic surgery. They have shown that the intraocular instrument-based OCT sensor could reliably measure the retinal layers comparable to preoperative OCT. Importantly, these measurements were not influenced by the inclination of the instrument and movement. Potentially, the OCT-based sensors can define the safety boundaries in manual and robotic surgeries.[5]
- *Combining with three-dimensional (3D) digital systems:* 3D large-screen display monitors can also be combined with OCT display.[6]
- *Shadow caused by metallic instruments:* Currently available metallic surgical instruments throw an absolute shadow on the underlying structures. Real-time OCT imaging of the area of interest is severely compromised by this shadowing. OCT-compatible instruments can

potentially reduce this issue.[7] Ehlers et al. have devised instruments made of plastic material that do not throw a shadow and permit the OCT image of the tissue–instrument interaction. However, there are challenges in adopting this technology to the whole spectrum of instrumentation needed for intraocular surgery.

CLINICAL EXPERIENCE WITH INTRAOPERATIVE OPTICAL COHERENCE TOMOGRAPHY

In 2014, the PIONEER (Prospective Intraoperative and Perioperative Ophthalmic Imaging with Optical Coherence Tomography) study was conducted to establish the utility of iOCT in both anterior and posterior segment surgeries. In 8% of cases, the surgeons reported the usefulness of the tool in this study.[8]

The same group followed upon the "PIONEER study" with the "DISCOVER (Determination of Feasibility and Utility of Microscope-integrated OCT During Ophthalmic Surgery) study." Several publications have come out of this study. The following is a distillate of their observations:

- In 38% of cases of lamellar keratoplasty, iOCT was found to be useful in detecting interface fluid and aiding the surgeon in decision-making in Descemet stripping automated endothelial keratoplasty (DSAEK) and Descemet membrane endothelial keratoplasty (DMEK).[9] In deep anterior lamellar keratoplasty (DALK), iOCT was found very useful in finding the depth of trephination in real time. Graft detachment could be identified and corrected by additional procedures due to iOCT. In glaucoma, iOCT was found useful in selecting a site for tube placement and verifying its location in relation to the cornea.
- In 19% of cases of posterior segment surgery where membrane peeling was done, iOCT information was at variance with the surgeon's clinical judgment in terms of completeness or otherwise of the membrane peeling and thus influenced additional surgical steps.[9]
- iOCT was found to give value addition in 36% of cases undergoing surgery for retinal detachment, while in 12% of cases, this tool changed the management plan. iOCT was found more useful in complex retinal detachment cases compared to simple cases (50% vs. 22%).[10]
- In a study comparing the outcomes after epiretinal membrane (ERM) removal using the conventional approach versus the iOCT-guided approach, the authors did not find any difference in the visual outcomes.[11] However, the authors found a larger reduction in central subfield thickness at 6 months in the iOCT group versus the conventional group. In the iOCT group, internal limiting membrane (ILM) peeling was not mandated and was peeled selectively guided by the iOCT. The authors believe that the avoidance of unwanted trauma has resulted in better anatomical result.

- In surgery on eyes with complications of proliferative diabetic retinopathy (PDR), the authors found iOCT to be useful in delineating:
  - The membrane plane for viscodissection
  - Completeness of membrane dissection in eyes with vitreoschisis
  - Confirmation/identification of the presence or lack of retinal holes
  - Differentiating between retinoschisis and retinal detachment which directly impacted the management.[12]
- In an eye with subfoveal perfluorocarbon liquid (PFCL),[13] iOCT was successfully used to:
  - Judge the behavior of the PFCL bubble (loculated within the retinal tissue or not) after the creation of a subretinal bleb of retinal detachment
  - Facilitate direct 41-gauge parafoveal entry and aspiration of the subfoveal PFCL bubble
  - Confirm the completeness of the removal of the subfoveal PFCL
- *Combining iOCT and 3D digital visualization for vitreoretinal sugery:*[6] In this integrated system, iOCT images are placed on the same 55" screen wherein 3D display is viewed by the surgeon and assistants. The perceived advantages are that the OCT image is large unlike the small image seen in the oculars of the microscope and, hence, permits visualization of subtle retinal anatomy. In addition, OCT can also be viewed by the assistant.

Parolini et al. have described their experience of using iOCT in a real-life setting on 265 eyes with different pathologies.[14] iOCT was found useful in excluding the presence of retinal breaks under retinal hemorrhages or air. It was easy to confirm the absence of any accidental macular hole creation while peeling ILM in eyes with lamellar macular holes or cysts.

The authors found iOCT to be especially useful while performing macular surgery in eyes with high myopia where there is poor contrast to visualize the ILM or ERM. While operating on macular holes, the authors found iOCT to be useful in assessing the location of ILM flap on the hole. In one case of failed macular hole surgery, the surgeon could use iOCT to assess the efficacy of maneuvers (aspirating under the edge of the hole or mobilizing the edges with a scrapper) to change the configuration of the hole.

In eyes with vitreous hemorrhage, often the status of the macula can only be assessed on the table after clearing the blood. This assessment is better done with iOCT than visual inspection. Other applications of iOCT in this series included verification of the relationship between macular buckle and macular hole, verification of the location of choroidal/retinal pigment epithelium (RPE) patch under the fovea after autograft placement, and discrimination of breaks and areas of schisis better in eyes with retinoschisis.

In a publication by Tan et al., iOCT was used during the creation of a retinal bleb (detachment) in nonhuman primates prior to the placement of donor RPE grafts. iOCT was able to assess the location of the bleb, as well

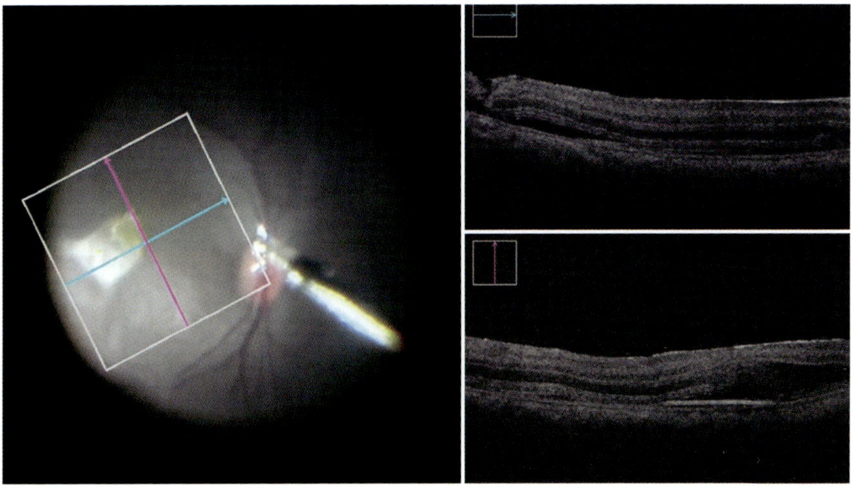

Fig. 14.2: iOCT of a nonhuman primate eye operated for subretinal implantation of scaffold with donor RPE. (iOCT: intraoperative optical coherence tomography; RPE: retinal pigment epithelium)

as the occurrence of any iatrogenic foveal tear which is a potential risk while inducing retinal detachment.[15] **Figure 14.2** demonstrates the location of the subretinally placed scaffold with an RPE graft that could be verified intraoperatively using iOCT.

CONCLUSION

Intraoperative optical coherence tomography is an upcoming tool that is being increasingly exploited for the benefit of vitreoretinal surgeons. The future should see this tool as a standard feature of operating microscopes. Based on the present experience, the following could be the potential applications during posterior segment surgery:

- Evaluation of the macula after clearing vitreous hemorrhage
- *Membrane peeling:*
  - Assessing the completeness of membrane peeling
  - Assisting membrane peeling in complex cases, such as eyes with poor visualization due to corneal edema, myopic macular schisis (poor contrast), and multiple layered vitreous schisis. In such complex cases, real-time OCT-guided peeling would be recommended
- *Retinal detachment surgery:*
  - Confirmation of absence of fluid under areas of white without pressure that were confused with shallow retinal detachment
  - Identifying residual membranes in proliferative vitreoretinopathy
  - Identifying the need for additional drainage of subretinal fluid
  - Confirming the presence of subretinal PFCL

- *Surgery for PDR:*
  - Differentiating between the fibrovascular tissue and retina in complex cases of PDR and assisting precise injection in viscodissection
  - Identifying the presence of retinal breaks under areas of retinal hemorrhage
  - Differentiating retinoschisis from retinal detachment
  - Helping to decide whether ILM peeling should be done in eyes with diabetic macular edema (ILM peeling is avoidable in eyes with grossly cystic macula and thin retina)
- *ROP:*
  - Helps to identify shallow macular detachment in stage 4 eyes
  - Postoperative macular attachment can be better defined
- *Coat's disease:* Permits macular evaluation in preverbal children who may not cooperate for routine OCT in the clinic
- *Surgery for macular diseases:*
  - Vitreomacular traction
  - Macular hole surgery to position ILM precisely
  - Myopic macular schisis for better visualization of ILM and assist in foveal sparing peeling
  - Potentially can reduce the use of dyes and thus the toxicity associated with the same
- *Submacular surgery:*
  - Guides in the creation of adequate retinal bleb
  - Verifies the location of submacular grafts of donor RPE/autografts of choroid and RPE

REFERENCES

1. Huang D, Swanson EA, Lin CP, Schuman JS, Stinson WG, Chang W, et al. Optical coherence tomography. Science. 1991;254(5035):1178-81.
2. Nguyen TP, Ni S, Liang G, Khan S, Wei X, Skalet A, et al. Widefield optical coherence tomography in pediatric retina: a case series of intraoperative applications using a prototype handheld device. Front Med (Lausanne). 2022;9:860371.
3. Toth CA, Carrasco-Zevallos O, Keller B, Shen L, Viehland C, Nam DH, et al. Surgically integrated swept source optical coherence tomography (SSOCT) to guide vitreoretinal (VR) surgery. Invest Ophthalmol Vis Sci. 2015;56(7):3512.
4. Balicki M, Han JH, Iordachita I, Gehlbach P, Handa J, Taylor R, et al. Single fiber optical coherence tomography microsurgical instruments for computer and robot-assisted retinal surgery. Med Image Comput Comput Assist Interv. 2009;12(1):108-15.
5. Cereda MG, Parrulli S, Douven YGM, Faridpooya K, van Romunde S, Hüttmann G, et al. Clinical evaluation of an instrument-integrated OCT-based distance sensor for robotic vitreoretinal surgery. Ophthalmol Sci. 2021;1(4):100085.
6. Ehlers JP, Uchida A, Srivastava SK. The integrative surgical theatre: combining intraoperative optical coherence tomography and 3D digital visualization for vitreoretinal surgery in the DISCOVER study. Retina. 2018;38(I):S88-96.

7. Ehlers JP, Uchida A, Srivastava SK. Intraoperative optical coherence tomography compatible surgical instruments for real time image-guided ophthalmic surgery. Br J Ophthalmol. 2017;101(10):1306-8.
8. Ehlers JP, Dupps WJ, Kaiser PK, Goshe J, Singh RP, Petkovsek D, et al. The prospective intraoperative and perioperative ophthalmic imaging with optical coherence tomography (PIONEER) study: 2-year results. Am J Ophthalmol. 2014;158(5):999-1007.
9. Ehlers JP, Goshe J, Dupps WJ, Kaiser PK, Singh RP, Gans R, et al. Determination of feasibility and utility of microscope integrated OCT during ophthalmic surgery: the DISCOVER study RESCAN results. JAMA Ophthalmol. 2015;133(10):1124-32.
10. Abraham JR, Srivastava SK, K Le T, Sharma S, Rachitskaya A, Reese JL, et al. Intraoperative OCT-assisted retinal detachment repair in the DISCOVER study: impact and outcomes. Ophthalmol Retina. 2020;4(4):378-83.
11. Tuifua TS, Sood AB, Abraham JR, Srivastava SK, Kaiser PK, Sharma S, et al. Epiretinal membrane surgery using intraoperative OCT aided membrane removal in the DISCOVER study versus conventional membrane removal. Ophthalmol Retina. 2021;5(12):1254-62.
12. Khan M, Srivastava SK, Reese JL, Shwani Z, Ehlers JP. Intraoperative OCT-assisted surgery for proliferative diabetic retinopathy in the DISCOVER study. Ophthalmol Retina. 2018;2(5):411-7.
13. Smith AG, Cost BM, Ehlers JP. Intraoperative OCT-assisted perfluorocarbon liquid removal in the DISCOVER study. Ophthalmic Surg Lasers Imaging Retina. 2015;46(9):964-6.
14. Parolini B, Ripa M, Frisina R, Matello V, Motta L. The role of the intraoperative optical coherence tomography for vitreoretinal surgery in a real-life setting. Life (Basel). 2023;13(9):1813.
15. Tan GSW, Liu Z, Ilmarinen T, Barathi VA, Chee CK, Lingam G, et al. Hints for gentle submacular injection in non-human primates based on intraoperative OCT guidance. Transl Vis Sci Technol. 2021;10(1):10.

15 CHAPTER

Recent Updates in Understanding and Management of Optic Neuritis

Abhipsa Sharma, Amol Bansal, Virender Sachdeva

ABSTRACT

Optic neuritis (ON) is one of the most common conditions that one comes across in the neuro-ophthalmological setting. Although the Optic Neuritis Treatment Trial (ONTT) provided initial guidelines for the treatment and management, the last two decades have seen significant new developments in the understanding of the condition. Since the discovery and widespread development of various biomarkers, such as aquaporin-4 (AQP-4) antibodies, myelin oligodendrocyte glycoprotein (MOG) antibodies, and glial fibrillary acidic protein (GFAP) antibodies, many characteristics of the disease have been developed. Recent years have also seen a greater understanding of the outcomes and generation of treatment guidelines for patients with acute ON.

This chapter focusses on the current understanding of the etiology, global trends of the final etiology, classification, and diagnostic criteria for multiple sclerosis (MS), neuromyelitis optica (NMO), and MOG-associated ON. Furthermore, a brief account of the recent recommendations for the workup and management of ON is presented.

Keywords: Optic neuritis, demyelinating, multiple sclerosis, neuromyelitis optica spectrum disorder, myelin oligodendrocyte glycoprotein-associated demyelination, glial fibrillary acidic protein astrocytopathy

INTRODUCTION

Optic neuritis (ON) literally refers to the inflammation of the optic nerve which might occur secondary to several underlying etiologies such as infections, inflammation, vaccination, and demyelination, but one of the most common etiologies is ON secondary to demyelinating diseases. It could be either idiopathic/postinfectious or postvaccination or as a part of the systemic neuroinflammatory disorders. Among the neuroinflammatory disorders, the most common and well-characterized conditions include multiple sclerosis (MS), neuromyelitis optica (NMO), myelin-oligodendrocyte glycoprotein (MOG)-associated ON, and acute disseminated encephalomyelitis (ADEM).[1] As our understanding of these diseases has increased, it is understood that each one of them has a different course, tendency to cause irreversible damage and recurrence, suggesting that a different time course and treatment guidelines will be needed for each one of them. Furthermore, while the Optic Neuritis Treatment Trial (ONTT) provided treatment guidelines,[2] current understanding suggests that this works best for idiopathic/MS-associated/postinflammatory and postvaccination-associated ON. These are currently referred to as *typical optic neuritis*. In contrast, patients with other forms of ON have a different clinical profile and clinical course and, therefore, are also labeled to have an *atypical optic neuritis*.[3]

The following section briefly describes the current ways to subclassify ON.

CLASSIFICATION

Optic neuritis can be classified based on the etiology, the segment of optic nerve involvement, and clinical features.

- *Based on clinical features:*
  - **Typical ON:**
    Clinical features that suggest typical forms of ON are as follows:
    - Predominantly affects females
    - Age group of 15–45 years
    - Acute and often painful loss of vision over hours to days
    - Retro-orbital pain which is worse on eye movements
    - Peak vision loss within 2 weeks
    - Visual loss is subtle to complete which improves over a few weeks
    - Relative afferent pupillary defect (RAPD), color vision, and contrast vision loss is common
    - Fundus might be normal in retrobulbar neuritis or might show hyperemic swollen disk in papillitis
    - Visual fields can show any type of defect, but the most common is generalized depression

    As mentioned above, this description usually refers to patients with idiopathic/postinflammatory/MS/postvaccination-associated ON.

    The ONTT showed that the visual prognosis in patients with typical ON is excellent and around 72% of patients maintained visual acuity of 20/20 in both eyes at 15 years of follow-up.[3]
  - **Atypical ON:**
    Clinical features that suggest atypical forms of ON are as follows:
    - Very poor presenting visual acuity such as no light perception vision
    - No female preponderance
    - Can occur in extremes of age
    - Optic disk or retinal hemorrhages
    - Severe optic disk swelling
    - Macular exudates

    - Absence of pain/pain persisting for many weeks
    - Presence of uveitis
    - Bilateral visual loss
    - Recurrent disease

  As mentioned above, the final etiology in these patients often tends to be non-MS demyelinating conditions, such as neuromyelitis optica spectrum disorders (NMOSDs) and MOG-associated ON, and nondemyelinating autoimmune conditions, such as autoimmune ON and ON in systemic lupus erythematosus (SLE).

- *Based on the etiology:*
  - **Demyelinating ON:**
    - MS
    - NMOSD
    - MOG-associated demyelination disorder (MOGAD)
    - Autoimmune GFAP astrocytopathy
    - Double seronegative ON
    - ADEM
    - Postvaccination
  - **Systemic inflammatory disorders:**
    - *Granulomatous diseases:* Sarcoidosis and granulomatous polyangiitis
    - *Autoimmune diseases:* SLE and Sjogren syndrome
  - **Paraneoplastic diseases:**
    - Collapsin response-mediator protein (CRMP) immunoglobulin G (IgG) mediated
  - **Other seronegative ON:**
    - Autoimmune optic neuropathy (AON)
    - Chronic relapsing inflammatory optic neuropathy (CRION)
    - Relapsing isolated optic neuritis (RION)
  - **Infectious ON:**
    - *Viral:* Varicella zoster virus, human immunodeficiency virus (HIV), West Nile virus
    - *Bacterial:* Tuberculosis, syphilis, *Borrelia*, *Bartonella*, toxoplasma

CURRENT LITERATURE ABOUT THE DISTRIBUTION OF VARIOUS ETIOLOGIES

As per the currently available literature, the most common underlying etiology of ON is demyelinating disease. Among these, the distribution of the final underlying etiology varies in various regions.

Adult Optic Neuritis

In the Western world, a recent prospective study analyzed the prevalence of ON in Rochester.[4] They reported that the prevalence of ON was about four cases/100,000 population in the Olmsted County. The most common final etiological diagnosis was MS in 57%, idiopathic in 29%, MOGAD in 5%, and aquaporin-positive-IgG4 NMOSD in 3%. Other causes were rare: Infectious (2%), sarcoidosis (2%), and seronegative NMOSD (1%).[4]

In contrast, a large study of 203 adult and pediatric patients with ON from a tertiary eye care center in South India again reported that the most common form of ON was demyelination.[5] However, the distribution of final etiological diagnosis was MOG: 28%, MS: 9.8%, NMO: 5.1%, and double seronegative: 56.1%. Double seronegative ON is a broad term that describes patients with features suggestive of demyelinating ON, but not positive for AQP-4 and MOG antibodies. This will be briefly described later.

Pediatric Optic Neuritis

In children, the final most common etiological diagnosis is usually postinfectious/postvaccination demyelinating ON. However, with the advent of biomarkers, MOG ON has been increasingly recognized. In a recent prospective trial by the Pediatric Eye Disease Investigator Group (PEDIG),[6] it was reported that the final etiological diagnosis at 6-month follow-up was still idiopathic in 48%, followed by MOG ON in 18%, ADEM in 16%, MS in 11%, and NMO in 7%. Other causes accounted for the remaining minority of the cases.

Details of Specific Etiologies

Although it is beyond the scope of this chapter to describe in detail each etiology, we present in brief the current advances in the understanding of common demyelinating conditions.

Multiple Sclerosis

Multiple sclerosis is one of the most well-understood demyelinating diseases. ON often is a presenting feature or occurs sometime during the disease. As per the existing literature, up to 20% of patients with MS have ON as the initial clinical presentation and 75% of patients have at least one episode throughout the course of their life time.[7] Most patients present with a monocular painful vision loss over hours to days and lasts a few weeks. Visual acuity loss can range from mild to severe; in ONTT, 10% of patients had 20/20, 25% recorded 20/30–20/40, 29% were between 20/50 and 20/200, and 36% showed 20/200 or worse vision.[8] 92% of patients experience orbital pain which is worse with extraocular movements. Dyschromatopsia is reported in 88% (best assessed by red desaturation).[8] Diminished contrast sensitivity, visual field loss (most commonly central scotoma), and an RAPD are often also present in unilateral cases. Optic disk swelling can be present in one third of the patients, although majority of them have retrobulbar neuritis at presentation.

While diagnostic criteria for the diagnosis of MS have been defined for many years, revised in 2017.[9] Basically, the diagnosis of MS requires dissemination of attacks in space (meaning two different white matter tracts are affected) and time (the episodes are separated in time by at least 30 days), either clinically or radiologically. Furthermore, a clinical attack is defined as a neurological symptom that is a manifestation of MS and lasts for a minimum of 24 hours. In the case of evidence of only one site having a prior episode, evidence of another site can be made based on the presence of an additional lesion on magnetic resonance imaging (MRI)/cerebrospinal fluid (CSF) analysis revealing oligoclonal bands. MRI can help by both revealing another lesion (e.g., one involving the white matter areas of the brain and another involving the spinal cord) and showing lesions of different ages. As regards finding lesions of different ages, active lesions show contrast enhancement, while older lesions usually are hypointense on T2-weighted images and do not show any active contrast enhancement.

Neuromyelitis Optica Spectrum Disorder

Neuromyelitis optica spectrum disorder refers to the spectrum of the conditions that we see in patients with NMO. NMOSD commonly presents as a bilateral or unilateral ON along with simultaneous or sequential transverse myelitis.[10] It is an astrocytopathy characterized by antibodies against AQP-4 proteins which are water channels located at the foot processes of astrocytes that help in facilitating water movement across the cell membrane. These channels are present in high numbers in the brain, spinal cord, and optic nerves.[10] The antibodies against AQP-4 activate the complement system that leads to the damage of astrocytes, which further leads to demyelination.[11,12]

Current literature suggests that the incidence of NMOSD is more frequent in Asian and African populations, with high mortality rates reported in the African population.[13,14] Like MS, female preponderance is reported, with the female:male ratio varying from 3:1 to 9:1.[15,16] The average age of onset is around 30–40 years.[17]

In the past, it was also called Devic's disease (ON and transverse myelitis). It is now understood that these patients might present with only ON or myelitis alone, and the concurrent presentation of both ON and longitudinally extensive transverse myelitis (LETM) is seen only in 15–40% of cases.[18] However, classically, NMO affects more than three contiguous spinal cord segments, which is called LETM. Often, these lesions are located in the cervical and thoracic/lumbar spine.

Other clinical syndromes that have been recognized with NMO are area postrema syndrome characterized by intractable hiccups and vomiting, seen in 4% of cases, and uncommonly narcolepsy, which constitute the classical presentation.[19]

Vision in NMOSD: There is usually a rapid and profound visual loss, with two thirds of the patients presenting with severe vision loss [presenting best-corrected visual acuity (BCVA) of worse than 20/200].[19] Similarly, the visual prognosis is also poor, with about 50–60% of patients regaining BCVA of <20/200.[19] Similarly, the relapse rate is also high, especially in seropositive patients.

Autoimmune diseases such as myasthenia gravis, SLE, and Sjogren's syndrome have also been reported in association with AQP-4-ON.[20-22] Therefore, the manifestation of acute vision loss, prolonged vomiting, and acute neurological problems in patients with known rheumatological disorders should raise concern about NMOSD and should be tested early for AQP-4-IgG antibody.

Recent advances in the diagnosis of NMOSD: While in the past, diagnosis of NMOSD was challenging, the discovery and widespread availability of AQP antibodies have led to a greater understanding of the disease. Current accepted criteria of disease are based on the guidelines proposed by the International Panel of Neurological Diseases (IPND) in 2015.[23] These criteria take into consideration the clinical presentation, serological results, and the MRI findings of the patients. MRI findings are especially important in patients with negative or unknown AQP-4 antibody results.[23]

While it may not be possible to put in detail these guidelines here, a brief summary is presented here:

- A diagnosis of seropositive NMOSD is considered when we have at least one of the core clinical criteria, positive serology, and an exclusion of other alternative diagnoses.[23]

  The following manifestations are considered as the core clinical characteristics: ON, acute myelitis, area postrema syndrome, and symptomatic narcolepsy.[23] Also, the presence of an acute diencephalic syndrome/focal cerebral symptom along with a corresponding lesion is considered as the core clinical characteristic.[23]
- As per the panel recommendations, a diagnosis of seronegative NMOSD/unknown serological status is considered if two of the core clinical criteria and the presence of additional MRI criteria are established in the absence of any other alternative diagnosis.

  The following are the additional MRI criteria relevant to the clinical presentation and as defined by the panel:[23]
  - In the setting of acute ON, the following criteria should be noted:
    - Nonspecific white matter lesions or normal findings in the brain
    - Optic nerve MRI with contrast-enhancing lesion involving more than half of the optic nerve length or optic chiasm. This is also referred to as *longitudinally extensive optic neuritis.*

- Acute myelitis requires an associated intramedullary lesion involving *more than three contiguous segments (LETM)* or more than three contiguous segments of focal spinal cord atrophy compatible with a history of acute myelitis.
- Area postrema syndrome requires the presence of a lesion in the dorsal medulla or an area postrema lesion.
- Acute brainstem syndrome requires the presence of a periependymal brainstem lesion.

Myelin Oligodendrocyte Glycoprotein-associated Optic Neuritis

This is a relatively newly diagnosed demyelinating disorder. It has a different pathological mechanism of demyelination which is distinct from MS and anti-AQP-4 antibody-mediated disease. MOG antibodies are directed against the glycoprotein located on the oligodendrocyte and myelin sheath.[24] The reported pathophysiological mechanisms of optic nerve damage are complement-mediated cytotoxicity, antibody-dependent cell-mediated phagocytosis and cytotoxicity, and antigen presentation in MOGAD.[24]

While the disease can affect all ages, this is the most commonly reported etiology among children. Among adults, it affects a similar age group as other demyelinating disorders (31–37 years).[25] However, unlike other autoimmune disorders, there is no gender predilection.[25]

Course and clinical features of ON in MOGAD ***(Fig. 15.1)****:* In MOGAD, 80% of patients present with isolated ON.[26] Another distinct clinical feature is the occurrence of diffuse central nervous system (CNS) involvement, such as myelitis and encephalomyelitis. Many patients might therefore have prodromal symptoms (fever, vomiting, and generalized illness prior to the onset of vision loss), and new-onset neurological symptoms, such as ataxia and seizures.[26] Therefore, the spectrum of manifestations is often referred to as MOG-associated ON, encephalitis, and myelitis (MONEM). Due to the wide spectrum, it is also called MOGAD.[26]

Visual loss in MOG-ON is often bilateral, severe, and painful. Nearly half of the patients present with disk edema as compared to AQP-4-ON and MS-ON. Visual prognosis is mostly excellent, and a majority of patients gain good visual acuity (BCVA >20/30).[26] The MRI features of MOGAD-ON include longitudinal lesions of the intraorbital optic nerve segments, with perineural enhancement and orbital fat stranding.

The recurrence rate of ON in MOG-positive cases has been reported to be 50–80% in various studies.[25-29]

Diagnosis is usually established by the presence of classical imaging findings and positive serological findings. However, serological testing has a low sensitivity and specificity. Therefore, it is recommended that we should consider live cell-based assays for serological testing.

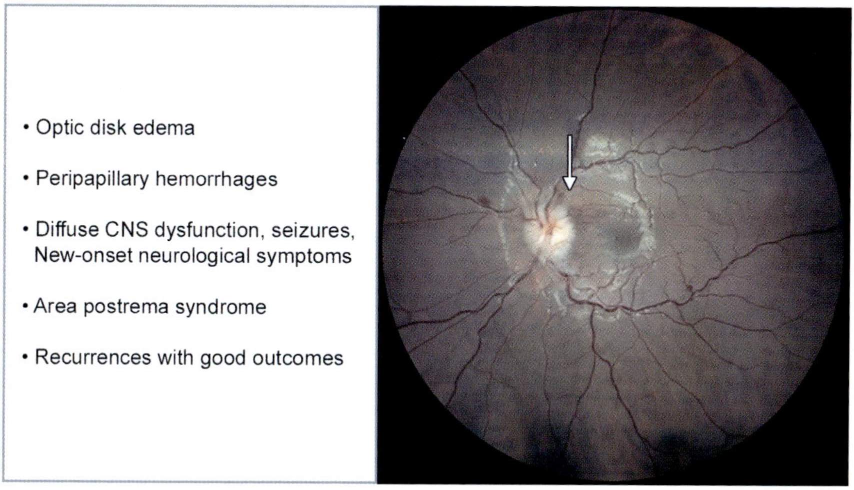

Fig. 15.1: Clinical features of myelin oligodendrocyte antibody-associated ON (arrow showing optic disk edema with hemorrhages in the left eye in a patient with MOG-associated ON). (CNS: central nervous system; MOG: myelin oligodendrocyte glycoprotein; ON: optic neuritis)

Recently, Banwell et al. described the international proposed panel criteria for the diagnosis of MOGAD, which were published in 2024.[30] According to the international panel, the following recommendations may be made:

- *Definite diagnosis requires* the presence of a core clinical demyelinating event, a positive serological test, and exclusion of other diagnoses including MS. The following constitute the core clinical criteria:
  - ON
  - Myelitis
  - ADEM
  - Cerebral mono- or polyfocal deficits
  - Brainstem or cerebellar deficits
  - Cerebral cortical encephalitis, often with seizures
- As regards the serological testing, the panel recommended the use of live cell-based assays. They also recommended regarding the interpretation as follows:
  - Clear positives for a live cell-based assay mean that the values are more than at least two doubling dilutions above the assay cutoff.
  - *Low positive:* Results are considered to be low positives if the titers are less than the doubling values for individual live cell-based assay. Similarly for the fixed cell-based assay results positive for dilutions less than 1:100 are considered as low positive.
  - *The panel recommended that in the presence of one of the core clinical features and clear positive serological tests and the absence of any other alternate diagnosis, the diagnosis of ON is clearly established.*[31]

However, in the absence of these, additional supportive imaging criteria are needed.

These are again according to the presentation of the patient:[30]

In patients with ON, MRI shows the following features:

- Bilateral simultaneous clinical involvement
- Longitudinal optic nerve involvement extending more than half of the length
- Perineural involvement (perineuritis)
- Optic disk edema

In patients with myelitis:

- Longitudinally extensive myelitis
- Central cord or H-shaped lesion
- Conus lesions

In patients with brain, brainstem, or cerebral syndrome:

- Multiple ill-defined T2 hyperintense lesions in supratentorial and/or infratentorial white matter
- Deep gray matter involvement
- Ill-defined hyperintensities in the pons, middle cerebral peduncle, or medulla
- Cortical lesions with or without lesional and overlying meningeal enhancement

Having described the common etiologies of ON, **Table 15.1** summarizes the key differences in the major demyelinating disorders of the CNS.

Glial Fibrillary Acidic Protein Antibody-associated Optic Neuritis

Among the well-defined neuroinflammatory syndromes, GFAP antibody-associated astrocytopathy is the most recent neuroinflammatory condition. It often presents as meningoencephalitis with various other signs of CNS involvement which can include movement disorders, seizures, brainstem attacks, and myelitis.[31-33]

There is a paucity of literature and experience about this condition due to the limited availability of serological testing. However, as per the published literature, MRI brain usually shows a characteristic radial perivascular enhancement. However, another leptomeningeal enhancement pattern has also been described.[34,35]

The diagnosis is established by the presence of the GFAP-IgG antibodies. They can be detected in the serum/CSF; however, positivity in the serum is nonspecific.[36] Therefore, CSF examination is reportedly very important. CSF analysis shows prominent pleocytosis in most patients.[31]

Course of disease and ON: As per the available literature, ON in this condition is monophasic in up to 89% of patients.[31] 25% of patients have visual

TABLE 15.1: Differences between demyelinating disorders of optic nerve.

Characteristics	*MS*	*AQP-4 IgG+ NMOSD*	*MOGAD*
Demographics	• Age of onset is 15–50 years • F > M (after puberty) • No racial preponderance	• Any age of onset • F >> M • More in white race	• Any age of onset • F = M • Predominantly white
Clinical features and MRI features			
ON	• Visual acuity mild to moderately impaired with good initial recovery • Clinically normal disk or mild hyperemia and mild optic disk edema in 1/3rd of cases	• Severely impaired visual acuity with risk for poor recovery • Edema and optic disk hemorrhage are less common	• Moderate, often severely impaired visual acuity with good recovery in most cases • Moderate-to-severe edema is typical and can be associated with hemorrhage
	MRI: Typically unilateral, short optic nerve lesions without involvement of optic nerve sheath	*MRI:* Unilateral or bilateral, long-segment optic nerve lesions with posterior nerve involvement and chiasm involvement	*MRI:* Frequently bilateral, long-segment optic nerve involvement with optic nerve sheath involvement
Spinal cord	• Initial deficits are mild to moderate with a risk of motor impairment in the progressive phase of the disease • Risk of bladder impairment during the progressive phase of the disease	• Initial deficit is severe with a risk of poor recovery with relapses • Variable residual bladder impairment after an attack	• Initial deficit is severe with excellent recovery with treatment • Risk of residual sphincter and erectile dysfunction despite good recovery
	MRI: Often, multiple focal cord lesions, often posterior, and involving only a portion of the cross-sectional area of the cord, and conus is rarely involved	*MRI:* Central cord lesion with >50% cord involvement, usually LETM (≈85%), the so-called *bright spotty lesions* and T1-hypointense lesions	*MRI:* Central cord lesion with >50% cord involvement, LETM in ≈75%, conus medullaris involvement in ≈40%, axial "H" sign, and sagittal T2-hyperintense line, less cord edema and enhancement than with AQP-4-positive NMOSD

Contd...

Contd...

Characteristics	*MS*	*AQP-4 IgG+ NMOSD*	*MOGAD*
Brain	Focal or polyfocal neurological deficits common; encephalopathy or seizures are rare	Area postrema symptoms, hiccups, hypersomnolence, or focal neurological deficits	Encephalopathy, seizures, focal deficits, and cerebral cortical encephalitis can occur
	MRI: Ovoid, periventricular, Dawson-finger-like, and U fiber lesions, ring or open ring enhancement; corpus callosum is the typical area of involvement	*MRI:* Large, confluent, unilateral or bilateral subcortical or deep white matter lesions, cloud-like enhancement; medulla oblongata and area postrema are typical areas of involvement	*MRI:* Fluffy or poorly demarcated T2 lesions, white matter, deep gray matter, middle cerebellar peduncle, large brainstem, and confluent cortical are typical areas of involvement, and cerebellar peduncle lesions are present in children

(AQP-4: aquaporin-4; IgG: immunoglobulin G; MRI: magnetic resonance imaging; MS: multiple sclerosis; NMOSD: neuromyelitis optica spectrum disorder; ON: optic neuritis)

symptoms, and the most common symptoms are blurred vision or transient visual obscuration; central visual acuity is often preserved.[31,37] As per the published literature, patients usually have bilateral optic disk swelling, which is reportedly asymptomatic in more than half of the patients.[37] The etiology of optic disk edema is unclear. Most visual symptoms are noted in patients with a relapsing disease course, and these patients might require chronic immunosuppression.[37]

Animal studies have shown that GFAP is crucial for blood–brain barrier integrity,[38] and fluorescein angiography studies on human patients show prominent venular leakage.[39] This suggests the source of inflammation in GFAP astrocytopathy to be a primary venular or perivenular inflammatory process.[39] ON is a rare visual manifestation in GFAP astrocytopathy, accounting for 24% of patients with visual involvement.[37] Acute treatment with intravenous (IV) steroids suffices in most patients, although some cases may be refractory and require plasma exchange (PLEX) and IV immunoglobulins.[31]

GFAP antibodies have also been associated with another, rarer phenotype: Bilateral ON with severe visual impairment and limited response to acute-phase treatment. Studies suggest that an axonal pattern of damage that has a resemblance to AQP-4 ON has been seen in visual evoked potential (VEP) and optical coherence tomography (OCT) findings.[40]

Collapsin Response-mediator Protein-5 Antibody-associated ON and Paraneoplastic ON

This is a relatively recently described optic neuropathy seen in patients in relation to various tumors. It presents as myelopathy, cranial neuropathy, polyneuropathy with painless mixed axonal demyelinating patterns, and basal ganglionitis.[41] The pathogenesis of this condition revolves around the formation of antibodies against CRMP5-IgG which have been identified as the markers of a wide range of neurological paraneoplastic autoimmunity. The hallmark manifestation is a complex phenotype of ON and retinitis with vitreous inflammatory cells, invariably associated with optic disk edema.[42] In this disease, a middle- or older-aged individual typically presents with a painless, bilateral or sequential, subacute vision loss of mild-to-moderate entity. The median high-contrast visual acuity (HCVA) at presentation is 20/40, although it can range from 20/20 to counting fingers vision.

Orbit MRI lacks any pattern of contrast enhancement and is unremarkable.[43] Fluorescein angiography shows optic nerve head hyperfluorescence and occasionally subretinal edema. Electroretinogram (ERG) is often abnormal, due to the inflammatory retinal involvement.

Reports suggest that small-cell lung cancer (SCLC) and less commonly thymoma are associated with CRMP5-IgG-related optic neuropathy. It is also reported that up to two thirds of patients develop this paraneoplastic syndrome before diagnosis of the underlying neoplasm.[41,44] It is therefore mandatory to screen thoroughly for possible tumors upon diagnosis, especially SCLC and mediastinal masses.

Prior reports suggest that autopsy may show that CD8 T lymphocytes infiltrate the optic nerve and spinal cord.[44]

The radiological features are not specific; however, it can be difficult to distinguish from the cancer-related leptomeningeal invasion of the optic nerves or radiation-induced damage on orbital MRI studies.[45] Researchers therefore recommend that it is advisable that adult patients with subacute painless loss of vision, optic disk edema, and posterior vitritis should be tested for CRMP5-IgG in the CSF. Treatment involves treating the underlying tumor and adjunctive therapy with IV steroids, PLEX, and immunoglobulins.[46]

Chronic Relapsing Inflammatory Optic Neuropathy

It was described for the first time by Kidd et al. in a seminal report in 2003.[47] Patients present with unilateral or bilateral, subacute loss of vision, where pain is a prominent feature,[48,49] which can be severe and persistent and can precede visual loss by a few days, and it worsens upon the visual deficit onset.[48,49] Visual loss is severe, and as per the prior reports, two thirds of patients usually have a severe vision loss of about 20/200.[47]

The reported pathology is believed to be demyelination, as indicated by VEP findings, showing prolonged latencies without amplitude reduction or conduction blocks in more severe cases; however, ERG is normal. As per the existing literature, there is good initial response to acute, high-dose steroid treatment: Visual acuity improves substantially, and pain eventually subsides, although it can sometimes prove refractory.[47-49] However, the hallmark of the disease is relapses and steroid dependency. The condition usually relapses as the doses of the steroids are reduced, thereby necessitating a prolonged oral steroid course after the acute event, to help complete the healing process and prevent relapses.[47]

Furthermore, clinically, this disease is difficult to distinguish from other causes, suggesting the need for an extensive workup to rule out other causes of ON.[47] It is necessary to look for signs of systemic sarcoidosis. CSF analysis should be done to rule out oligoclonal bands. In a study, up to 66% of CRION patients were found to have MOG antibody positivity and were therefore diagnosed with MOG antibody-associated disorder (MOGAD).[50]

Treatment involves IV and oral steroids and PLEX in refractory cases. As per the existing literature, CRION patients have a threefold higher risk of a relapsing course compared with idiopathic ON.[48] Therefore, patients should be carefully followed up to promptly identify the need for chronic immunosuppression with agents, such as azathioprine, mycophenolate mofetil (MMF), and methotrexate.[51]

Optic Neuritis Associated with Other Systemic Autoimmune Disorders

SLE rarely presents with isolated ON. However, if SLE patients present with acute visual loss and pain, AQP-4 antibodies should be checked. In these patients, AQP-4-IgG seropositivity is common who present with NMOSD, LETM, and recurrent ON.[52] One should remember that an ischemic optic neuropathy might occur in SLE secondary to vasculitis.

- *Sjogren syndrome* uncommonly presents with CNS involvement which is reported in about 4% of Sjogren patients having ON.[53] However, as per previous reports, the visual loss resembles that of NMOSD, and hence, AQP-4 antibodies should be checked.[53]
- *Behcet's disease* presents with ocular features of anterior uveitis with hypopyon and vaso-occlusive retinal vasculitis.[54,55] A retrospective case series showed that patients with optic neuropathy in Bechet's disease might present with a subacute, progressive loss of vision with optic disk edema and minimal retro-orbital pain.[56] Corticosteroids improve symptoms and two thirds of patients return to their normal vision.[56] Adjunctive immunosuppressive therapy may be needed because of the primary systemic disorder.
- *Granulomatosis with polyangiitis* has ocular involvement in 30% of patients which commonly includes scleritis, conjunctivitis, and peripheral ulcerative keratitis.[57] Rarely, retrobulbar ON and optic perineuritis have been reported. These patients present with severe visual loss.[57]

Though we do not have much experience of this condition, management of the condition might require treatment with high-dose IV steroids as well as strong immunosuppressive agents.

Sarcoidosis-associated Optic Neuritis

As per the reports, CNS gets involved in around 5–10% of cases of sarcoidosis,[55] and the most common manifestation is seventh nerve palsy, followed by other cranial neuropathies, including ON and aseptic meningitis.[58]

As regards ON, a subacute ON is reportedly the most common manifestation. Patients complain of subacute to rapidly progressive visual loss, which is generally less painful than typical ON. The degree of vision loss is severe.[58,59] Although optic disk swelling is most common, patients can have retrobulbar ON.[59] Reports suggest that one-third of patients with sarcoidosis-associated ON have associated signs of ocular inflammation, such as anterior uveitis, panuveitis, vitritis, nerve fiber layer infarcts, macular exudates, and retinal vasculitis, accompanied with "candle wax drippings" which are perivascular infiltrates and are characteristic of sarcoidosis.[60] There may not be specific clues, but radiological findings might show optic chiasm involvement, optic perineuritis, and meningeal thickening.

Role of biopsy: Sarcoidosis diagnosis is made on the pathologic evidence of noncaseating granulomas[61] on biopsy, which can be identified through whole-body imaging, such as chest CT or fludeoxyglucose positron emission tomography (FDG-PET).[61] Reports suggest that serum angiotensin-converting enzyme (ACE) is elevated in 50% of patients at the time of diagnosis.

Treatment is with oral steroids and gives good improvement. However, long-term immunosuppression is required in most cases.[58,59]

To summarize, optic nerve involvement due to sarcoidosis should be suspected in all patients with a slowly developing visual loss which is only slightly painful and is initially steroid responsive, especially when associated with signs of ocular inflammation in the anterior chamber. Other manifestations include perineuritis and orbital inflammation and optic nerve head granulomas.

Infectious Optic Neuritis

Although not common, various infections have been reported to cause ON, such as syphilis, tuberculosis, Lyme disease, *Bartonella*, herpetic disease, West Nile virus, and HIV.[1,3]

The diagnosis can be established with a preceding history of fever, exposure to infective organisms, and travel to endemic areas. The other features of infective etiology that can point to the diagnosis include meningitis, encephalitis, meningoencephalitis, retinitis, vitritis, and infective uveitis **(Flowchart 15.1)**. These patients require extensive laboratory workup and CSF analysis to confirm the diagnosis.

Flowchart 15.1: Summary of key features of the newer less frequent etiologies of ON.

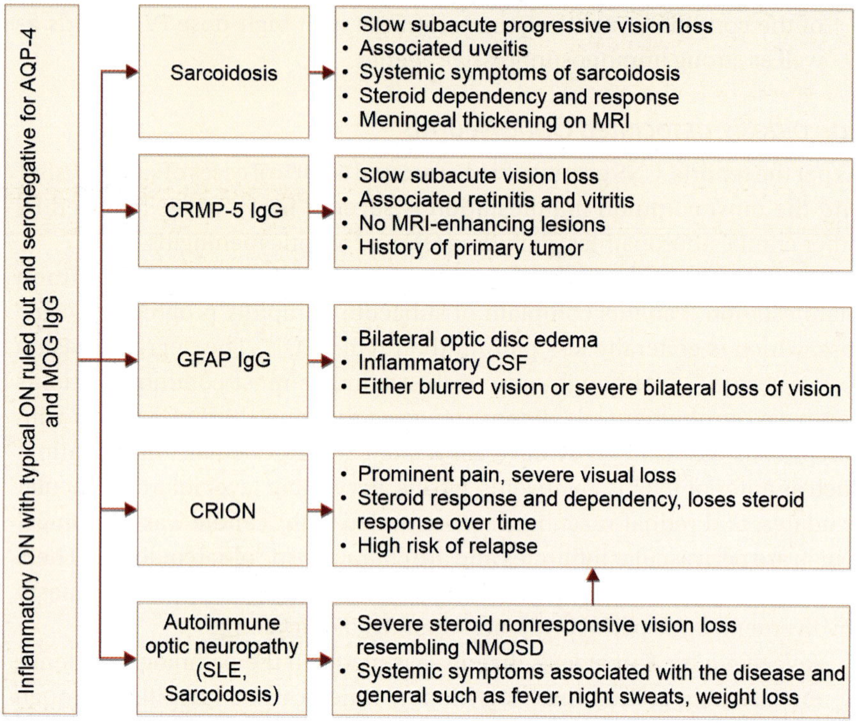

(AQP-4: aquaporin-4; CRION: chronic relapsing inflammatory optic neuropathy; CRMP-5 IgG: collapsin response-mediator protein-5 immunoglobulin G; CSF: cerebrospinal fluid; MOG IgG: myelin oligodendrocyte glycoprotein immunoglobulin G; MRI: magnetic resonance imaging; NMOSD: neuromyelitis optica spectrum disorder; ON: optic neuritis; SLE: systemic lupus erythematosus)

DIAGNOSIS OF OPTIC NEURITIS

Apart from doing a thorough history taking and clinical examination, neuroimaging and serology also play a pivotal role in diagnosing the underlying etiology. The necessary workup of a patient can be summarized as given in the following text.

Ocular Investigations

- *Visual acuity* is invariably reduced in the affected eye and can range from 20/20 to no perception of light.
- *Color vision and contrast visual acuity* are usually reduced in the affected eye.
- *Visual field testing* is essential in patients with ON. Multiple kinds of visual field defects are possible. In the acute phase, many patients show a generalized depression of sensitivity. As per the reports in the late phases, the most common visual field defect in affected eyes is a central scotoma

BOX 15.1: Characteristic VEP changes in ON.[63]

- Preserved waveforms, with reduced amplitudes but prolonged P100/P2 latencies
- Intereye latency difference of more than 10 ms
- Extinguished pattern VEP in the acute phase

(ON: optic neuritis; VEP: visual evoked potential)

(41%) followed by nerve fiber layer bundle defects (29%) and paracentral scotomas (14%).[62] The fellow eyes in monocular ON can have normal visual fields in 65% of cases; however, 21% of fellow eyes show nerve fiber layer bundle defects and 9% have diffuse visual field loss.[62]

- *VEPs* may show definite changes in a patient with acute ON. These are summarized in **Box 15.1** and **Figure 15.2A and B**; however, currently, VEP is being less commonly utilized in the acute phase as the changes can be nonspecific and variable. These might still be very helpful in a patient with subacute ON and whenever the MRI does not show classical lesions. It can also serve as ancillary evidence in the evaluation of a patient with postneuritic optic atrophy and provide evidence of optic nerve involvement in a patient with established MS.

  It is important to note that the latency alterations could persist even after the full recovery of visual acuity. The contralateral eye might also show increased latency in a case affecting one eye clinically. This shows the presence of subclinical alterations of the conduction of the impulse along the optic nerve, even before clinical signs or symptoms of nerve involvement manifest. Therefore, it is useful in detecting a subclinical ON in the contralateral eye in unilateral manifest disease.
- OCT is not helpful in identifying the cause of ON but can be used to assess the damage to the neurons in the anterior visual pathway. Retinal nerve fiber layer (RNFL) and macular ganglion cell-inner plexiform layer (GC-IPL) analysis is useful in assessing the damage to the optic nerve. RNFL thickness can be increased in acute stages of ON if associated with disk edema, and its decline over the follow-up shows the damage to the nerve fiber layer which is clinically apparent as optic atrophy **(Figs. 15.3A and B)**.

Optic neuritis often causes central field loss that primarily affects the papillomacular bundle, and this is reflected as thinning in the GC-IPL more than RNFL thinning.

As optic atrophy ensues, GC-IPL thickness also reduces. In a prospective evaluation of OCT in ON, Kupersmith et al.[64] found that GC-IPL thinning can be seen as early as 2 weeks after ON, which becomes more prominent at 1 month, while the RNFL stays normal or slightly thick even at this stage. Others have also found that GC-IPL is more robust in detecting early ON.[65-67] As a result, GC-IPL is favored over RNFL in detecting ON within 3 months. As per the recent understanding, a few generalizations can be made regarding the role of OCT in the diagnosis and management of ON **(Table 15.2)**.

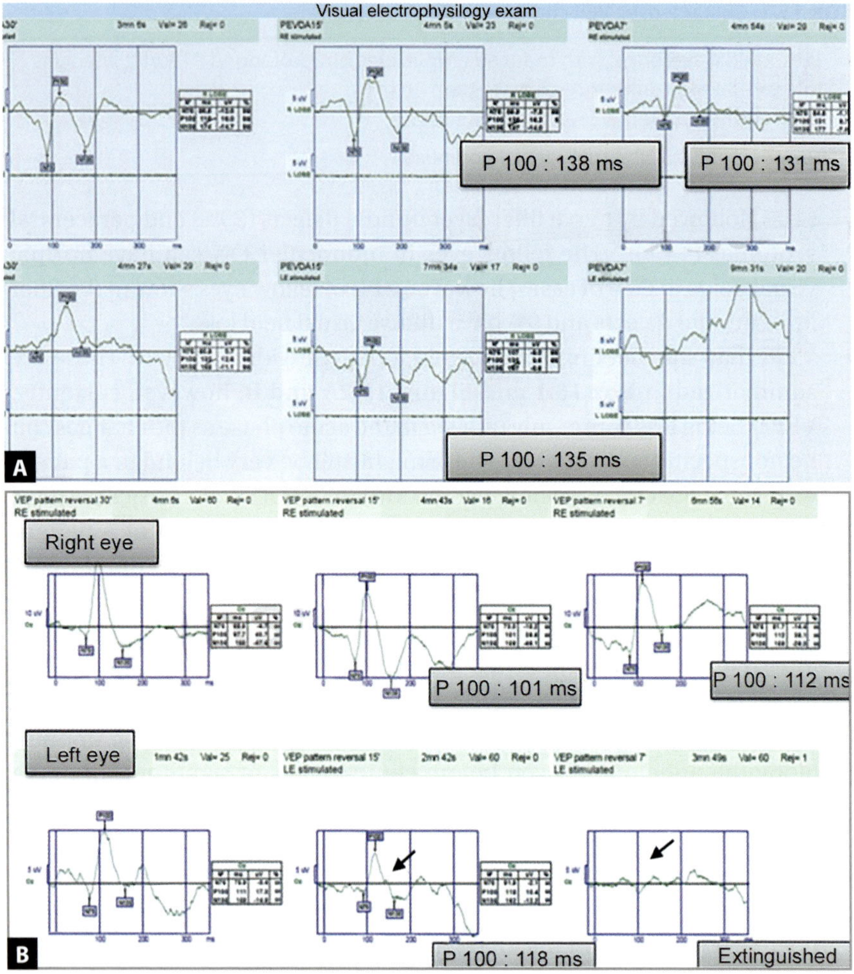

Figs. 15.2A and B: Key abnormalities on the VEP in a patient with optic neuritis. (A) Pattern VEP in acute optic neuritis showing reproducible waveforms for small sizes and prolonged P 100 implicit times; (B) Pattern VEP in subclinical optic neuritis showing extinguished waveform in the left eye for 7-minute stimulus and an intereye difference of 17 ms, suggestive of acute demyelination in the left eye. (VEP: visual evoked potential)

Neuroimaging

Currently, neuroimaging is the most important investigation in a patient with ON. The recommended imaging in a case of demyelinating ON is a contrast-enhanced MRI of the brain, orbit, and spine with fat suppression or fluid-attenuated inversion recovery (FLAIR) sequence. Imaging is important to diagnose the disease as well as fulfill the criteria for AQP-4-NMOSD, MS, and MOG-associated disease. It also helps in prognosticating the patient.

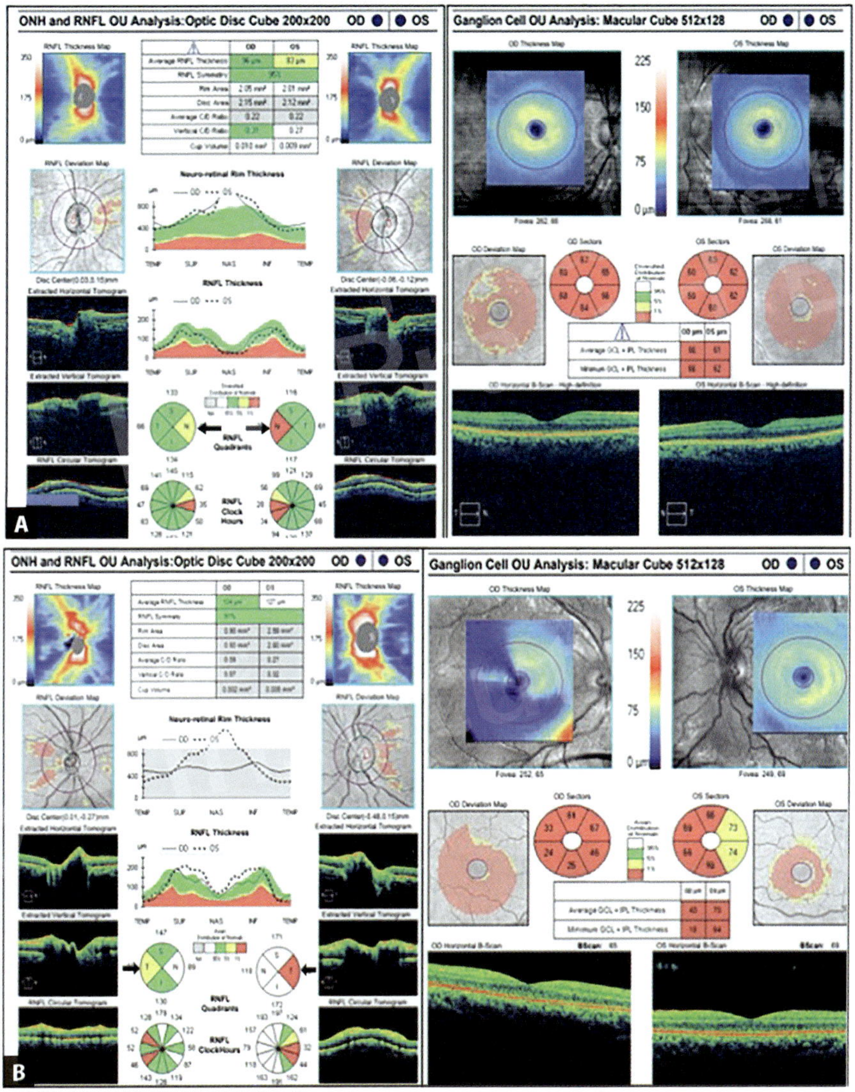

Figs. 15.3A and B: OCT findings in a patient with optic neuritis. (A) OCT of the peripapillary RNFL and mGCL of a patient with multiple sclerosis who never had a clinical attack showing mGCL thinning in both eyes, suggestive of a previous subclinical attack; (B) OCT of a patient with acute optic neuritis in the left eye showing RNFL edema with mGCL thinning more in the nasal than the temporal quadrant. Note temporal RNFL thinning and severe mGCL thinning in the right eye (uninvolved eye), suggestive of a previous attack of optic neuritis. (mGCL: macular ganglion cell layer; MS: multiple sclerosis; OCT: optical coherence tomography; RNFL: retinal nerve fiber layer)

Multiple Sclerosis

Acute ON shows a T2 hyperintense lesion which enhances on postcontrast images. The lesion is usually focal and retrobulbar but can also involve

TABLE 15.2: Role of OCT in ON.

Role	*Explanation*
Differentiate ON associated with MS, NMOSD, and MOG ON	• After an acute episode, there is nearly 28–30 µm loss of RNFL in NMO/MOG ON, while there is only about 12–14 µm loss in MS-related ON • The presence of microcystic macular edema in the inner nuclear layer of retina is seen more commonly with NMOSD as compared to MS and can be associated with poor vision[68]
Prognostic marker	RNFL and mGCL thinning is correlated with worse visual function[69–71]
Evidence of optic nerve involvement	In a patient with known neuroinflammatory syndrome, RNFL and mGCL thinning would suggest the evidence of optic nerve involvement
Evidence of NEDA in patients with MS	• In a patient with proven MS/other diseases, stable OCT parameters would suggest the evidence of stable disease • Thinning of the RNFL or GC-IPL has been shown to occur in patients with MS, even in the absence of clinically overt ON[69,72]

(mGCL: macular ganglion cell layer; MOG: myelin oligodendrocyte glycoprotein; MS: multiple sclerosis; NEDA: no evidence of disease activity; NMO: neuromyelitis optica; NMOSD: neuromyelitis optica spectrum disorder; OCT: optical coherence tomography; ON: optic neuritis; RNFL: retinal nerve fiber layer)

intracanalicular and intracranial segments.[73] The demyelinating lesions seen on MRI brain are characteristically T2 hyperintense, typically discrete, ovoid, at least 3 mm long, and classically located in the periventricular and infratentorial areas but also in the juxtacortical and subcortical areas (known as *Dawson's fingers*).[73] Acute lesions show enhancement which is ovoid, ring, or open ring enhancing with contrast, while older lesions are nonenhancing (also called *black holes*). The spinal cord lesions in MS tend to be peripheral and shorter, i.e., involving less than three segments. They are often multiple focal cord lesions, are often posterior, and involve only a portion of the cross-sectional area of the cord; the conus is rarely involved.[73]

The ONTT showed that the presence of demyelinating lesions on baseline brain MRI can predict conversion to clinically defined MS after the initial attack of ON.[1,3] Presence of lesions on MRI is the strongest predictor of the development of MS for patients with acute typical ON: 72% of patients with at least one demyelinating lesion on baseline brain MRI developed clinically definite MS at 15 years as compared to 25% of those who did not have any demyelinating lesions on baseline scan **(Figs. 15.4A to D)**.[1,3]

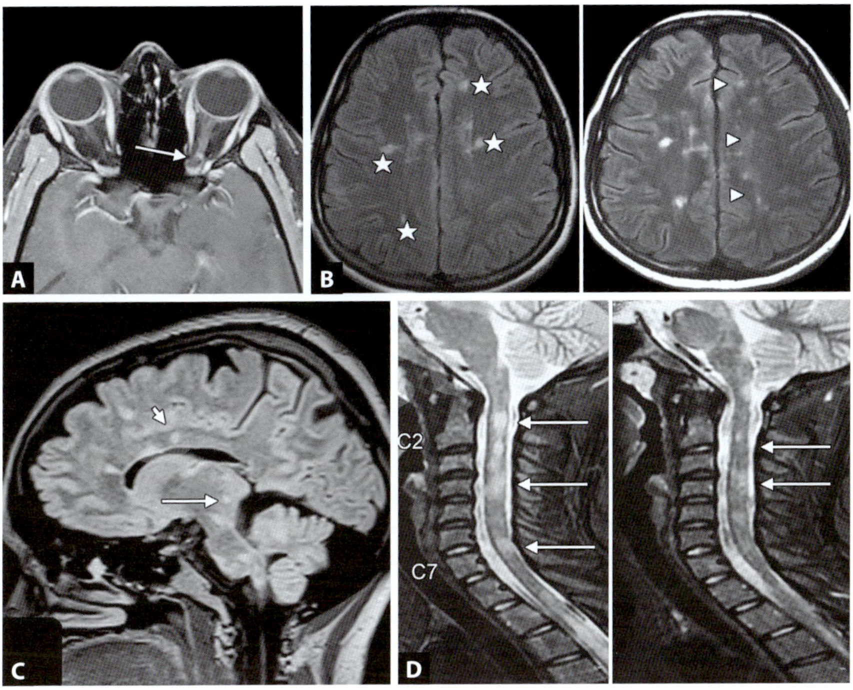

Figs. 15.4A to D: Representative images showing MRI findings in patients with multiple sclerosis. (A) Postcontrast T1-weighted axial MRI scan showing a focal lesion with postcontrast hyperintense enhancement in the posterior optic nerve in a patient with multiple sclerosis; (B) Axial T2-weighted MRI scan showing T2 hyperintensities in the white matter of a patient with multiple sclerosis 2 years apart. Note the sequential scans, one on the left side showing lesions in the deep white matter (marked with asterisk) and in the newer scans, the arrowheads showing new areas of hyperintensities 2 years later. The scans show new lesions, suggestive of lesions disseminated in time; (C) Sagittal FLAIR scan showing typically discrete, ovoid lesions located in the periventricular white matter, suggestive of Dawson's fingers in a case of multiple sclerosis. Note also the oval lesions noted in the brainstem; (D) T2-weighed sagittal MRI scan showing multiple, discrete, short T2 hyperintense lesions involving the cervical and thoracic cord of a patient with multiple sclerosis. (FLAIR: fluid-attenuated inversion recovery; MRI: magnetic resonance imaging)

Neuromyelitis Optica Spectrum Disorder

Optic nerve lesions may be unilateral or bilateral with increased T2 signal or T1 gadolinium enhancement within the optic nerve or optic chiasm. It is important to note that relatively long lesions (e.g., those extending more than half the length of the optic nerve) and those involving the posterior aspects of the optic nerves or the chiasm are frequent in NMOSD.[75-79]

On spine MRI, we see a LETM; that is, in the acute phase, there is an increased signal on sagittal T2-weighted images extending over three or more complete vertebral segments.[74,80,81] The lesions also tend to involve the central spinal cord in over 70% of the patients. Other characteristic features that may

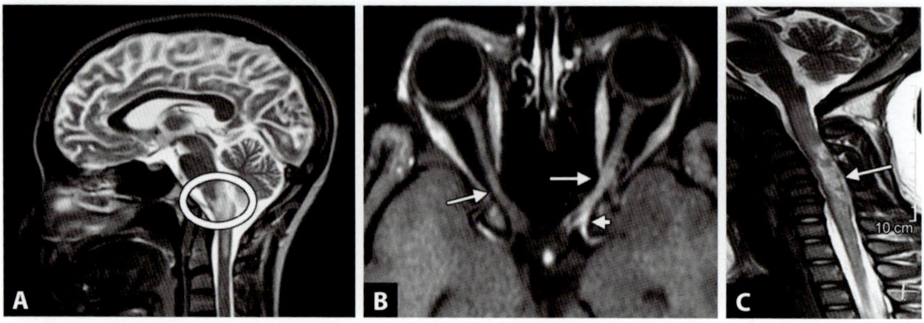

Figs. 15.5A to C: Representative images show MRI findings in patients with multiple NMOSD. (A) T2-weighted sagittal MRI image showing T2 hyperintensity in the posterior aspect of the pons and medulla (area postrema, white circle) extending into the cervical cord in a patient with NMOSD; (B) Axial T1 postcontrast MRI image showing a hyperintense lesion with enhancement in the posterior intraorbital and intracanalicular portions of the optic nerve (arrow) extending into the optic chiasm (arrow) in a patient with NMOSD. Also note thinning of the optic nerve on the right side with faint hyperintensity suggestive of optic atrophy, suggestive of prior involvement; (C) Sagittal MRI image of the spinal cord showing T2 hyperintensity involving three contiguous segments of the thoracic spinal cord, suggestive of LETM in a patient with NMOSD. (LETM: longitudinally extensive transverse myelitis; MRI: magnetic resonance imaging; NMOSD: neuromyelitis optica spectrum disorder)

be present are the extension of the lesion into the brainstem and there may also be spinal cord expansion/swelling.[74,80,81] Existing literature suggests that MRI brain may show the following features:[26,79,82]

- Lesions involving the brainstem especially in the dorsal medulla (especially the area postrema). These may be small and localized but are often bilateral or contiguous with an upper cervical spinal cord lesion.
- Lesions involving periependymal surfaces of the fourth ventricle in the brainstem/cerebellum
- Lesions involving the hypothalamus, thalamus, or periependymal surfaces of the third ventricle
- Long (one half of the length of the corpus callosum or greater), diffuse, heterogeneous, or edematous corpus callosum lesions[26]
- Large, confluent, unilateral, or bilateral subcortical or deep white matter lesions
- Long corticospinal tract lesions, unilateral or bilateral, contiguously involving the internal capsule and cerebral peduncle

These MRI features are important in establishing the diagnosis of NMOSD, especially in patients who are seronegative **(Figs. 15.5A to C)**.

Myelin Oligodendrocyte-associated Demyelinating Disorder

MRI findings in MOGAD show features that are similar to NMOSD but still are characteristically different.

MRI of the orbits typically shows the following features:

- *Optic nerve involvement* implicates optic nerve parenchyma. The affected nerve is usually edematous, enlarged, and tortuous. The length of the optic nerve involvement might be short or long segment. However, it predominantly involves the anterior segments of the optic nerve and typically spares the optic chiasm and retrochiasmal pathways.
- *Perineuritis* occurs in the form of involvement of the optic nerve sheath which is frequent and a common feature.
- *Orbital fat stranding* (inflammation spreading to the adjoining orbital fat) is present in 50–80% of patients with MOGAD.[24,83]

MRI of the brain may show the following features:

- Lesions are usually bilateral, T2 hyperintense, three or less in number, and distributed in the white matter areas. It is important to note that lesions in MOGAD might be poorly demarcated and fluffy in appearance.[84]
- Children more commonly have bilateral, large, brainstem, and deep gray nuclei lesions, which resemble those of ADEM.[84,85] Cerebellar peduncle lesions are typical of MOGAD in children.[86]
- MOGAD encephalomyelitis or encephalitis resembles an ADEM-like pattern with diffuse signal abnormality in the cortical gray matter, subcortical white matter, deep white matter, deep gray matter, or a combination of these locations.[87]
- Lesions in the basal ganglia as well as brainstem may be seen. It is reported that patients with MOGAD have a higher occurrence of thalamic (18.4% vs. 0%) and pontine (34.7% vs. 4.5%) lesions as compared to AQP-4 disease.[82]
- Cortical lesions and leptomeningeal enhancement have also been recently reported in MOGAD.[88,89]

Note: The last 2 described lesions are reported but are still less common patterns of brain involvement in MOGAD.

MRI of the spine may show the following features:

- Abnormal T2 hyperintense lesions involving both white and gray matter and >50% of the axial section of the cord and LETM involving more than three cord segments. Conus medullaris is more frequently involved in MOGAD.[90-92]
- *H sign* refers to central T2 hyperintensity with faint surrounding T2-hyperintense signal confined to cord gray matter with no gadolinium enhancement. It is seen in 28% of MOGAD cases and 8% of NMOSD cases but not in MS cases **(Figs. 15.6A to D)**.[93,94]

Cerebrospinal Fluid Analysis

The role of CSF analysis in each patient with demyelinating ON is to help in establishing the diagnosis. CSF analysis may show the presence of oligoclonal

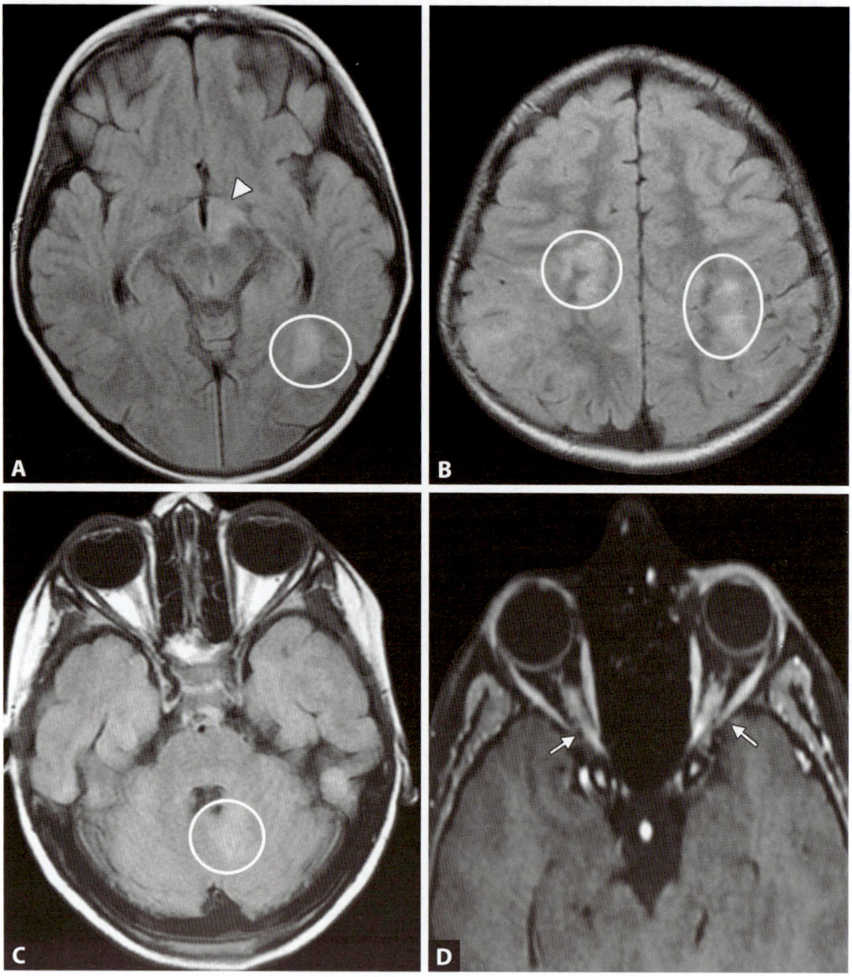

Figs. 15.6A to D: Representative images show the MRI findings in a patient with MOG-associated optic neuritis (MOGAD); (A) Axial T2-weighted MRI image showing a hyperintense lesion at the posterior horn of the lateral ventricle in the left temporoparietal cortex in a patient with MOGAD (white circle) and also inflammation along the left optic tract (white arrowhead); (B) Axial T2-weighted image showing poorly demarcated, fluffy, hyperintense lesions in the deep white matter in the temporoparietal lobe in a patient with MOGAD; (C) Axial T1-weighted MRI image showing a hyperintense lesion in the left cerebellum around the fourth ventricle in a child with MOGAD; (D) T1 postcontrast axial MRI scan showing intensely enhancing intraorbital and intracanalicular segments of both optic nerves. Note also the optic nerve sheath enhancement and mild swelling of the perineural fat stranding. (MRI: magnetic resonance imaging)

bands, pleocytosis, and biomarkers (CSF AQP-4, MOG, GFAP antibodies, and others such as CSF ACE levels). It can also help in ruling out other causes, such as infectious and paraneoplastic ON. Although CSF analysis was initially not recommended as an essential part of the workup of demyelinating ON, currently, in view of the increased spectrum of the etiologies understood, CSF analysis is gaining more importance.

Ideally, it should be performed in all patients, but it MUST be performed for patients showing the following features:

- Suspicion of MS
- Recurrent ON
- Suspected atypical ON
- High suspicion of ON in sarcoidosis, GFAP, paraneoplastic optic neuropathy, neurosyphilis, etc.

The following generalizations may be made as to the utility of the CSF abnormalities:

- *CSF oligoclonal bands'* presence is seen in 90% of MS patients as compared to 20% of patients with NMOSD.[95] It is important to note that a comparison should be done with the serum oligoclonal bands, and the presence of CSF oligoclonal bands without the presence of similar bands in serum is characteristic of demyelination.
- *CSF pleocytosis,* i.e., increased leukocytes in the CSF, is noted in many etiologies. CSF pleocytosis with >50 leukocytes/mL (observed approximately in 35% of NMOSD cases) or the presence of neutrophils or eosinophils (observed in 44% and 10% of patients with NMOSD, respectively, in attack-associated samples) is particularly useful in distinguishing NMOSD from MS.[96-98]

Cerebrospinal fluid analysis can also rule out infections and shows pleocytosis, high protein, and low glucose levels. It is important to do a microbiological examination to rule out infection in general.

In GFAP astrocytopathy, the presence of GFAP IgG in the CSF of patients with typical clinical presentation and MRI findings is confirmatory.[99] However, it is important to note that this is elevated only for a short period of time following an attack.[96,100]

Serology

Serological examination for various antibodies is needed and essential in every case of suspected ON in today's scenario. Serum testing is generally more sensitive than CSF for APQ-4 and MOG antibodies.[101,102]

The type of assay used for the detection of these antibodies determines the sensitivity and specificity for the detection of AQP-4 and MOG antibodies. The current recommendation is to use live cell-based assays. Existing literature suggests that assays based on the cell line of HEK293 are the most sensitive (77%), while cell-binding assays with fixed cells have a sensitivity of 73%, enzyme-linked immunosorbent assay (ELISA) assay has a sensitivity of 60%, and green fluorescent protein (GFP)-AQP-4 fluorescence immunoprecipitation assay is sensitive at 53%.[97,103] As already highlighted,

Flowchart 15.2: Suggested ocular and systemic workup of a patient with ON covering the major demyelinating diseases.

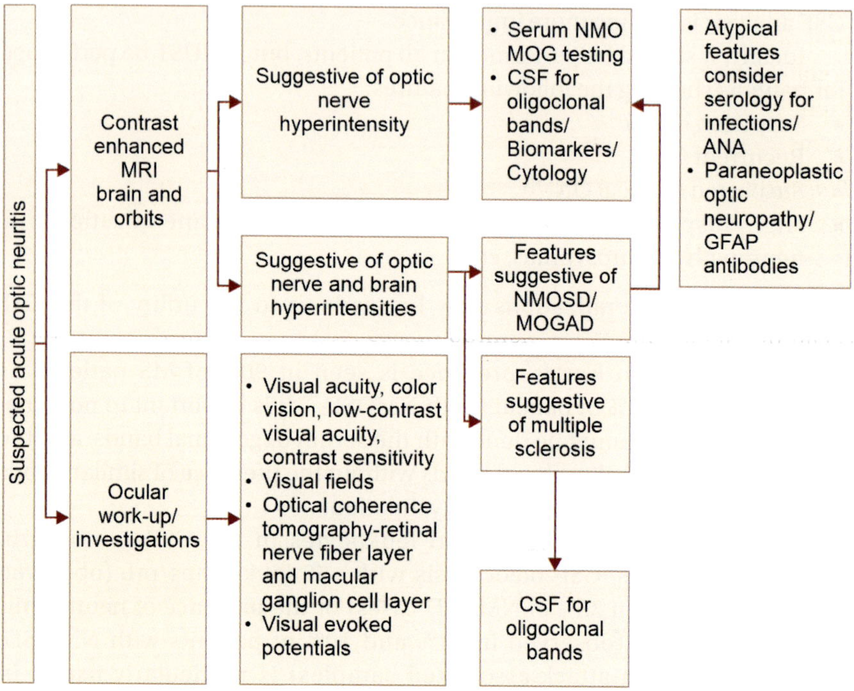

(CSF: cerebrospinal fluid; mGCL: macular ganglion cell layer; MOG: myelin oligodendrocyte glycoprotein; MRI: magnetic resonance imaging; MS: multiple sclerosis; NMO: neuromyelitis optica; NMOSD: neuromyelitis optica spectrum disorder; OCT: optical coherence tomography; ON: optic neuritis; RNFL: retinal nerve fiber layer; VEP: visual evoked potential)

particularly in the cases of AQP-4-ON, coexisting autoantibodies such as antinuclear antibody, antidouble-stranded deoxyribonucleic acid (DNA), anti-Ro, and anti-La may be seen in a substantial number of cases.

Serological tests to rule out infective causes should be done according to the suspected etiology **(Flowchart 15.2)**.

TREATMENT OF OPTIC NEURITIS

Acute Phase

Steroids: The evidence of using steroids was first shown by the ONTT,[1] where they showed that recurrence of ON was noted to be maximum after using oral steroids as compared to IV steroids or placebo. Following IV methylprednisolone (IVMP), a short rapid taper of oral steroids was given for 11 days. The authors also reported that there was no difference in the final visual acuity among the three groups. This study was done in the case of typical ON.[104] The most frequently used IV steroid is methylprednisolone, which is given at the dosage of 16–30 mg/kg body weight (about 1 g/day for 60 kg adults) for 3–5 days. This is followed by the prolonged taper of oral steroids. IV dexamethasone 200 mg/kg has also been shown to be equally effective as 1 g of IVMP. A Cochrane review by Gal et al. reported that there is no significant benefit in using IVMP or oral steroids in typical ON in terms of visual acuity, contrast sensitivity, and visual field.[105]

Plasmapheresis: It is generally used in patients who fail to respond to IVMP, especially in the case of NMOSD. It has been shown that plasmapheresis is associated with better visual outcomes, when used earlier.[106] It works on the principle of removing the inciting antibodies from the serum to prevent further damage to the neurons. It is most effective in cases of NMOSD in which AQP-4 antibodies are "sieved" from the serum.

Intravenous immunoglobulins (IVIGs): IVIGs are known to produce remyelination in cases of demyelination. It was postulated by Rodriguez that the presence of IgG in areas of demyelination has the potential to cause myelin repair.[107] It has been shown to be effective in cases of ON that are refractory to steroids. However, this study only analyzed its effects on ON due to MS.[108] Another study showed that IVIG can be useful in cases of NMOSD with recurrent ON.[109] Currently, the following are considered to be the indications for the use of IVIG in the acute phase: MOGAD especially syndromic presentations with meningoencephalitis, poor visual recovery in MOGAD, and recurrent MOGAD disease.[86,103] IVIG might be considered even in refractory cases of NMOSD but plasmapheresis has a better outcome.

Chronic Phase

Long-term treatment of ON includes disease-modifying drugs for patients in the chronic phase of ON.

Various disease-modifying agents have been tested for MS-related ON. Interferon beta-1a and 1b, which are given as subcutaneous injections, have been shown to reduce relapses in clinically defined MS.[110,111] Glatiramer acetate and dimethyl fumarate have also been shown to reduce relapses in cases of MS.[112,113] However, clinically, these drugs are uncommonly used by ophthalmologists alone and must be used in conjunction with a neurologist.

In cases of NMOSD, it is critical to start immunosuppressive therapy as the first-line therapy along with acute management with steroids or plasmapheresis, to prevent relapses. *Azathioprine* has been shown to reduce relapses by 75%.[114,115] It should be started at the time of oral steroids as the peak effect of this drug takes 3 months. Hence, by the time steroids are tapered, azathioprine begins to act. The dose used is 2.5–3 mg/kg/day. If a patient is on this drug, 3-monthly monitoring of liver function tests and blood counts should be done as this drug is hepatotoxic and can cause bone marrow suppression.

Mycophenolate mofetil is an alternative to azathioprine which has also been shown to reduce relapses in NMOSD. Some studies suggest that MMF might be even more effective than azathioprine in managing these patients. This too, like azathioprine, is hepatotoxic and can cause bone marrow suppression. In addition, it also has renal toxicity for which renal function tests should be done routinely.[115]

The above-mentioned drugs are expensive and, hence, not commonly used in Indian settings. *Methotrexate* is a cheaper alternative to these drugs. Some studies suggest that it can reduce the recurrence rates by 86%. It is started at a dose of 7.5 mg once weekly that can be built up successively. It is a relatively well-tolerated drug but not considered as the first-line drug in the management of demyelinating ON.[116]

NEWER TREATMENT OPTIONS

Mesenchymal stem cell research is being investigated for the treatment of ON. A review by Aneesh et al. has summarized the utility of mesenchymal stem cell-based extracellular vehicles for their anti-inflammatory effect and remyelination of optic nerves in ON, based on studies primarily done in animals.[116,117]

Eculizumab is a newer humanized C5 monoclonal antibody that has been tried in cases with NMOSD **(Table 15.3)**. It is used previously in paroxysmal nocturnal hemoglobinuria as well as refractory myasthenia gravis. Studies by Pittock et al. have shown that it reduces relapses in these cases. The drawback with this drug is that there is a high risk of meningococcal meningitis for which it is recommended to take vaccination against the same before starting the treatment.[118]

Satralizumab is another monoclonal antibody being explored for NMOSD. It is believed to work against the interleukin (IL)-6 signaling pathways, which then reduces the inflammation.[119] SAkuraStar and SAkuraSky are two randomized controlled trials that have shown the efficacy of this drug in NMOSD.[120]

A humanized afucosylated monoclonal antibody, known as *inebilizumab*, has been developed. It targets the B cells that express CD-19. The N-Momentum study evaluated the efficacy of this drug in NMOSD patients and showed reduced recurrences in such patients.[121]

TABLE 15.3: Monoclonal antibodies used for the treatment of NMOSD.

Drugs	*Type of antibody*	*Clinical trial*
Eculizumab	C5 monoclonal antibody	PREVENT
Satralizumab	Anti-IL-6 monoclonal antibody	SAkuraStar and SAkuraSky
Inebilizumab	Anti-CD-19 monoclonal antibody	N-Momentum

(IL: interleukin; NMOSD: neuromyelitis optica spectrum disorder)

PEDIATRIC OPTIC NEURITIS

Optic neuritis in the pediatric population is different from ON in adults, as it is more commonly bilateral, steroid-sensitive, and steroid-dependent and usually preceded by a viral infection/vaccination. In all cases, complete blood picture and antibody tests for NMO and MOG should be done, in addition to MRI brain and orbit with contrast. Children are also more likely to have ADEM/meningoencephalitis-like presentation as compared to adults, where the disease usually presents as a monofocal CNS disease. One more differentiating feature of pediatric ON is that it tends to have a better visual recovery than ON in adults. As in adults, IVMP is the first line of treatment, given at a dose of 16–30 mg/kg/body weight. Definite treatment does depend upon the underlying final etiology.

In general, the following suggestions might be considered:[86,122]

- Clinically isolated syndrome/postinfectious case/idiopathic ON: No immunosuppressive agents are needed.
- If the child has MS, then the first-line therapy would include interferon beta and glatiramer acetate.
- In cases of NMOSD, rituximab is the first choice.
- In MOG-associated ON, IVIG is considered as the first-line drug for the treatment of recurrent disease/severe disease with ADEM/ meningoencephalitis-like presentation.

CONCLUSION

To summarize, currently, a lot of advances have taken place in the understanding of ON. Currently, it is best recognized as a syndrome of acute vision loss (or disturbance), usually associated with pain and dyschromatopsia, occurring commonly due to an underlying demyelinating ON. The most common etiologies are isolated demyelination, MS, NMOSD, and MOGAD; however, many biomarkers and their characteristics are being identified. Therefore, it is essential to establish the underlying etiology. Workup involves ocular investigations, neuroimaging of brain and spine, serological investigations to identify biomarkers, and CSF analysis. Each of these conditions has a different clinical course and chances of recurrence. Treatment should be tailor-made according to the final etiology, and multidisciplinary care is often needed.

REFERENCES

1. Optic Neuritis Study Group. The clinical profile of optic neuritis. Experience of the optic neuritis treatment trial. Arch Ophthalmol. 1991;109(12):1673-8.
2. Beck RW. The optic neuritis treatment trial: three-year follow-up results. Arch Ophthalmol. 1995;113(2):136-7.
3. Optic Neuritis Study Group. Visual function 15 years after optic neuritis: a final follow-up report from the optic neuritis treatment trial. Ophthalmology. 2008;115(6):1079-82.

4. Hassan MB, Stern C, Flanagan EP, Pittock SJ, Kunchok A, Foster RC, et al. Population-based incidence of optic neuritis in the era of aquaporin-4 and myelin oligodendrocyte glycoprotein antibodies. Am J Ophthalmol. 2020;220:110-4.
5. Ambika S, Durgapriyadarshini S, Padmalakshmi K, Noronha V, Arjundas D. Clinical profile, imaging features and short-term visual outcomes of Indian optic neuritis patients with and without seromarkers for myelin oligodendrocyte glycoprotein and neuromyelitis optica. Indian J Ophthalmol. 2022;70(1):194-200.
6. Writing Committee for the Pediatric Eye Disease Investigator Group (PEDIG); Pineles SL, Repka MX, Liu GT, Waldman AT, Borchert MS, Khanna S, et al. Assessment of pediatric optic neuritis visual acuity outcomes at 6 months. JAMA Ophthalmol. 2020;138(12):1253-61.
7. Miller D, Barkhof F, Montalban X, Thompson A, Filippi M. Clinically isolated syndromes suggestive of multiple sclerosis, part I: natural history, pathogenesis, diagnosis, and prognosis. Lancet Neurol. 2005;4(5):281-8.
8. The clinical profile of optic neuritis. Experience of the optic neuritis treatment trial. Optic Neuritis Study Group. Arch Ophthalmol. 1991;109(12):1673-8.
9. Thompson AJ, Banwell BL, Barkhof F, Carroll WM, Coetzee T, Comi G, et al. Diagnosis of multiple sclerosis: 2017 revisions of the McDonald criteria. Lancet Neurol. 2018;17(2):162-73.
10. Lennon VA, Wingerchuk DM, Kryzer TJ, Pittock SJ, Lucchinetti CF, Fujihara K, et al. A serum autoantibody marker of neuromyelitis optica: distinction from multiple sclerosis. Lancet. 2004;364(9451):2106-12.
11. Hinson SR, Pittock SJ, Lucchinetti CF, Roemer SF, Fryer JP, Kryzer TJ, et al. Pathogenic potential of IgG binding to water channel extracellular domain in neuromyelitis optica. Neurology. 2007;69(24):2221-31.
12. Pittock SJ, Lucchinetti CF. Neuromyelitis optica and the evolving spectrum of autoimmune aquaporin-4 channelopathies: a decade later. Ann N Y Acad Sci. 2016;1366(1):20-39.
13. Mealy MA, Kessler RA, Rimler Z, Reid A, Totonis L, Cutter G, et al. Mortality in neuromyelitis optica is strongly associated with African ancestry. Neurol Neuroimmunol Neuroinflamm. 2018;5(4):e468.
14. Huda S, Whittam D, Bhojak M, Kneen R. Neuromyelitis optica spectrum disorders. Clin Med. 2019;19(2):169-76.
15. Quek AM, McKeon A, Lennon VA, Mandrekar JN, Iorio R, Jiao Y, et al. Effects of age and sex on aquaporin-4 autoimmunity. Arch Neurol. 2012;69(8):1039-43.
16. Bove R, Elsone L, Alvarez E, Borisow N, Cortez MM, Mateen FJ, et al. Female hormonal exposures and neuromyelitis optica symptom onset in a multicenter study. Neurol Neuroimmunol Neuroinflamm. 2017;4(3):e339.
17. Pereira WL, Reiche EM, Kallaur AP, Kaimen-Maciel DR. Epidemiological, clinical, and immunological characteristics of neuromyelitis optica: a review. J Neurol Sci. 2015;355(1-2):7-17.
18. Pandit L. Neuromyelitis optica spectrum disorders: an update. Ann Indian Acad Neurol. 2015;18(Supp 1):S11-5.
19. Hansapinyo L, Vivattanaseth C. Clinical characteristics, treatment outcome and predictive factors in optic neuritis. Open Ophthalmol J. 2018;12:247-55.
20. Pittock SJ, Lennon VA, de Seze J, Vermersch P, Homburger HA, Wingerchuk DM, et al. Neuromyelitis optica and non-organ specific autoimmunity. Arch Neurol. 2008;65(1):78-83.

21. Jacob S, Zarei M, Kenton A Allroggen H. Gluten sensitivity and neuro-myelitis optica: two case reports. J Neurol Neurosurg Psychiatry. 2005;76(7):1028-30.
22. Leite MI, Coutinho E, Lana-Peixoto M, Apostolos S, Waters P, Sato D, et al. Myasthenia gravis and neuromyelitis optica spectrum disorder: a multicenter study of 16 patients. Neurology. 2012;78(20):1601-7.
23. Wingerchuk DM, Banwell B, Bennett JL, Cabre P, Carroll W, Chitnis T, et al. International panel for NMO diagnosis. International consensus diagnostic criteria for neuromyelitis optica spectrum disorders. Neurology. 2015;85(2): 177-89.
24. De Lott LB, Bennett JL, Costello F. The changing landscape of optic neuritis: a narrative review. J Neurol. 2022;269(1):111-24.
25. Weber MS, Derfuss T, Metz I, Brück W. Defining distinct features of anti-MOG antibody associated central nervous system demyelination. Ther Adv Neurol Disord. 2018;11:1-15.
26. Chen JJ, Flanagan EP, Jitprapaikulsan J, López-Chiriboga AS, Fryer JP, Leavitt JA, et al. Myelin oligodendrocyte glycoprotein antibody-positive optic neuritis: clinical characteristics, radiologic clues, and outcome. Am J Ophthalmol. 2018;195:8-15.
27. Di Pauli F, Berger T. Myelin oligodendrocyte glycoprotein antibody-associated and disorders: toward a new spectrum of inflammatory demyelinating CNS disorders? Front Immunol. 2018;9:2753.
28. Ramanathan S, Mohammad S, Tantsis E, Nguyen TK, Merheb V, Fung VS, et al. Clinical course, therapeutic and responses and outcomes in relapsing MOG antibody-associated demyelination. J Neurol Neurosurg Psychiatry. 2018;89(2):127-37.
29. Satukijchai C, Mariano R, Messina S, et al. Factors associated with relapse and treatment of myelin oligodendrocyte glycoprotein antibody-associated disease in the United Kingdom. JAMA Netw Open. 2022;5(1):e2142780.
30. Banwell B, Bennett JL, Marignier R, Kim HJ, Brilot F, Flanagan EP, et al. Diagnosis of myelin oligodendrocyte glycoprotein antibody-associated disease: international MOGAD panel proposed criteria. Lancet Neurol. 2023;22(3):268-82.
31. Gravier-Dumonceau A, Ameli R, Rogemond V, Ruiz A, Joubert B, Muñiz-Castrillo S, et al. Glial fibrillary acidic protein autoimmunity: a French Cohort Study. Neurology. 2022;98(6):e653-68.
32. Kunchok A, Zekeridou A, McKeon A. Autoimmune glial fibrillary acidic protein astrocytopathy. Curr Opin Neurol. 2019;32(3):452-8.
33. Fang B, McKeon A, Hinson SR, Kryzer TJ, Pittock SJ, Aksamit AJ, Lennon VA. Autoimmune glial fibrillary acidic protein astrocytopathy: a novel meningoencephalomyelitis. JAMA Neurol. 2016;73(11):1297-307.
34. Azzolini F, Farina A, Gastaldi M, Barilaro A, Scotti V, Falchetti G, et al. Leptomeningeal gadolinium enhancement in autoimmune GFAP astrocytopathy. Neurology. 2022;98(17):720-2.
35. Tewkesbury G, Song JW, Perrone CM. Magnetic resonance imaging of autoimmune GFAP astrocytopathy. Ann Neurol. 2021;90(4):691-2.
36. Dubey D, Hinson SR, Jolliffe EA, Zekeridou A, Flanagan EP, Pittock SJ, et al. Autoimmune GFAP astrocytopathy: prospective evaluation of 90 patients in 1 year. J Neuroimmunol. 2018;321:157-63.
37. Greco G, Masciocchi S, Diamanti L, Bini P, Vegezzi E, Marchioni E, et al. Visual system involvement in glial fibrillary acidic protein astrocytopathy:

two case reports and a systematic literature review. Neurol Neuroimmunol Neuroinflamm. 2023;15;10(5):e200146.

38. Liedtke W, Edelmann W, Bieri PL, Chiu FC, Cowan NJ, Kucherlapati R, et al. GFAP is necessary for the integrity of CNS white matter architecture and long-term maintenance of myelination. Neuron. 1996;17(4):607-15.
39. Chen JJ, Aksamit AJ, McKeon A, Pittock SJ, Weinshenker BG, Leavitt JA, et al. Optic disc edema in glial fibrillary acidic protein autoantibody-positive meningoencephalitis. J Neuroophthalmol. 2018;38(3):276-81.
40. Utley WJ, El-Dieb A, Chancellor AM. Anti-GFAP neuroinflammation with synchronous bilateral papillitis and characteristic imaging. Pract Neurol. 2020;002805.
41. Dubey D, Lennon VA, Gadoth A, Pittock SJ, Flanagan EP, Schmeling JE, et al. Autoimmune CRMP5 neuropathy phenotype and outcome defined from 105 cases. Neurology. 2018;90(2):e103-10.
42. Cohen DA, Bhatti MT, Pulido JS, Lennon VA, Dubey D, Flanagan EP, et al. Collapsin response-mediator protein 5-associated retinitis, vitritis, and optic disc edema. Ophthalmology. 2020;127(2):221-9.
43. Igarashi N, Sawamura H, Kaburaki T, Aihara M. Anti-collapsing response-mediating protein-5 antibody-positive paraneoplastic perioptic neuritis without typical neurological symptoms. Neuroophthalmology. 2016;41(1):24-9.
44. Cross SA, Salomao DR, Parisi JE, Kryzer TJ, Bradley EA, Mines JA. Paraneoplastic autoimmune optic neuritis with retinitis defined by CRMP-5-IgG. Ann Neurol. 2003;54(1):38-50.
45. Arés-Luque A, García-Tuñón LA, Saiz A, Cabezas BC, Hernández-Echebarría LE, Franco M, et al. Isolated paraneoplastic optic neuropathy associated with small-cell lung cancer and anti-CV2 antibodies. J Neurol. 2007;254(8):1131-2.
46. Durrani A, Shah RJ, Kim SJ. Successful long-term treatment of paraneoplastic optic neuropathy with mycophenolate mofetil, prednisone, and plasmapheresis. Am J Ophthalmol Case Rep. 2017;8:31-4.
47. Kidd D, Burton B, Plant GT, Graham EM. Chronic relapsing inflammatory optic neuropathy (CRION). Brain. 2003;126(2):276-84.
48. Benoilid A, Tilikete C, Collongues N, Arndt C, Vighetto A, Vignal C, et al. Relapsing optic neuritis: a multicenter study of 62 patients. Mult Scler. 2014;20(7):848-53.
49. Petzold A, Plant GT. Chronic relapsing inflammatory optic neuropathy: a systematic review of 122 cases reported. J Neurol. 2014;261(1):17-26.
50. Liu H, Zhou H, Wang J, Xu Q, Wei S. Antibodies to myelin oligodendrocyte glycoprotein in chronic relapsing inflammatory optic neuropathy. Br J Ophthalmol. 2019;103(10):1423-8.
51. Frohman L, Dellatorre K, Turbin R, Bielory L. Clinical characteristics, diagnostic criteria and therapeutic outcomes in autoimmune optic neuropathy. Br J Ophthalmol. 2009;93(12):1660-6.
52. Asgari N, Jarius S, Laustrup H, Skejoe HP, Lillevang ST, Weinshenker BG, et al. Aquaporin-4-autoimmunity in patients with systemic lupus erythematosus: a predominantly population-based study. Mult Scler. 2018;24(3):331-9.
53. Baughman RP, Weiss KL, Golnik KC. Neuro-ophthalmic sarcoidosis. Eye Brain. 2012;4:13-25.
54. Cunningham ET Jr, Tugal-Tutkun I, Khairallah M, Okada AA, Bodaghi B, Zierhut M. Behçet Uveitis. Ocul Immunol Inflamm. 2017;25(1):2-6.

55. Arepalli SR, Thomas AS. Occlusive retinal vasculitis: novel insights into causes, pathogenesis and treatment. Curr Opin Ophthalmol. 2022;33(3):147-56.
56. Kidd DP. Optic neuropathy in Behçet's syndrome. J Neurol. 2013;260(12):3065-70.
57. Comarmond C, Cacoub P. Granulomatosis with polyangiitis (Wegener): clinical aspects and treatment. Autoimmun Rev. 2014;13(11):1121-5.
58. Kidd DP, Burton BJ, Graham EM, Plant GT. Optic neuropathy associated with systemic sarcoidosis. Neurol Neuroimmunol Neuroinflamm. 2016;3(5):e270.
59. Kidd DP. Neurosarcoidosis: clinical manifestations, investigation and treatment. Pract Neurol. 2020;20(3):199-212.
60. Iannuzzi MC, Rybicki BA, Teirstein AS. Sarcoidosis. N Engl J Med. 2007;357(21): 2153-65.
61. Grunewald J, Grutters JC, Arkema EV, Saketkoo LA, Moller DR, Müller-Quernheim J. Sarcoidosis. Nat Rev Dis Primers. 2019;5(1):45.
62. Nevalainen J, Krapp E, Paetzold J, Mildenberger I, Besch D, Vonthein R, et al. Visual field defects in acute optic neuritis-distribution of different types of defect pattern, assessed with threshold-related supraliminal perimetry, ensuring high spatial resolution. Graefes Arch Clin Exp Ophthalmol. 2008;246(4):599-607.
63. Holder GE. Electrophysiological assessment of optic nerve disease. Eye (Lond). 2004;18(11):1133-43.
64. Kupersmith MJ, Garvin MK, Wang JK, Durbin M, Kardon R. Retinal ganglion cell layer thinning within one month of presentation for optic neuritis. Mult Scler. 2016;22:641-8.
65. Behbehani R, Al-Moosa A, Sriraman D, Alroughani R. Ganglion cell analysis in acute optic neuritis. Mult Scler Relat Disord. 2016;5:66-9.
66. Fukuchi M, Kishi S, Li D, Akiyama H. Acute ganglion cell loss during rapid visual recovery in optic neuritis. Graefes Arch Clin Exp Ophthalmol. 2016;254(12):2355-60.
67. Huang-Link YM, Al-Hawasi A, Lindehammar H. Acute optic neuritis: retinal ganglion cell loss precedes retinal nerve fiber thinning. Neurol Sci. 2015;36(4): 617-20.
68. Fisher JB, Jacobs DA, Markowitz CE, Galetta SJ, Volpe NJ, Nano-Schiahvi et al. Relation of visual function to retinal nerve fiber layer thickness in multiple sclerosis. Ophthalmology. 2006;113(2):324-32.
69. Petzold A, de Boer JF, Schippling S, Vermersch P, Kardon R, Green A, et al. Optical coherence tomography in multiple sclerosis: a systematic review and meta-analysis. Lancet Neurol. 2010;9(9):921-32.
70. Saidha S, Syc SB, Durbin MK, Eckstein C, Oakley JD, Meyer SA, et al. Visual dysfunction in multiple sclerosis correlates better with optical coherence tomography derived estimates of macular ganglion cell layer thickness than peripapillary retinal nerve fiber layer thickness. Mult Scler. 2011;17(12):1449-63.
71. Pillay G, Ganger A, Singh D, Bhatia R, Sharma P, Menon V, et al. Retinal nerve fiber layer and ganglion cell layer changes on optical coherence tomography in early multiple sclerosis and optic neuritis cases. Indian J Ophthalmol. 2018;66(1): 114-9.
72. Bennett JL, de Seze J, Lana-Peixoto M, Palace J, Waldman A, Schippling S, et al. Neuromyelitis optica and multiple sclerosis: seeing differences through optical coherence tomography. Mult Scler. 2015;21(6):678-88.
73. Hemond CC, Bakshi R. Magnetic resonance imaging in multiple sclerosis. Cold Spring Harb Perspect Med. 2018;8(5):a028969.

74. Kim W, Park MS, Lee SH, Kim SH, Jung IJ, Takahashi T, et al. Characteristic brain magnetic resonance imaging abnormalities in central nervous system aquaporin-4 autoimmunity. Mult Scler. 2010;16(10):1229-36.
75. Merle H, Olindo S, Jeannin S, Hage R, Donnio A, Richer R, et al. Visual field characteristics in neuromyelitis optica in absence of and after one episode of optic neuritis. Clin Ophthalmol. 2013;7:1145-53.
76. Li Y, Xie P, Lv F, Mu J, Li Q, Yang Q, et al. Brain magnetic resonance imaging abnormalities in neuromyelitis Optica. Acta Neurol Scand. 2008;118(4):218-25.
77. Storoni M, Davagnanam I, Radon M, Siddiqui A, Plant GT. Distinguishing optic neuritis in neuromyelitis optica spectrum disease from multiple sclerosis: a novel magnetic resonance imaging scoring system. J Neuroophthalmol. 2013;33(2):123-7.
78. Jarius S, Ruprecht K, Wildemann B, Kuempfel T, Ringelstein M, Geis C, et al. Contrasting disease patterns in seropositive and seronegative neuromyelitis optica: a multicenter study of 175 patients. J Neuroinflammation. 2012;9:14.
79. Pittock SJ, Lennon VA, Krecke K, Wingerchuk DM, Lucchinetti CF, Weinshenker BG. Brain abnormalities in neuromyelitis optica. Arch Neurol. 2006;63(3):390-6.
80. Wingerchuk DM, Hogancamp WF, O'Brien PC, Weinshenker BG. The clinical course of neuromyelitis optica (Devic's syndrome). Neurology. 1999;53(5):1107-14.
81. Flanagan EP, Weinshenker BG, Krecke KN, Lennon VA, Lucchinetti CF, McKeon A, et al. Pittock SJ. Short myelitis lesions in aquaporin-4-IgG-positive neuromyelitis optica spectrum disorders. JAMA Neurol. 2015;72(1):81-7.
82. Pittock SJ, Weinshenker BG, Lucchinetti CF, Wingerchuk DM, Corboy JR, Lennon VA. Neuromyelitis optica brain lesions localized at sites of high aquaporin 4 expression. Arch Neurol. 2006;63(7):964-8.
83. Nakamura M, Misu T, Fujihara K, Miyazawa I, Nakashima I, Takahashi T, et al. Occurrence of acute large and edematous callosal lesions in neuromyelitis optica. Mult Scler. 2009;15(6):695-700.
84. Jurynczyk M, Geraldes R, Probert F, Woodhall MR, Waters P, Tackley G, et al. Distinct brain imaging characteristics of autoantibody-mediated CNS conditions and multiple sclerosis. Brain. 2017;140(3):617-27.
85. Cobo-Calvo Á, Ruiz A, D'Indy H, Poulat AL, Carneiro M, Philippe N, et al. MOG antibody-related disorders: common features and uncommon presentations. J Neurol. 2017;264(9):1945-55.
86. Hacohen Y, Mankad K, Chong WK, Barkhof F, Vincent A, Lim M, et al. Diagnostic algorithm for relapsing acquired demyelinating syndromes in children. Neurology. 2017;89(3):269-78.
87. Salama S, Khan M, Pardo S, Izbudak I, Levy M. MOG antibody-associated encephalomyelitis/encephalitis. Mult Scler. 2019;25(11):1427-33.
88. Cobo-Calvo A, Ruiz A, Maillart E, Audoin B, Zephir H, Bourre B, et al; OFSEP and NOMADMUS Study Group. Clinical spectrum and prognostic value of CNS MOG autoimmunity in adults: the MOGADOR study. Neurology. 2018;90(21):e1858-69.
89. Numa S, Kasai T, Kondo T, Kushimura Y, Kimura A, Takahashi H, et al. An adult case of anti-myelin oligodendrocyte glycoprotein (MOG) antibody-associated multiphasic acute disseminated encephalomyelitis at 33-year Intervals. Intern Med. 2016;55(6):699-702.

90. Kitley J, Leite MI, Küker W, Quaghebeur G, George J, Waters P, et al. Longitudinally extensive transverse myelitis with and without aquaporin 4 antibodies. JAMA Neurol. 2013;70(11):1375-81.
91. Pekcevik Y, Mitchell CH, Mealy MA, Orman G, Lee In H, Newsome Scott D, et al. Differentiating neuromyelitis optica from other causes of longitudinally extensive transverse myelitis on spinal magnetic resonance imaging. Mult Scler. 2016;22(3):302-11.
92. Kitley J, Waters P, Woodhall M, Leite MI, Murchison A, George J, et al. Neuromyelitis optica spectrum disorders with aquaporin-4 and myelin-oligodendrocyte glycoprotein antibodies: a comparative study. JAMA Neurol. 2014;71(3):276-83.
93. Ogawa R, Nakashima I, Takahashi T, et al. MOG antibody-positive, benign, unilateral, cerebral cortical encephalitis with epilepsy. Neurol Neuroimmunol Neuroinflamm. 2017;4(2):e322.
94. Lana-Peixoto MA, Talim N. Neuromyelitis optica spectrum disorder and anti-MOG syndromes. Biomedicines. 2019;7(2):42.
95. Bergamaschi R, Tonietti S, Franciotta D, Candeloro E, Tavazzi E, Piccolo G, et al. Oligoclonal bands in Devic's neuromyelitis Optica and multiple sclerosis: differences in repeated cerebrospinal fluid examinations. Mult Scler. 2004;10(1):2-4.
96. Takano R, Misu T, Takahashi T, Sato S, Fujihara K, Itoyama Y. Astrocytic damage is far more severe than demyelination in NMO: a clinical CSF biomarker study. Neurology. 2010;75(3):208-16.
97. Reindl M, Schanda K, Woodhall M, Tea F, Ramanathan S, Sagen J, et al. International multicenter examination of MOG antibody assays. Neurol Neuroimmunol Neuroinflamm. 2020;7(2):e674.
98. Jarius S, Pellkofer H, Siebert N, Korporal-Kuhnke M, Hümmert MW, Ringelstein M, et al. Cerebrospinal fluid findings in patients with myelin oligodendrocyte glycoprotein (MOG) antibodies. Part 1: results from 163 lumbar punctures in 100 adult patients. J Neuroinflammation. 2020;17(1):261.
99. Flanagan EP, Hinson SR, Lennon VA, Fang B, Aksamit AJ, Morris PP, et al. Glial fibrillary acidic protein immunoglobulin G as biomarker of autoimmune astrocytopathy: analysis of 102 patients. Ann Neurol. 2017;81(2):298-309.
100. Misu T, Takano R, Fujihara K, Takahashi T, Sato S, Itoyama Y. Marked increase in cerebrospinal fluid glial fibrillar acidic protein in neuromyelitis optica: an astrocytic damage marker. J Neurol Neurosurg Psychiatr. 2009;80(5):575-7.
101. Majed M, Fryer JP, McKeon A, Lennon VA, Pittock SJ. Clinical utility of testing AQP4-IgG in CSF: guidance for physicians. Neurol Neuroimmunol Neuroinflamm. 2016;3(3):e231.
102. Pace S, Orrell M, Woodhall M, Palace J, Leite MI, Irani SR, et al. Frequency of MOG-IgG in cerebrospinal fluid versus serum. J Neurol Neurosurg Psychiatry. 2022;93(3):334-5.
103. Marchionatti A, Hansel G, Avila GU, Sato DK. Detection of MOG-IgG in clinical samples by live cell-based assays: performance of immunofluorescence microscopy and flow cytometry. Front Immunol. 2021;12:642272.
104. Beck RW, Cleary PA, Anderson MM Jr, Keltner JL, Shults WT, Kaufman DI, et al. A randomized, controlled trial of corticosteroids in the treatment of acute optic neuritis. The Optic Neuritis Study Group. N Engl J Med. 1992;326(9):581-8.

105. Gal RL, Vedula SS, Beck R. Corticosteroids for treating optic neuritis. Cochrane Eyes and Vision Group, editor. Cochrane Database Syst Rev. [online] Available from https://pubmed.ncbi.nlm.nih.gov/26273799/ [Last accessed September, 2024].
106. Chen JJ, Flanagan EP, Pittock SJ, Stern NC, Tisavipat N, Bhatti MT, et al. Visual outcomes following plasma exchange for optic neuritis: an international multicenter retrospective analysis of 395 optic neuritis attacks. Am J Ophthalmol. 2023;252:213-24.
107. Rodriguez M, Lennon VA. Immunoglobulins promote remyelination in the central nervous system. Ann Neurol. 1990;27(1):12-7.
108. Tselis A, Perumal J, Caon C, Hreha S, Ching W, Din M, et al. Treatment of corticosteroid refractory optic neuritis in multiple sclerosis patients with intravenous immunoglobulin. Eur J Neurol. 2008;15(11):1163-7.
109. Altunrende B, Akdal G, Soylev Bajin M, Yaman A, Kocaslan M, Nalbantoglu M, et al. Intravenous immunoglobulin treatment for recurrent optic neuritis. Noro Psikiyatri Arsivi. [online] Available from http://www.noropsikiyatriarsivi.com/crossref?doi=10.5152/npa.2017.20577 [Last accessed September, 2024]
110. Jacobs LD, Beck RW, Simon JH, Kinkel RP, Brownscheidle CM, Murray TJ, et al. Intramuscular interferon beta-1A therapy initiated during a first demyelinating event in multiple sclerosis. N Engl J Med. 2000;343(13):898-904.
111. Kappos L, Freedman MS, Polman CH, Edan G, Hartung HP, Miller DH, et al. Effect of early versus delayed interferon beta-1b treatment on disability after a first clinical event suggestive of multiple sclerosis: a 3-year follow-up analysis of the BENEFIT study. Lancet. 2007;370(9585):389-97.
112. Fox RJ, Miller DH, Phillips JT, Hutchinson M, Havrdova E, Kita M, et al. Placebo-controlled phase 3 study of oral BG-12 or glatiramer in multiple sclerosis. N Engl J Med. 2012;367(12):1087-97.
113. Khan O, Rieckmann P, Boyko A, Selmaj K, Zivadinov R, GALA Study Group. Three times weekly glatiramer acetate in relapsing–remitting multiple sclerosis. Ann Neurol. 2013;73(6):705-13.
114. Costanzi C, Matiello M, Lucchinetti CF, Weinshenker BG, Pittock SJ, Mandrekar J, et al. Azathioprine: tolerability, efficacy, and predictors of benefit in neuromyelitis Optica. Neurology. 2011;77(7):659-66.
115. Jacob A, Matiello M, Weinshenker BG, Wingerchuk DM, Lucchinetti C, Shuster E, et al. Treatment of neuromyelitis Optica with mycophenolate mofetil. Arch Neurol. 2009;66(9):1128-33.
116. Kitley J, Elsone L, George J, Waters P, Woodhall M, Vincent A, et al. Methotrexate is an alternative to azathioprine in neuromyelitis Optica spectrum disorders with aquaporin-4 antibodies. J Neurol Neurosurg Psychiatry. 2013;84(8):918-21.
117. Aneesh A, Liu A, Moss HE, Feinstein D, Ravindran S, Mathew B, et al. Emerging concepts in the treatment of optic neuritis: mesenchymal stem cell-derived extracellular vesicles. Stem Cell Res Ther. 2021;12(1):594.
118. Pittock SJ, Lennon VA, McKeon A, Mandrekar J, Weinshenker BG, Lucchinetti CF, et al. Eculizumab in AQP4-IgG-positive relapsing neuromyelitis optica spectrum disorders: an open-label pilot study. Lancet Neurol. 2013;12(6):554-62.

119. Traboulsee A, Greenberg BM, Bennett JL, Szczechowski L, Fox E, Shkrobot S, et al. Safety and efficacy of satralizumab monotherapy in neuromyelitis optica spectrum disorder: a randomized, double-blind, multicenter, placebo-controlled phase 3 trial. Lancet Neurol. 2020;19(5):402-12.
120. Sudhakar P, Abusamra K, Thandampallayam M, Kini A. New advancements in the management of neuromyelitis optica spectrum disease: literature review. Front Ophthalmol. 2023;3:1130971.
121. Cree BAC, Bennett JL, Kim HJ, Weinshenker BG, Pittock SJ, Wingerchuk DM, et al. Inebilizumab for the treatment of neuromyelitis optica spectrum disorder (N-MOmentum): a double-blind, randomized placebo-controlled phase 2/3 trial. Lancet. 2019;394(10206):1352-63.
122. Borchert M, Liu GT, Pineles S, Waldman AT. Pediatric optic neuritis: what is new. J Neuroophthalmol. 2017;37(Suppl 1):14-22.

16 CHAPTER

Management of Orbital Hemangioma

Rajendra Prakash Maurya, Sneha Gupta, Dipankar Das, Abdullah S Al-Mujaini

ABSTRACT

There is a wide variety of orbital tumors described in the literature, with hemangiomas emerging as the most prevalent benign vascular neoplasms. Cavernous hemangioma is the most common benign orbital tumor in adults, while capillary hemangioma is the most common vascular tumor in infancy. Over the past decade, diagnostic and treatment modalities for oculo-orbital hemangiomas have significantly advanced. State-of-the-art, noninvasive techniques such as time-resolved magnetic resonance angiography (MRA) offer intricate visualization of vascular orbital mass lesions. Treatment options for infantile capillary hemangiomas include systemic, intralesional, and topical corticosteroids; oral and intralesional propranolol; interferon-alpha; vincristine; and pulse dye laser (PDL) or carbon dioxide laser. Surgery is reserved solely for cases where infantile hemangiomas pose a threat to life or vision. Surgical excision remains the cornerstone of cavernous hemangioma treatment. Recent reports have highlighted successful applications of innovative techniques, such as intralesional pingyangmycin (bleomycin A5) as sclerotherapy and stereotactic fractional radiotherapy for cavernous hemangioma situated at the orbital apex. This chapter delineates the current understanding of the etiopathogenesis and pathophysiology of orbital hemangiomas, alongside recent advancements in diagnosis and management.

Keywords: Vascular tumor, cavernous venous malformations, orbital hemangioma, capillary hemangioma, infantile hemangioma, Kasabach–Merritt syndrome, sclerotherapy, oral propranolol, pulse dye laser

INTRODUCTION

Vascular anomalies encompass a spectrum of disorders characterized by abnormal blood vessel growth, presenting as identifiable vascular lesions. These anomalies commonly manifest in the pediatric age group. Among vascular anomalies, hemangiomas represent the most prevalent type, distinguished by endothelial cell proliferation.

In 1982, Mulliken and Glowacki introduced a *"biological classification scheme,"* categorizing vascular lesions into two primary groups: (1) Hemangiomas and (2) vascular malformations, depending on their clinical and histological features.[1] This classification labeled cavernous hemangioma as a benign neoplasm, but it is, in fact, a non-neoplastic condition occurring exclusively in adults. Cavernous hemangiomas neither proliferate nor involute and do not respond to systemic corticosteroids or beta-blockers.

Rootman later refined the classification of vascular anomalies into three categories: (1) Malformations, (2) shunts, and (3) new growths/neoplasms.[2,3] Vascular neoplasms, characterized by endothelial proliferation, are not present at birth and are more prevalent in females and individuals of Caucasian ethnicity. Infantile hemangiomas (IHs) gradually involute over time. In contrast, vascular malformations are present at birth, exhibit no proliferation or involution, and grow slowly in tandem with the individual's growth through ectasia and hypertrophy **(Table 16.1)**. However, factors such as trauma, hormonal fluctuations, and respiratory infections can trigger rapid expansion.[4,5] Vascular malformations show no predilection for gender or ethnicity. Shunts are abnormal communication between arterial and venous systems, such as caroticocavernous fistula (high flow) and dural fistula (low flow).

In 1999, the Orbital Society proposed a novel classification of vascular lesions based on their hemodynamic behavior, categorizing them into three types: Type I (no-flow lesions, e.g., lymphatic malformations), type II (low-flow lesions, e.g., venous malformations), and type III (high-flow lesions, e.g., arteriovenous malformations).[6]

In 2014, the International Society for the Study of Vascular Anomalies (ISSVA) revised the classification of vascular lesions, including IH among vascular neoplasms.[7] Infantile hemangiomas proliferate through mitosis, involuting over time, and respond to systemic steroids and beta-blockers. Many vascular lesions consist of multiple histological components; for

TABLE 16.1: Comparison of hemangiomas and vascular malformations.

Hemangiomas	*Vascular malformations*
Absent at birth	Present at birth
Independent life cycle	Relentless progression
Rapid proliferation (+ mitosis)	Slow expansion (hypertrophy)
Slow involution	Never involute
Female preponderance	No gender predilection
More common in Caucasian people	No racial predilection
Histology varies with the stage of lesion	Blood and lymphatic histology consistent over time

example, IHs may contain predominantly capillary components with some cavernous components. Hence, some experts consider capillary hemangiomas and cavernous hemangiomas as "vascular hamartomatous lesions."[6]

CAVERNOUS HEMANGIOMA

Cavernous hemangioma [also known as *cavernous venous malformation* (CVM)] stands as the most prevalent benign noninfiltrative vascular lesion encountered in the adult orbit. It constitutes 3.1–9% of all histopathologically confirmed orbital tumors.[8-12] CVM exhibits a predilection for females, with a ratio of 2:1, and typically manifests in the third or fifth decade of life.[13-15] The term "cavernous hemangioma" is considered obsolete due to the lesion's non-neoplastic behavior, characterized by the absence of active proliferation and mitosis of endothelial cells. Instead, it is referred to as cavernous venous malformation, reflecting normal endothelial cell turnover.[6]

Pathogenesis

The precise origin of CVM remains unclear; however, some studies suggest that it may arise from pre-existing capillary hemangioma or other congenital anomalies, with enlargement and budding of endothelial cells from interstitial vascular spaces followed by ensheathment by myofibroblast cells.[6,16] The growth of CVM is stimulated by various factors, including local hemodynamic disturbances, hypoxia, and hormonal changes.[6,15-17] Hood proposed that tumor growth does not stem from vascular element proliferation but rather from canalization and blood flow into pre-existing vascular malformations, secondary to systemic hemodynamic alterations.[18] Its enlargement during puberty and pregnancy suggests a role for hormone- or cytokine-mediated angiogenic factors. The high expression of progesterone receptors in the epithelial cells of CVM could underpin its female preponderance.[14,19]

Clinical Features

Cavernous venous malformations predominantly occur in the adult orbit, with rare manifestations in children due to their low proliferative tendencies. In instances where they do occur in children, they may be associated with systemic conditions, such as Maffucci syndrome (characterized by multiple enchondromas and soft-tissue hemangiomas) and blue rubber bleb nevus syndrome (featuring bluish cutaneous and mucosal hemangiomas, along with enteric hemangiomas, leading to gastrointestinal bleeding).[20,21] The clinical presentation of CVMs varies depending on their location within the orbit. Typically, over 90% of CVMs are situated in the lateral aspect of the intraconal space, with extraconal and medial locations being uncommon (<10% occurrence).[6,22] Rare occurrences include CVM presenting as a lacrimal gland mass or an intraosseous tumor.[23-25] The classical presentation of orbital CVMs involves a slowly progressive, nonpulsatile, painless unilateral proptosis **(Figs. 16.1A to D)**.

Other relatively less common presentations include hyperopia, gaze-induced amaurosis fugax (due to ischemia of the optic nerve), and diplopia.[19,26] Larger CVMs, particularly those located at the orbital apex, may lead to diffuse neuralgia, restriction of extraocular movement, visual field defects, and visual impairment or blindness.[27,28] Larger lesions, due to their mass effect, can cause bone remodeling, compressive optic neuropathy, and hyperdynamic disturbances in the surrounding soft tissue. Ophthalmoscopic signs commonly observed include choroidal folds, optic disc edema,

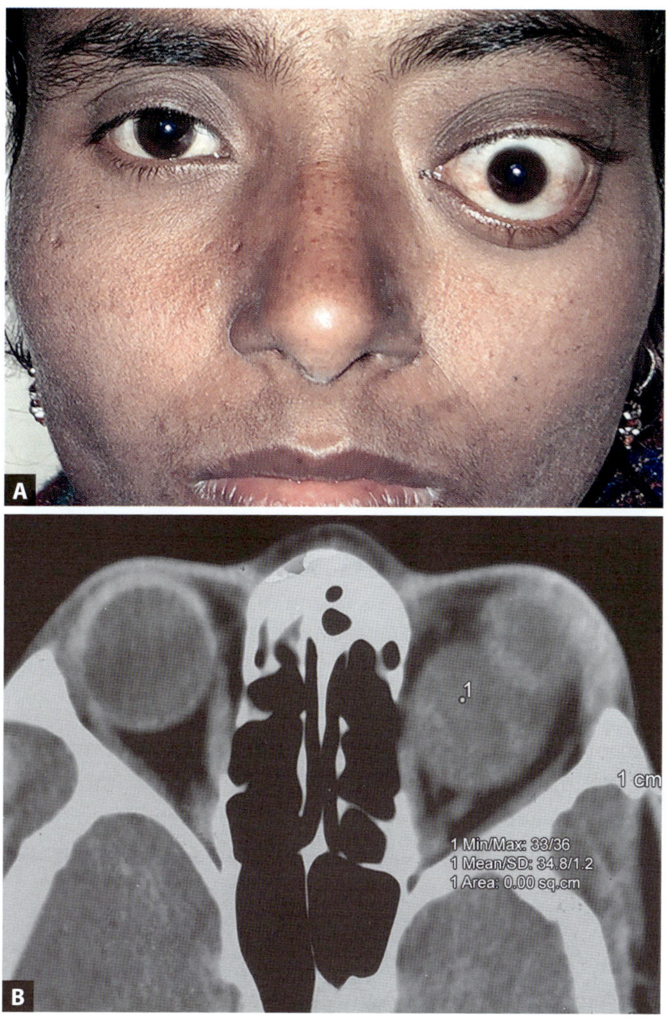

Figs. 16.1A and B

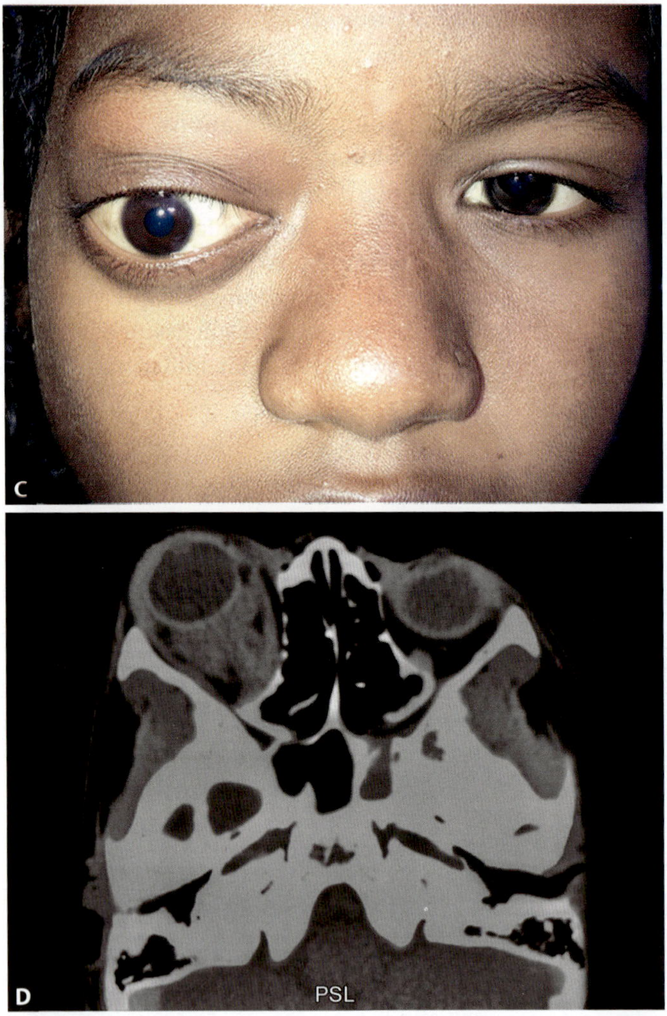

Figs. 16.1C and D

Figs. 16.1A to D: Cavernous hemangioma: (A and C) Clinically presented with slowly progressive unilateral proptosis due to an intraconal lesion; (B and D) CT scan axial views of patients showing well-defined intraconal mass lesion causing proptosis.

and optic atrophy. While a solitary unilateral CVM is the most common presentation, multiple unilateral and bilateral cavernous tumors have also been reported.[6,20,29] Multiple orbital CVMs may present as sporadic lesions or be associated with Maffucci syndrome and blue rubber bleb nevus syndrome.

Imaging

Ultrasonography (USG), computed tomography (CT) scanning, and magnetic resonance imaging (MRI) are valuable imaging tools for investigating CVMs. USG demonstrates a well-defined, round lesion with sharp borders (attributed to a pseudocapsule), medium-to-high internal echo reflectivity, and an accentuated angle kappa. Lesions often exhibit heterogenicity with a honeycomb-like structure representing low reflective vascular spaces and high reflective connective tissue septi.[6] USG aids in distinguishing CVMs from other intraconal lesions, such as gliomas, schwannomas/solitary neurofibromas, and lymphangiomas.[19,22,30] Contrast-enhanced CT scanning of the orbit remains the diagnostic modality of choice, particularly its coronal view, which facilitates surgical planning by demonstrating the extent of the lesion and revealing the anatomical relationship and bony landmark.[6,28] CVM appears as well-circumscribed, homogeneously hyperattenuating round-to-ovoid intraconal lesions on CT scans, displacing the optic nerve laterally and potentially indenting the globe **(Figs. 16.1 and 16.2)**.[31] Bone remodeling may also be evident on CT scans. Delayed contrast enhancement on CT is suggestive of a lack of feeding vessels.

On MRI, the tumor is typically isointense to extraocular muscle on T1-weighted images and hypointense to muscle and isointense to vitreous on T2-weighted images, with gadolinium administration revealing progressive filling and enhancement. CVM typically exhibits a characteristic pattern of contrast enhancement, initially appearing patchy and gradually becoming homogeneous due to pooling of contrast in the cavernous space.[28,31-34] CT and MRI also provide insight into the degree of vascularization of hemangiomas; hyperdense areas represent vascular regions, while heterogeneous images correspond to areas of reduced vascularization due to thrombosis or hemorrhage.[29,35] Carotid angiography is indicated in high-flow hemangiomas but is not useful in CVMs due to the small caliber of their feeding vessels. It is not possible to identify the feeding vessels of a cavernous hemangioma via CT angiography and MRA.[36] Orbital phlebography may be utilized to differentiate CVMs from true varices, occasionally demonstrating the local

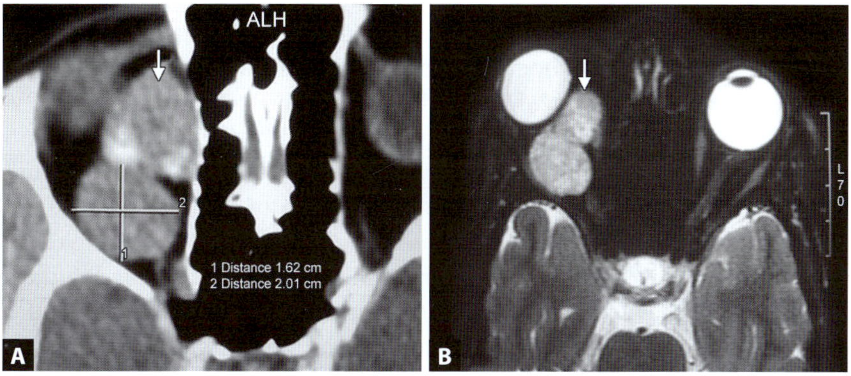

Figs. 16.2A and B: (A) CT scan axial view showing dumbbell-shaped cavernous hemangioma in the right orbit; (B) MRI axial view showing contrast enhancement of the lesion.

draining veins of the malformations, although it is rarely employed nowadays due to the availability of superior alternatives such as color Doppler.[37]

Differential Diagnosis

Distinguishing cavernous hemangioma of the orbit from other solid orbital tumors such as schwannoma, solitary neurofibroma, optic nerve sheath meningioma, solitary fibrous tumor, lymphoma, hemangiopericytoma, and angiofibroma is crucial.[38-42] Optic nerve sheath meningiomas and optic nerve gliomas can be differentiated from cavernous hemangiomas by their characteristic growth patterns and early diminution or loss of vision.[40] When observed via CT and MRI, cavernous hemangiomas typically present as well-differentiated, moderately enhancing mass lesions, while orbital lymphomas manifest as diffuse infiltrative masses often accompanied by periorbital edema.[43] Distinguishing between cavernous lymphangiomas and hemangiomas based on CT imaging features can be challenging. However, on MRI, cavernous hemangiomas appear hyperintense on T2-weighted images, while neurofibromas and schwannomas exhibit heterogeneity and are hypointense on T2-weighted images.[25] Cavernous lymphangiomas tend to be more diffuse and occur at a younger age than cavernous hemangiomas.[22] CVMs display a horizontal disposition, whereas oval cavernous lymphangiomas have their vertex directed toward the orbital apex.[25]

Pathology

Cavernous hemangiomas manifest as well-circumscribed mass lesions with an outer fibrous pseudocapsule formed by progressively condensed collagen during tumor growth. The lesion appears purple or dark red in color with a sponge-like consistency. Multiple dilated vascular spaces **(Figs. 16.3A and B)** elevating its capsule lead to the formation of fine bosselations on the tumor surface.[44] On the cut surface, numerous ecstatic cavernous spaces are evident, separated by connective tissue septa. In younger patients, the cavernous component predominates over the connective tissue, resulting in a more spongy consistency. Histopathologically, cavernous hemangiomas consist of large congested vascular channels lined by flattened epithelium and separated by thin fibrous septae **(Fig. 16.3C)**. Inflammatory cell and macrophages may be present in the interstitium of the tumor, although lymphocytic infiltrations are usually absent, unlike in orbital lymphangiomas where multiple foci of lymphocytes are common.[7,15] The vascular channels frequently contain sedimented erythrocytes or intraluminal thrombi, and secondary changes such as calcifications and phleboliths may occur.[16] Common diagnostic immunohistochemical markers are endothelial cell expression of glucose transporter type (GLUT-1) (erythrocyte glucose transporter), CD31, and CD34 **(Fig. 16.3D)**.

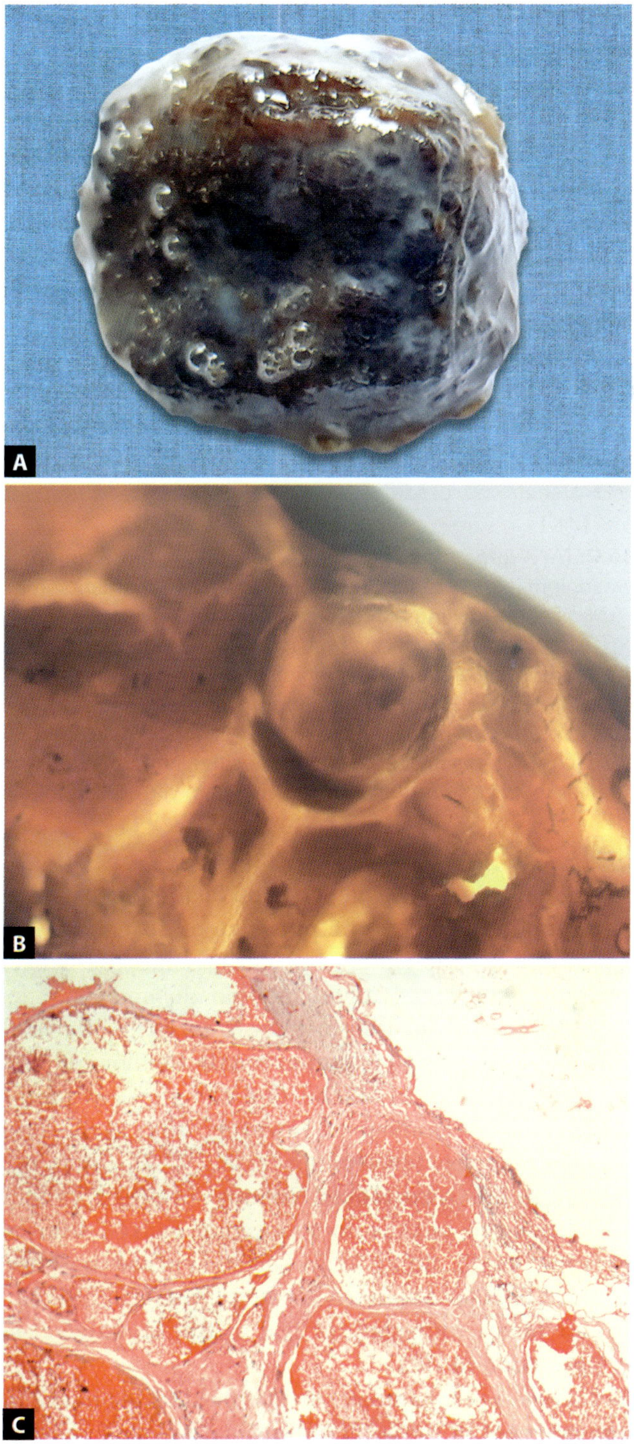

Figs. 16.3A to C

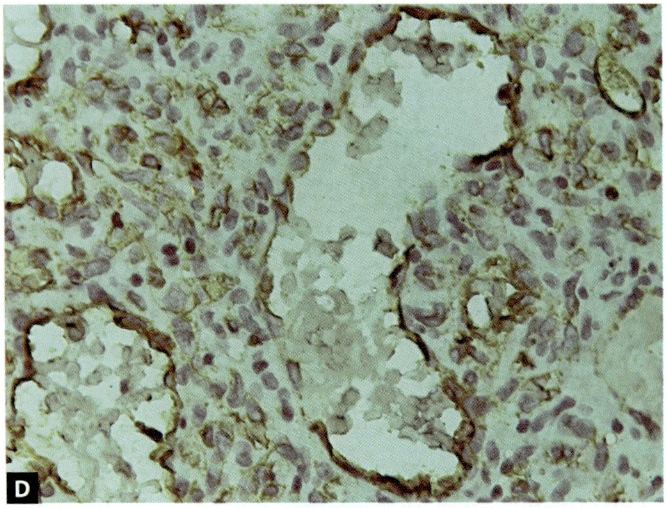

Fig. 16.3D

Figs. 16.3A to D: (A) A large reddish-black orbital mass in gross confirmed later as cavernous hemangioma; (B) Slice section of gross cavernous hemangioma enhanced by a drop of 70% alcohol showing blood-filled spaces under compound microscope's objective, 10×; (C) Histopathology of cavernous hemangioma having large blood-filled spaces lined by endothelial cells with intervening fibrous septa. Portion of the capsule is visible in the section (H&E, 20×); (D) Immunohistochemistry showing CD34-stained endothelial cells in cavernous hemangioma (ScyTek Laboratories, Logan, UTAH, USA; 20×). All positive controls showed appropriate positive immunostaining. Negative control slide did not show immunostaining. (H&E: hematoxylin and eosin)

Management

The approach to managing CVMs depends on factors, such as the size and location of the tumor as well as the presence or absence of symptoms. Small asymptomatic lesions situated posteriorly may be conservatively observed for signs of compressive optic neuropathy and vision loss, while large symptomatic lesions located in the orbital apex often necessitate surgical excision.[6,7,19] Surgical intervention is indicated for conditions, such as hyperopia, diplopia, pain, headache, optic neuropathy, proptosis, and bothersome cosmesis.[19,26] Complete excision is possible as the tumor is well encapsulated with relatively few feeding vessels.[45,46] However, incomplete excision can lead to late recurrence.[9] Various surgical approaches have been proposed depending on the tumor's location, with CT scans and MRIs, particularly coronal views, aiding in the selection of the most appropriate surgical approach. Smaller anteriorly located CVMs can often be excised through anterior/fornix transconjunctival or transcutaneous lid crease approaches **(Figs. 16.4 and 16.5)**.

Excision of larger hemangiomas (15–20 mm) located in the intraconal or lateral compartment of the orbit and orbital apex may require lateral orbitotomy with or without osteotomy.[3] Managing large orbital apex tumors

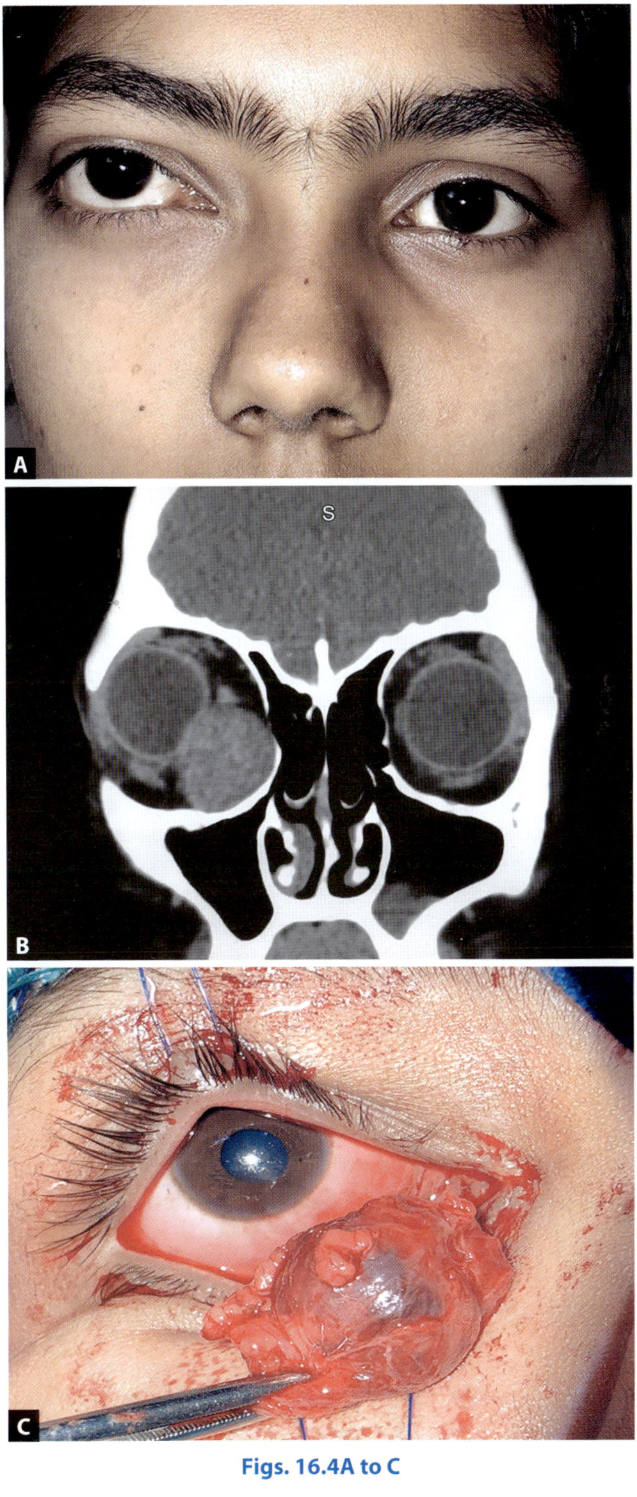

Figs. 16.4A to C

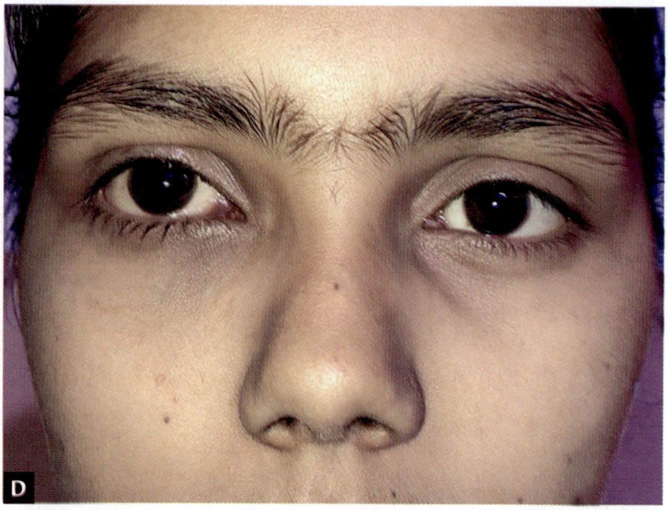

Fig. 16.4D

Figs. 16.4A to D: Cavernous hemangioma: (A) 22-year-old female with an inferomedially located lesion in the right orbit producing upward and outward displacement of the globe; (B) Coronal CT image showing a well-defined oval mass with pressure effect on the adjacent orbital bone and abutting the globe; (C) Complete excision of the tumor through a transconjunctival approach; (D) Postoperative appearance of the patient showing no residual globe displacement.

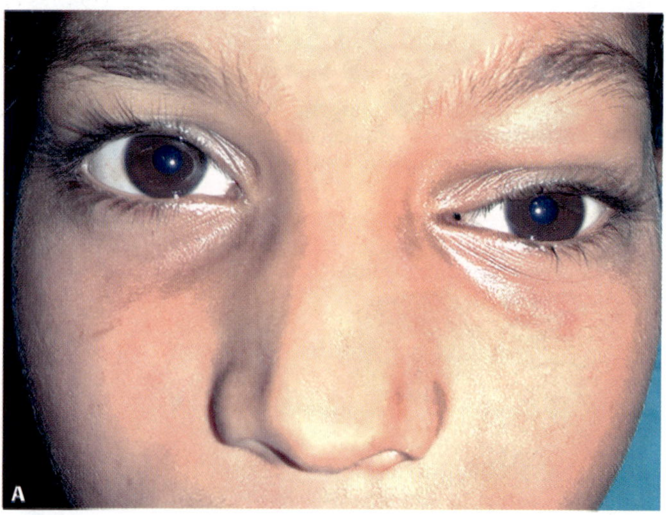

Fig. 16.5A

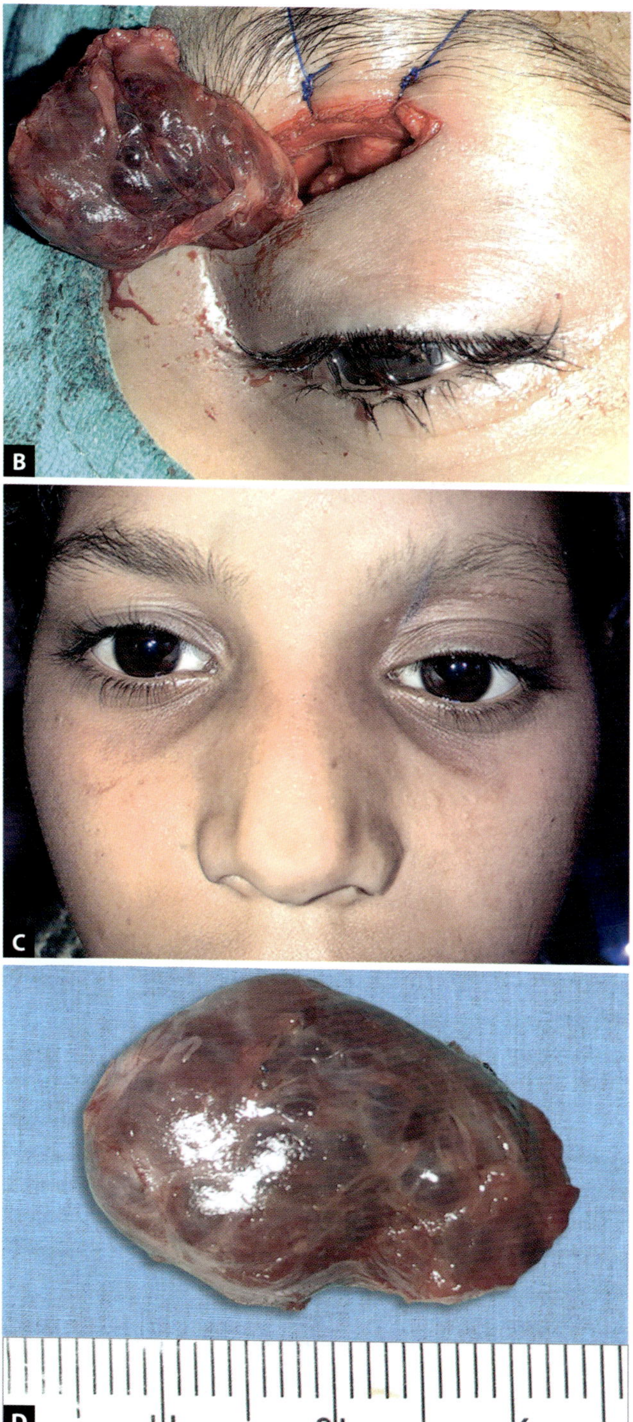

Figs. 16.5B to D

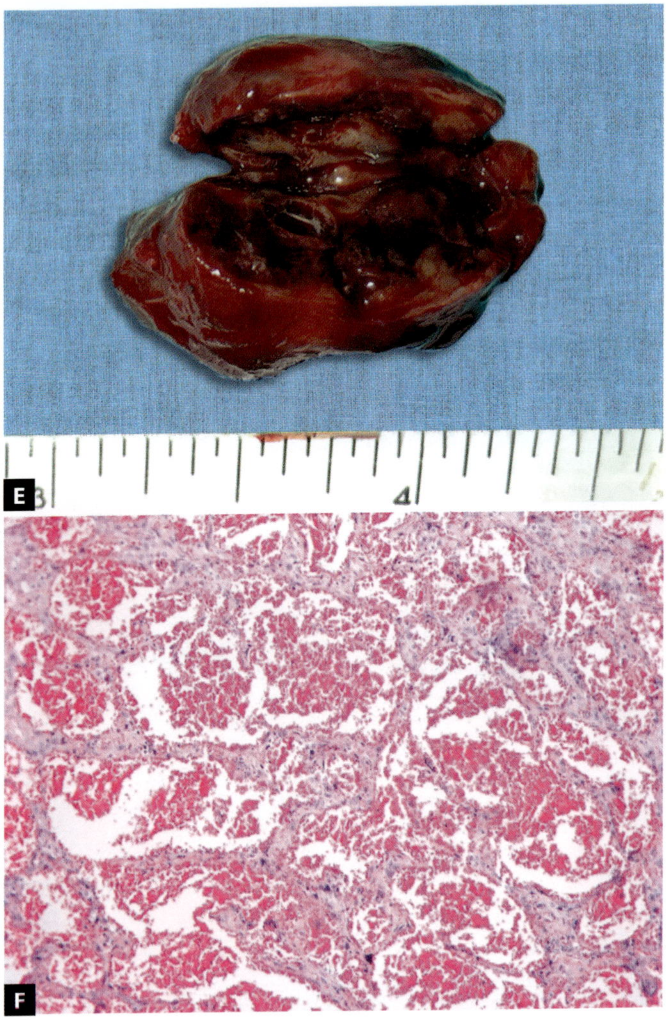

Figs. 16.5E and F

Figs. 16.5A to F: (A) 19-year-old female having cavernous hemangioma involving the left superomedial orbit showing nonaxial proptosis (outward and downward); (B) The lesion was excised completely through transcutaneous anterior orbitotomy (sub-brow incision); (C) Postoperative photograph of the patient; (D and E) Gross specimen after surgical excision showing a reddish-blue encapsulated lesion and cut section showing blood filled chambers; (F) Histopathology (H&E, 40×) showing multiple cavernous spaces separated by fibrous septae, with most of the cavernous spaces filled with blood. (H&E: hematoxylin and eosin)

is particularly challenging and may necessitate a transcranial approach.[13,19] Some hemangiomas in the orbital apex may be adherent to adjacent tissues such as muscle and the optic nerve sheath, and traction during surgery can lead to vascular spasm and rupture, resulting in posterior orbital hemorrhage and optic nerve infarction. In cases where complete dissection is not possible, partial resection or tumor amputation is recommended. Surgeons operating in the intraconal space and orbital apex must exercise caution and be less aggressive, with intraoperative assessment of the pupil being mandatory; any mydriasis suggests optic nerve injury.

Some surgeons prefer to excise large hemangiomas through small orbitotomy after decompressing or deflating the tumor by draining blood. Deep medially located tumors can be resected using minimally invasive orbital surgery via an endoscopic transethmoidal approach.[47,48] Other surgical approaches employed for the excision of posteriorly located tumors affecting the optic canal include the orbitozygomatic approach, transorbital craniotomy, and transnasal approach.[49-51] Stereotactic fractionated radiotherapy has been reported as a treatment option for orbital CVMs that are not easily amenable to surgical excision, such as lesions located at the orbital apex.[3] Multisession gamma knife resection is an effective treatment modality for circumscribed orbital apex tumors.[52-54] Sclerotherapy, involving intralesional injection of pingyangmycin (bleomycin A5), is a newer technique used in the treatment of orbital CVMs and lymphangiomas. Bleomycin induces mild inflammation, fibrosis, and reduced vasculature of the malformations.[55]

CAPILLARY HEMANGIOMA

Capillary hemangiomas of the eyelid and orbit rank among the most common vascular tumors in childhood. They represent 0.7–2.2% of all histopathologically proven orbital space-occupying lesions.[10,11] These hemangiomas can be classified as either superficial (cutaneous or subcutaneous) or deep, with deep capillary hemangiomas situated behind the orbital septum, potentially leading to proptosis or displacement of the globe. Superficial capillary hemangiomas, also known as *infantile hemangiomas* **(Figs. 16.6A to D)**, are most prevalent, affecting approximately 2–3% of all neonates and 10% of white infants under the age of 1 year.[56,57]

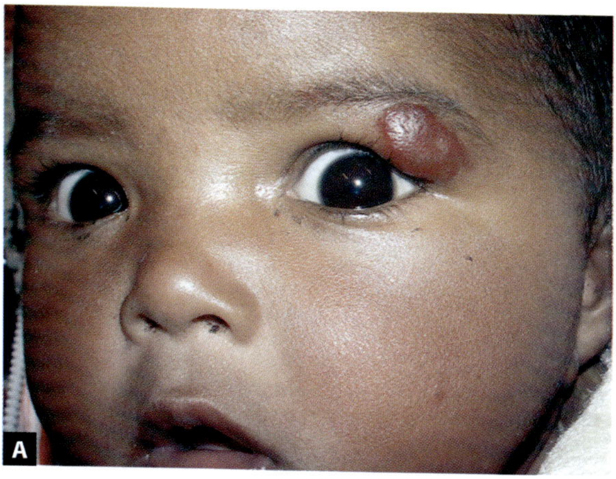

Fig. 16.6A

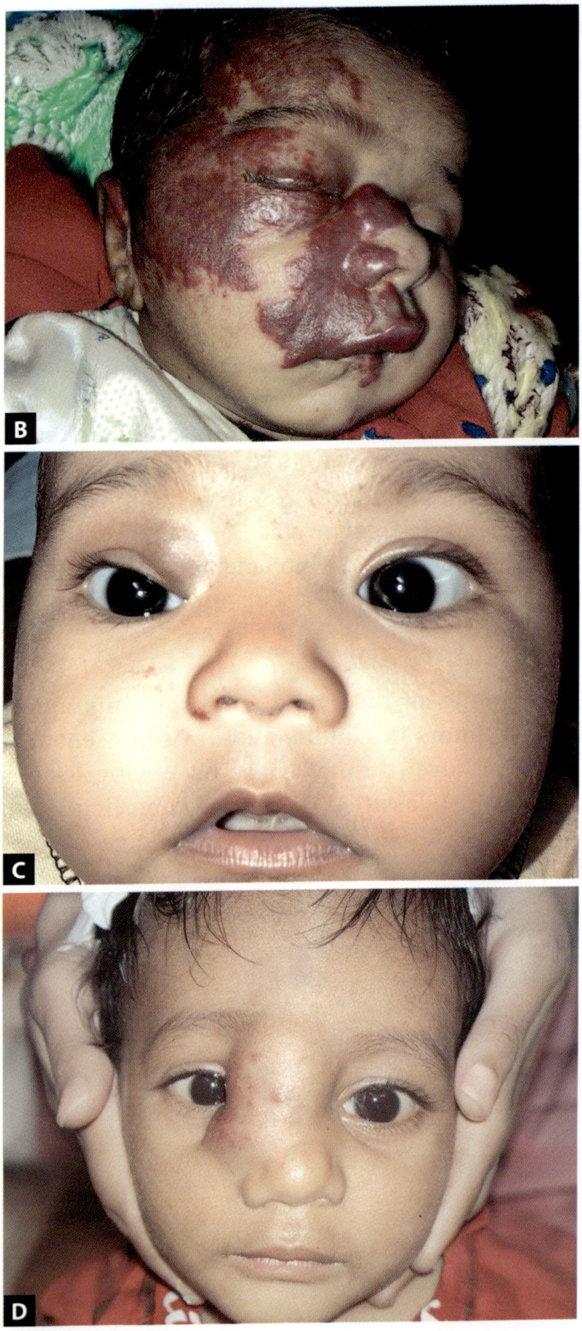

Figs. 16.6B to D

Figs. 16.6A to D: Infantile capillary hemangioma: (A) Focal superficial hemangioma involving the temporal aspect of the left upper eyelid; (B) Segmental mid-facial hemangioma; (C) Subcutaneous capillary hemangioma of the right superior nasal quadrant without involvement of skin; (D) Mixed capillary hemangioma of the naso-orbital part.

Infantile hemangiomas are more common among female infants, with a female-to-male ratio ranging from 3:2 to 5:1.[58,59] Low birth weight (LBW) is a major risk factor for this, with preterm infants weighing <1 kg having an incidence of 22–30%.[60,61] Every 500 g reduction in birth weight results in a 25% increase in the risk of developing an IH.[62] Other risk factors include Caucasian race, maternal age, multiparity, placenta previa, pre-eclampsia, gestational diabetes, maternal use of fertility drugs, and chorionic villus sampling.[60,63]

Pathogenesis

The pathogenesis of IH is not fully understood, but several theories have been proposed:

- *Placenta theory:* This theory suggests that fetal endothelial progenitor cells, released due to placenta disruption during gestation or birth, and released placental tissues embolize to fetal cutaneous vessels. Molecular markers of placental tissues such as GLUT-1, indolamine 2,3 deoxygenase, and type III iodothyronine deiodinase have been observed in hemangioma, supporting this hypothesis.[64]
- *Metastatic theory:* According to this theory, secretagogues produced by the fetal portion of the placenta prepare a site for the precursor cells of hemangioma, which migrate through neuromesenchyme at the site.
- *Progenitor cell theory:* This theory suggests that hemangiomas arise from the somatic maturation and clonal expansion of progenitor cells.[65]
- *Extrinsic factor theory:* This theory proposes that hypoxia plays a significant role in IH development. Local ischemia may create a hypoxic environment, leading to the release of chemokines like stromal cell-derived factor-1 alpha (SDF-1α) and vascular endothelial growth factor (VEGF), promoting IH development.[66]

Clinical Features

The clinical presentation of capillary hemangioma varies depending on its location, size, extent, and stage of the life cycle. IHs exhibit unique biological behavior, growing rapidly, regressing slowly, and never recurring. IHs follow a predictable life cycle consisting of three stages:

1. *Proliferation phase (01 year of age):* This is characterized by rapid enlargement of the lesion due to endothelial hyperplasia. Growth may be biphasic, with maximum growth occurring within the 1st month, followed by rapid growth at 6 months, and a typical plateau in growth noticed by 10–12 months.
2. *Involuting phase (1–5 years of age):* This is characterized by spontaneous, steady regression with fibrosis and fat deposition.
3. *Involuted phase (>5 years of age):* More than 70% of IHs fully resolve, leaving behind residual telangiectasia, redundant skin depigmentation, or scar. Deep IHs appear later and grow longer than their superficial counterparts.

Superficial dermal lesions appear bright red with a strawberry-like appearance during the growth phase and dark gray discoloration during involution, while deeply located hemangiomas appear slightly raised with a bluish hue. IHs involving the eyelid can lead to cosmetic disfigurement, mechanical ptosis, and deprivational amblyopia.[67] Orbital capillary hemangiomas can result in proptosis, diplopia, compressive optic neuropathy, and strabismic amblyopia.[68] Left untreated, large intraorbital hemangiomas can lead to orbital expansion.

Systemic Associations

Occasionally, IHs are associated with congenital anomalies and systemic disorders. Two commonly reported syndromes associated with capillary hemangiomas are Kasabach–Merritt syndrome (KMS) and PHACE (posterior fossa anomalies, hemangioma, arterial anomalies, cardiac anomalies, and eye anomalies) syndrome. KMS primarily affects children with large IHs and is characterized by thrombocytopenia and consumptive coagulopathy due to platelet sequestration in large vascular lesions.[69] PHACE syndrome is characterized by posterior fossa malformation, large segmental hemangioma of the head, face, or neck, optic nerve hypoplasia, coloboma, and peripapillary staphyloma.[70,71]

Investigations

Clinical evaluation is often sufficient for diagnosing superficial capillary hemangiomas. However, radio imaging such as USG, contrast-enhanced CT scans, and MRI are necessary for deeply located hemangiomas. USG aids in evaluating size and internal changes during the involution phase. CT scans typically reveal well-defined borders with internal heterogeneity. On MRI, capillary hemangiomas appear as well-defined, oval lesions, iso- to hyperintense on T1-weighted images and hyperintense on T2-weighted images compared to extraocular muscles **(Figs. 16.7A to C)**. MRI may also show high blood flow vessels as signal-void areas.[28]

Histopathological and Immunohistochemical Features

The histopathological findings of capillary hemangioma vary in each phase of evolution. In the proliferative phase, it appears as a well-defined mass with small blood vessel proliferations. Endothelial cells line the capillary walls **(Figs. 16.8A to C)**. The endothelium flattens as the lumen enlarges. End-stage lesions show a fibrofatty background with a mast cell count comparable with that of normal skin. No endothelial or pericyte mitotic activity remains.[72] Completely involuted hemangiomas show sponge-like structure with scattered thin-walled blood vessels lined by a flattened endothelium. The most vital and diagnostic immunohistochemical marker

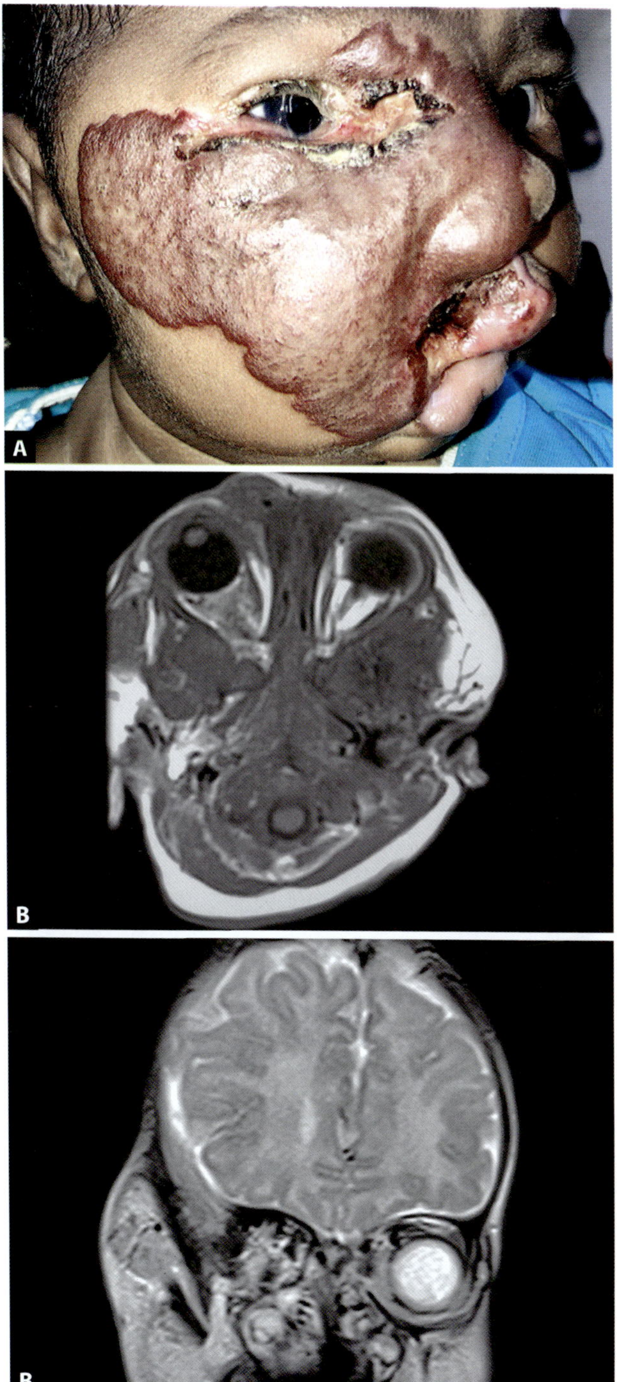

Figs. 16.7A to C: (A) Segmental facial IH with ulceration; (B) T1-weighted axial MRI; (C) T2-weighted coronal MRI images showing large facial IH. (IH: infantile hemangioma)

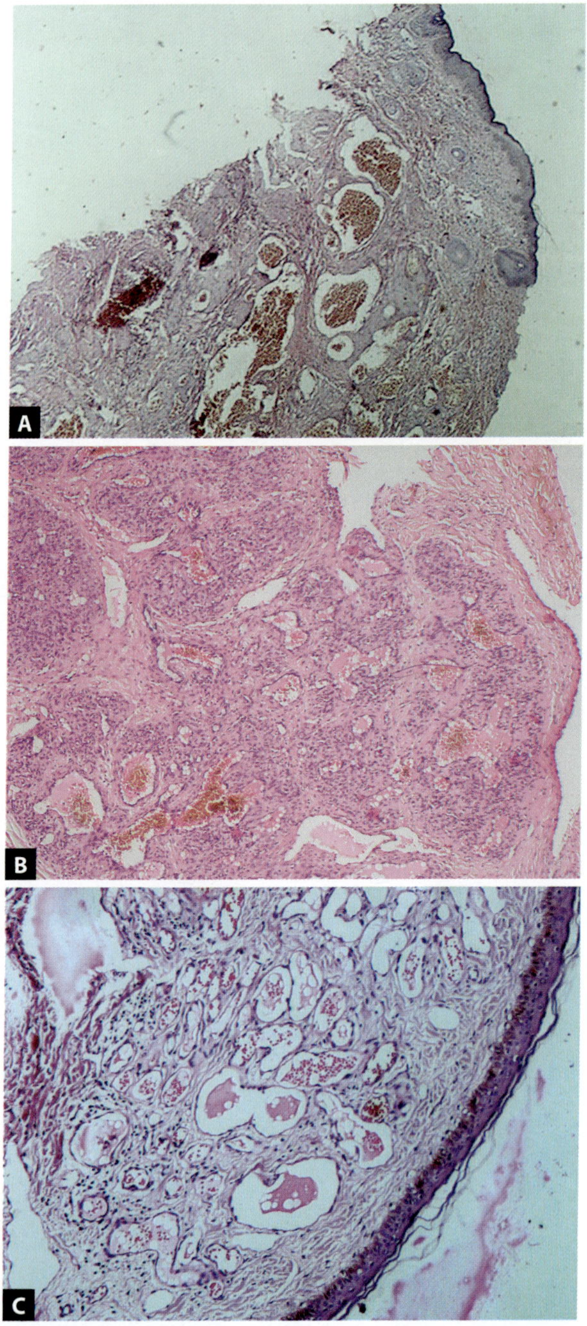

Figs. 16.8A to C: Histopathology of capillary hemangioma: (A) Microphotograph of lobular capillary hemangioma showing small- and medium-sized vessels separated by connective tissue septa (H&E, 10×); (B) Microphotograph showing a vascular tumor composed of capillaries, vascular buds, and lymphocytes (H&E, 10×); (C) Microphotograph showing proliferations of small-sized blood vessels in capillary hemangioma (H&E, 40×). (H&E: hematoxylin and eosin)

for IHs is the endothelial cell expression of GLUT-1 (erythrocyte glucose transporter). Other immunohistochemical markers expressed by IHs include CD31 and CD34, merosin, Lewis Y antigen, and FC-γ RII. While these markers are not specific to IHs, their presence supports the diagnosis of a vascular tumor.[73]

Management

The treatment of periocular IHs and orbital capillary hemangiomas depends on factors, such as anatomical location, lesion size, stage of growth, and the child's age. Close observation is warranted for involuting small hemangiomas or stable lesions in nonvital sites that do cause significant aesthetic or functional derangement. The growth of hemangiomas should be regularly observed, recorded, and photographed. Large oculofacial IHs require treatment before the child develops self-awareness of body image. Indications for the treatment of orbital and periocular capillary hemangiomas include large-sized lesions leading to astigmatism, globe deformity, obscuration of the visual axis, ptosis, exposure keratopathy, compressive optic neuropathy, and ulceration of the tumor. Capillary hemangioma has multimodal treatment such as pharmacological treatment, laser, radiation therapy, surgery, or combination therapy.

Medical Therapy

Propranolol: Propranolol, a nonselective beta-blocker, has become the first-line drug for the treatment of IHs. Léauté-Labrèze et al. first reported the use of propranolol for the treatment of proliferating IHs **(Figs. 16.9A to D)** in 2009.[72] The recommended dose of oral propranolol is 1–2 mg/kg/day, administered orally and divided into two doses. Baseline cardiac monitoring [blood pressure, pulse rate, electrocardiography (ECG), chest X-ray] should be performed before therapy initiation. The proposed mechanisms of action in IHs include (1) reduction of nitric oxide release and vasoconstriction, (2) inhibition of angiogenesis of hemangioma stem cells by blocking proangiogenic signals, and (3) induction of endothelial cell apoptosis in late stages of IHs. Common adverse effects of propranolol include sleep disturbance, transient hypoglycemia, hypotension, bradycardia, bronchospasm, and diarrhea. Propranolol is contraindicated in patients with hypotension, sinus bradycardia, heart failure, etc. Although topical propranolol (2% cream) is less effective, it is safer than oral propranolol.[74] Recently, oral atenolol has been used for problematic IHs (ulcerative IHs). Atenolol, being a selective beta-2 blocker, may reduce the risk of asthma, hypoglycemia, and sleep disturbance. Atenolol has a faster therapeutic effect, and the frequency of oral administration can be reduced due to its long half-life.[75,76]

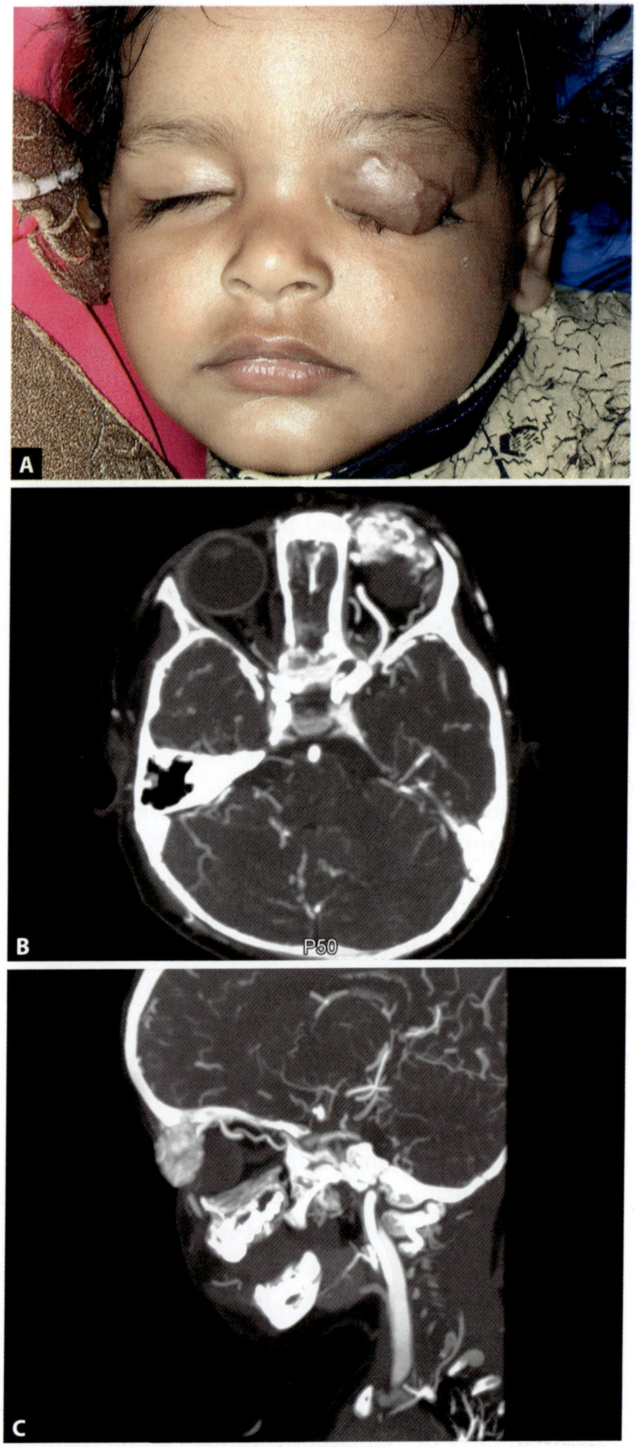

Figs. 16.9A to C

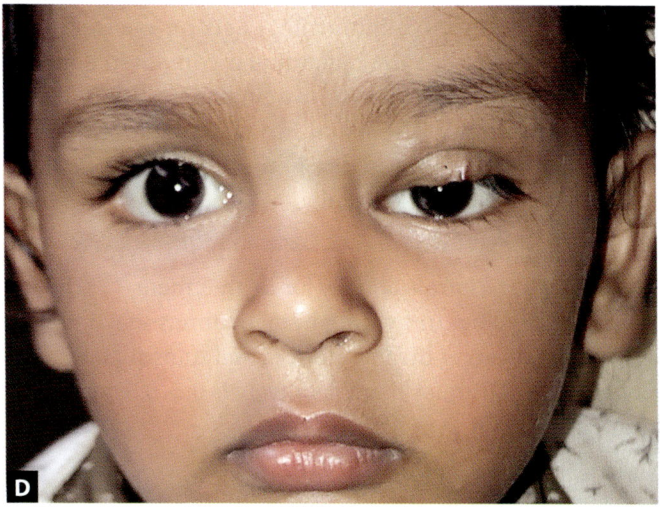

Fig. 16.9D

Figs. 16.9A to D: (A) Clinical photograph of a 14-month-old boy having focal capillary hemangioma of the left upper eyelid showing mechanical ptosis and prominent blood vessels on the skin surface; (B and C) Orbital CT angiogram, axial and sagittal views demonstrating feeding vessels to the eyelid hemangioma; (D) The lesion decreased in size 6 months after oral propranolol therapy.

Corticosteroids: These were the first-line treatment for IHs before the advent of propranolol. They are now reserved for patients who do not respond to beta-blockers or when beta-blockers are contraindicated. Corticosteroids can be administered orally, intravenously, intralesionally, and topically. The recommended dose of prednisone is 2–3 mg/kg/day for 4–12 weeks, followed by a gradual reduction until the patient reaches 9–12 months of age.[77] Long-term systemic use of corticosteroids may lead to adverse reactions, such as gastrointestinal discomfort, cushingoid appearance, growth retardation, irritability, and mental symptoms. Topical application of clobetasol propionate 0.05% ointment for small IHs is advantageous, safe, and effective.

Topical timolol: Topical timolol maleate (0.5% eye hydrogel twice daily) may be an effective treatment for superficial IHs. However, its application may lead to adverse reactions, such as eczema, ulceration, periocular rashes, and erythema.[78]

Interferon-α: Interferon α-2a and 2b, which have antiviral and antitumor effects, can be used for steroid-resistant IHs. They inhibit endothelial proliferation and promote apoptosis.[79] Common adverse reactions to interferon-α treatment include fever, malaise, anemia, and neutropenia. Intralesional injection of interferon-α is typically administered at a dosage of 1–3 million IU/m^2 weekly for 6 weeks.

Vincristine: This is a mitotic inhibitor that acts on microtubules. IHs are sensitive to vincristine due to the high tubular content in endothelial cells. It has been used to treat steroid-resistant hemangiomas and life-threatening hemangiomas with KMS.[80] The usual intravenous dose of vincristine is 1.5 mg/m^2 in infants weighing >10 kg. Common side effects include fever, headache, constipation, and neuropathy.

Bleomycin: Bleomycin and pingyangmycin are cytotoxic antitumor antibiotics that are used intralesionally for IH treatment.[81,82] The mechanism of intralesional bleomycin in treating hemangiomas may involve blocking the cell cycle and activating the apoptotic signal transduction pathway. The recommended dose of intralesional bleomycin is 0.3–0.5 mg/kg given under general anesthesia.

Imiquimod: Imiquimod, an imidazole quinolone amine, is a topical immunoresponse modifier drug commonly used in the treatment of basal cell carcinoma (BCC), squamous cell carcinoma in situ, and actinic keratosis. Topical 5% imiquimod cream has been recommended for the treatment of small-to-moderate-sized superficial IHs not involving the eyelid margin. However, it has no role in the treatment of mixed and deep IHs. The cream is applied topically once every other day for 3–5 months. Local irritation, crusting, or ulceration may occur with topical imiquimod.[83-85] Its mechanism of action involves enhancing innate immunity through the production of various cytokines, including interferon-α, interleukin (IL)-6, IL-12, and tumor necrosis factor-α (TNF-α). These cytokines enhance cell-mediated immunity, induce apoptosis, inhibit angiogenesis, and downregulate proangiogenic factors, such as matrix metallopeptidase 9 (MMP-9) and basic fibroblast growth factor (bFGF).[86,87]

Laser Therapy

Pulse dye laser (PDL): This has become the standard treatment for superficial proliferative hemangiomas (up to a depth of 1.2 mm) and residual lesions during or after involution. It may be used as adjunctive therapy with oral propranolol or intralesional steroids for deeper hemangiomas. PDL operates through selective photothermolysis, with light of 585 nm being absorbed by oxyhemoglobin, converting to heat that coagulates the endothelial cells of IHs. A standard treatment regimen involves PDL 585–895 nm with fluences of 9–12 J/cm^2, a pulse duration of 300–450 μs, and a spot size of 7–10 mm. Treatment is typically repeated at 6–8-week intervals for six or more sessions. Complications may include blistering, ulceration, crusting, scarring, and hyper- or hypopigmentations.[88-90]

Carbon dioxide laser: Previously, carbon dioxide laser resurfacing was used for atrophic scar after the involution of cutaneous hemangiomas and to revise surgical scars. However, standard CO_2 laser treatment has been largely replaced by nonablative fractional photothermolysis treatment.[91]

Surgical Treatment

Although surgical excision of IHs is complete, rapid, and definitive, surgery is still only considered in life- and sight-threatening conditions, as well as for IHs refractory to medical therapy and for end-stage reconstruction. Surgical excision is often associated with intraoperative or postoperative bleeding, necessitating strategic management. Early surgical excision is advantageous for better skin closure and easier reconstruction of lid defects **(Figs. 16.10A to F)**.[92] Embolization treatment for orbital capillary hemangiomas has been recommended as a sole treatment or prior to surgical excision.[93]

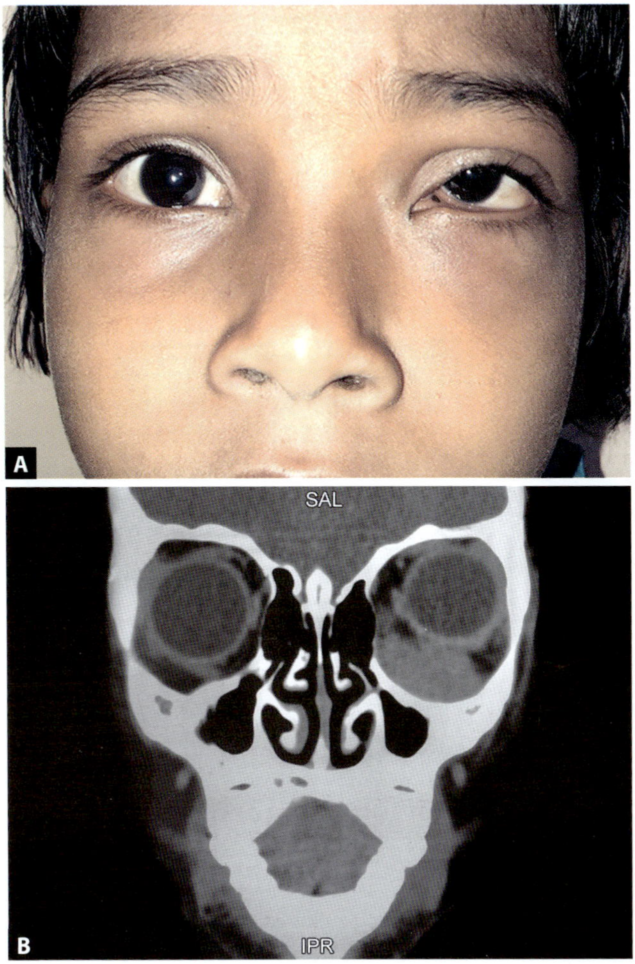

Figs. 16.10A and B

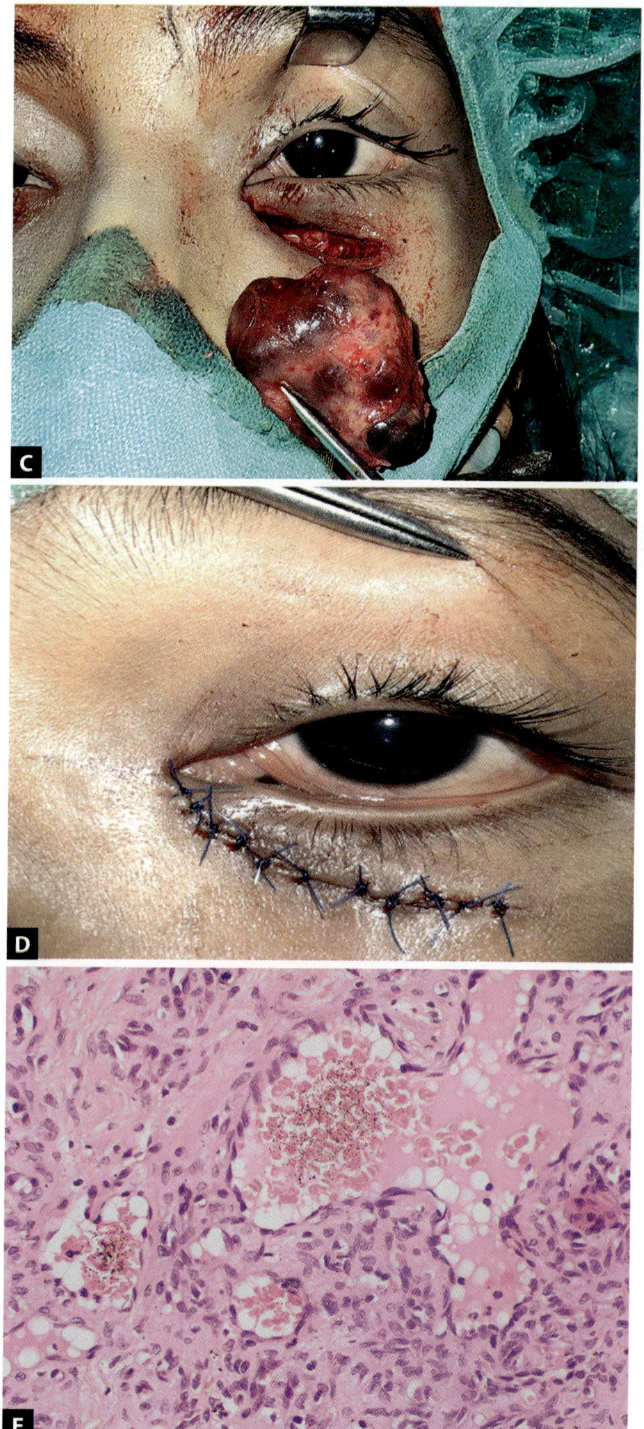

Figs. 16.10C to E

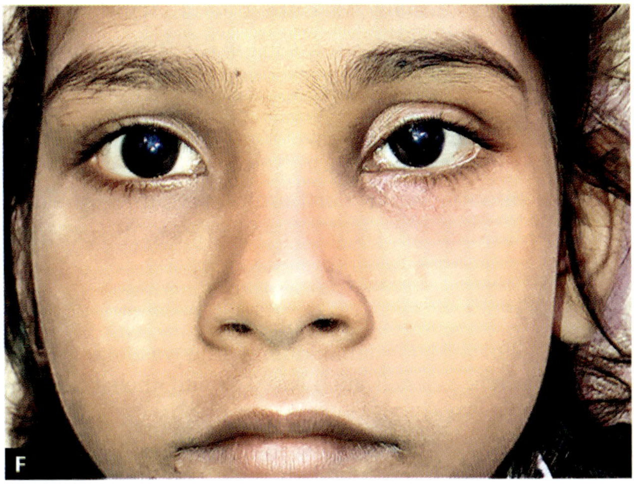

Fig. 16.10F

Figs. 16.10A to F: (A) A 5-year-old girl having deep capillary hemangioma of the left orbital floor without eyelid involvement leading to upward displacement of the left eyeball; (B) Coronal CT image with contrast showing a homogeneous mass with poorly defined borders, displacing the globe upward;(C and D) The tumor was excised completely through transcutaneous anterior orbitotomy approach; (E) Histopathology showing blood-containing capillaries lined by a single layer of endothelial cells (H&E, 40×); (F) Clinical photograph 6 months after surgery. (H&E: hematoxylin and eosin)

CONCLUSION

Orbital hemangiomas represent a significant category of orbital space-occupying lesions. Cavernous hemangioma, or CVM, is the most common vascular lesion in the adult orbit, typically presenting as a solitary unilateral tumor. It often manifests as a slowly progressive axial proptosis when located intraconally. Diagnosis of orbital cavernous hemangiomas relies on CT or MRI findings. Surgical excision remains the cornerstone of treatment, although incomplete excision may lead to recurrence after several years. In recent years, intralesional injection of bleomycin A5 as sclerotherapy has emerged as a newer treatment technique. Capillary hemangiomas of the eyelid and orbit are most commonly seen in infants and children. Managing IHs remains a challenge and requires individualized approaches. Treatment decisions hinge on factors such as size, location, depth, and growing stage of the hemangiomas. The overarching goals of treatment include preventing life- or sight-threatening complications, minimizing permanent disfigurement, treating ulceration to reduce scarring, and alleviating psychological stress for both patients and parents. Oral propranolol is the current first-line mainstay of treatment for IHs. In cases where first-line treatment proves ineffective or is contraindicated, corticosteroid therapy, topical application, intralesional injections of drugs, and surgical excision may be considered. Additionally, PDL and fractional photothermolysis offer options for improving residual lesions during the regression phase of IHs.

ACKNOWLEDGMENTS

We are thankful to Professor Virendra Pratap Singh, Chief, RIO, BHU, for his guidance and valuable input. Furthermore, we feel grateful to Drs Kokil Tiwari and PR Sen for their help and contributions to the work.

REFERENCES

1. Mulliken JB, Glowacki J. Hemangiomas and vascular malformations in infants and children: a classification based on endothelial characteristics. Plast Reconstr Surg. 1982;69:412-22.
2. Rootman J, Graeb DA. Vascular lesions. In: Rootman J (Ed). Diseases of the Orbit. A Multidisciplinary Approach. Philadelphia: Lippincott Williams & Wilkins; 1988. pp. 525-68.
3. Rootman J, Heran MK, Grab DA. Vascular malformations of the orbit: classification and the role of imaging in diagnosis and treatment strategies. Ophthal Plast Reconstr Surg. 2014;30:91-104.
4. Waner M, Suen JY. A classification of congenital vascular lesions. In: Waner M, Suen JY (Eds). Hemangiomas and vascular malformations of head and neck. New York: Wiley; 1999. pp. 1-12.
5. North PE, Mihm MC Jr. Histopathological diagnosis of infantile hemangiomas and vascular malformations. Facial Plast Surg Clin North Am. 2001;9:505-24.
6. Harris GJ, Jakobiec FA. Cavernous hemangioma of the orbit. J Neurosurg. 1979;51:219-28.
7. International Society for the Study of Vascular Anomalies (ISSVA). Classification. Available from: https://www.issva.org/classification [Last accessed September, 2024].
8. Shields JA, Bakewell B, Augsburger JJ, Flanagan JC. Classification and incidence of space-occupying lesions of the orbit. Arch Ophthalmol. 1984;102:1606-11.
9. Henderson JW, Campbell RJ, Farrow GM, Garrity JA. Clinical course of an incompletely removed cavernous hemangioma of the orbit. Ophthalmology. 1990;97:625-8.
10. Günalp I, Gündüz K. Biopsy-proven orbital lesions in Turkey. A survey of 1092 cases over 30 years. Orbit. 1994;13:67-79.
11. Seregard S, Sahlin S. Panorama of orbital space-occupying lesions. The 24-year experience of a referral center. Acta Ophthalmol Scand. 1999;77:91-8.
12. Sen DK. A etiological pattern of orbital tumors in India and their clinical presentations: a 20-year retrospective study. Orbit. 1990;9:299-302.
13. Fay A, Rand Rodgers I. Vascular anomalies of the eyelid and orbit. In: Albert DM, Miller JW, Azar DT, Young LH (Eds). Albert and Jakobiec's Principles and Practice of Ophthalmology. Philadelphia: Elsevier; 2008. p. 26.
14. Smoker WR, Gentry LR, Yee NK, Reede DL, Nerad JA. Vascular lesions of the orbit: more than meets the eye. Radiographic. 2008;28:185-204.
15. Gujar SK, Gandhi D. Congenital malformations of the orbit. Neuroimaging Clin N Am. 2011;21:585-602.

16. Osaki TH, Jakobiec FA, Mendoza PR, Lee Y, Fay AM. Immunohistological investigations of orbital infantile hemangiomas and adult encapsulated cavernous venous lesions (malformation versus hemangioma). Ophthalmic Plast Reconstr Surg. 2013;29:183-95.
17. Witschel MD, Font RL. Hemangioma of the choroid: a clinicopathologic study of 71 cases and a review of the literature. Surv Ophthalmol. 1976;20:415-31.
18. Hood CI. Cavernous hemangioma of the orbit. A consideration of pathogenesis with an illustrative case. Arch Ophthalmol. 1970;83:49-53.
19. Scheuerle AF, Steiner HH, Kolling G, Kunze S, Aschoff A. Treatment and long-term outcome of patients with orbital cavernomas. Am J Ophthalmol. 2004;138:237-44.
20. Sullivan TJ, Aylward GW, Wright JE, Moseley IF, Garner A. Bilateral multiple cavernous hemangiomas of the orbit. Br J Ophthalmol. 1992;76:627-9.
21. Mojon D, Odel JG, Rios R, Hirano M. Presumed orbital hemangioma associated with the blue rubber bleb nevus syndrome. Arch Ophthalmol. 1996;114: 618-9.
22. Davis KR, Hesselink JR, Dallow RL, Grove AS Jr. CT and ultrasound in the diagnosis of cavernous hemangiomas of the orbit. J Comput Tomogr. 1980;4:98-104.
23. Slem G, Ilçayto R. Hemangioma of the lacrimal gland in an adult. Ann Ophthalmol. 1972;4:77-8.
24. Madge SN, Simon S, Abidin Z, Ghabrial R, Davis G, McNab A, et al. Primary orbital intraosseous hemangioma. Ophthal Plast Reconstr Surg. 2009;25:37-41.
25. Sweet C, Silbergleit R, Mehta B. Primary intraosseous hemangioma of the orbit. CT and MR appearance. Am J Neuroradiol. 1997;18:379-81.
26. Missori P, Tarantino R, Deflfini R, Lunardi P, Cantore G. Surgical management of orbital cavernous angioma: prognosis for visual function after removal. Neurosurg. 1994;(1)35:34-8.
27. Costa e Silva I, Symon L. Cavernous hemangioma of the optic canal Report of two cases. J Neurosurg. 1984;60:838-41.
28. Bilaniuk LT. Orbital vascular lesions. Role of imaging. Radiol Clin North Am. 1999;37:169-83.
29. Fries PD, Char DH. Bilateral orbital cavernous hemangiomas. Br J Ophthalmol. 1988;72:871-3.
30. Iwamoto T, Jacobiec FA. Ultrastructural comparison of capillary and cavernous hemangiomas of the orbit. Arch Ophthalmol. 1979;97:1144-53.
31. Fries DP, Char HD, Norman D. MR imaging of orbital cavernous hemangioma. J Comput Assist Tomogr. 1987;11:418-21.
32. Ansari SA, Mafee MF. Orbital cavernous hemangioma: role of imaging. Neuroimag Clin North America. 2005;15:219-28.
33. Thorn-Kayny M, Arrué P, Delisle MB, Lacroix F, Lagarrigue J, Manelfe C. Cavenous hemangiomas of the orbit: MR imaging. J Neuroradiol. 1999;26:79-86.
34. Mafee MF, Putterman A, Valvassori GE, Campos M, Capek V. Orbital space-occupying lesions: role of computed tomography and magnetic resonance imaging. An analysis of 145 cases. Radiol Clin North Am. 1987;25:529-59.
35. De Potter, Dolinkskas C, Shields C, Shields J. Vascular tumors in MRI of the eye and orbit. Lippicott Co. 1995;159-81.
36. Khan SN, Sepahdari AR. Orbital masses CT and MRI of common vascular lesions, benign tumors and malignancies. Saudi J Ophthalmol. 2012;26:373-83.
37. Lloyd GAS. Pathological veins in the orbit. Br J Radiol. 1974;47:570-8.

38. Xian J, Zhang Z, Wang Z, Li J, Yang B, Chen Q, et al. Evaluation of MR imaging findings differentiating cavernous hemangiomas from schwannomas in the orbit. Eur Radiol. 2010;20:2221-8.
39. Savoiado M, Strada L, Passerini A. Cavernous hemangioma of the orbit: value of CT, Angiography and Phlebography. Am J Neuroradiol. 1983;4:741-4.
40. Byrd SE, Harwood-Nash DC, Fitz CR, Barry JF, Rogovitz DM. Computed tomography of intraorbital optic nerve gliomas in children. Radiology. 1978;129:73-8.
41. Westacott S, Garner A, Moseley IF, Wright JE. Orbital lymphoma versus reactive lymphoid hyperplasia: an analysis of the use of computed tomography in differential diagnosis. Brit J Ophthalmol. 1991;75:722-5.
42. Jacobiec FA, Zakka FR, Papakostas TD, Fay A. Angiomyofibroma of the orbit: a hybrid of vascular leiomyoma and cavernous hemangioma. Ophthal Plast Reconstr Surg. 2012;28:438-45.
43. Forbes GS, Earnest F 4th, Waller RR. Computed tomography of orbital tumors, including late-generation scanning techniques. Radiology. 1982;142(2):387-94.
44. Gunduz K, Karcioglu ZA. Vascular tumor. In: Karcioglu ZA (Ed), Orbital Tumor. New York: Springer; 2015; pp. 155-81.
45. Cheng JW, Wei RL, Cai JP, Li Y. Transconjunctival orbitotomy for orbital cavernous hemangiomas. Can J Ophthalmol. 2008;43:234-8.
46. Arai H, Sato K, Katsuta T, Rhoton AL, Jr. Lateral approach to intraorbital lesions: anatomic and surgical considerations. Neurosurgery. 1996;39:1157-62.
47. Chhabra N, Wu AW, Fay A, Metson R. Endoscopic resection of orbital hemangiomas. Int Forum Allergy Rhinol. 2014;4:251-5.
48. Castelnuovo P, Dallan I, Locatelli, Battaglia P, Farneti P, Tomazic PV, et al. Endoscopic trans nasal-intraorbital surgery: our experience with 16 cases. Eur Arch Otorhinolaryngol. 2012;269:1929-35.
49. Rohde V, Scaller K, Hassler W. The combined pterional and orbit zygomatic approach to extensive tumors of the lateral and latero-basal orbit and orbital apex. Acta Neurochir (Wien). 1995;132:127-30.
50. Maus M, Goldman HW. Removal of orbital apex hemangioma using new transorbital craniotomy through suprabrow approach. Ophthalmic Plast Reconstr Surg. 1999;15:166-70.
51. Santoro A, Salvati M, Vangelista T, Delfine R, Cantore GP. Fronto-temporo-orbito-zygomatic approach and variants. Surgical technique and indications. J Neurosurg Sci. 2003;47:141-7.
52. Kim JW, Im YS, Nam DH, Park K, Kim JH, Lee JI. Preliminary report of multi-session gamma knife radiosurgery for benign perioptic lesions: visual outcome in 22 patients. J Korean Neurosurg Soc. 2008;44:67-71.
53. Goh ASC, Kim YD, Woo KI, Lee JI. Benign orbital apex tumors treated with multisession gamma knife radiosurgery. Ophthalmology. 2013;120:635-41.
54. Young SM, Kim KH, Kim YD, Lang SS, Park JW, Woo KI, et al. Orbital apex venous cavernous malformation with optic neuropathy-treatment with multisession Gamma knife radiosurgery. Br J Ophthalmol. 2019;103:1453-9.
55. Yue H, Qian J, Elner VM, Guo J, Yuan YF, Zhang R, et al. Treatment of orbital vascular malformations with intralesional injection of pingyangmycin. Br J Ophthalmol. 2013;97:739-45.
56. Drolet BA, Esterly NB, Frieden IJ. Hemangiomas in children. N Engl J Med. 1999;341:173-81.

57. Jacobs AH, Walton RG. The incidence of birthmarks in the neonate. Pediatrics. 1976;58:218-22.
58. Hoornweg MJ, Smeulders MJ, Ubbink BT, van der Horst CM. The prevalence and risk factors of infantile hemangiomas: a case control study in the Dutch population. Paediatr Perinat Epidemiol. 2012;26:156-62.
59. Bowers RE, Graham EA, Tomlinson KM. The natural history of the strawberry hemangioma nexus. Arch Dermatol. 1960;82:667-80.
60. Haggstorm AN, Drolet BA, Baselga E, Chamlin SL, Garzon MC, Horii KA, et al. Prospective study of infantile hemangiomas: demographic, perinatal characteristics. J Pediatr. 2007;150:291-4.
61. Amir J, Metzker A, Kirkler R, Reisner SH. Strawberry hemangioma in preterm infants. Pediatr Dermatol. 1986;3:331-2.
62. Drolet BA, Swanson EA, Frieden IJ. Hemangioma Investigator group. Infantile hemangiomas: an emerging health issue linked to an increased rate of low birth weight infants. J Pediatr. 2008;163:712-5.
63. Li J, Chen X, Zhao S, Hu X, Chen C, Ouyang F, et al. Demographic and clinical characteristics and risk factors for infantile hemangioma: a Chinese case control study. Arch Dermatol. 2011;147:1049-56.
64. North PE, Waner M, Mizeracki A, Mrak RE, Nicholas R, Kincannon J, et al. A unique microvascular phenotype shared by juvenile hemangiomas and human placenta. Arch Dermatol. 2001;137:559-70.
65. Fay A, Santiago Y, Waner M. Infantile hemangiomas and other vascular neoplasms. In: Fay A, Dolman PJ (Eds). Diseases and Disorders of the Orbit and Ocular Adnexa. Philadelphia: Elsevier; 2017. pp. 473-96.
66. Lo K, Mihm M, Fay A. Current theories of the pathogenesis of infantile hemangioma. Semin Ophthalmol. 2009;24:172-7.
67. Schwartz SR, Blei F, Ceisler E, Steele M, Furlan L, Kodsi S. Risk factors for amblyopia in children with capillary hemangiomas of the eyelids and orbit. J AAPOS. 2006;10:262-8.
68. Halk BG, Jacobiec FA, Ellsworth RM, Jones IS. Capillary hemangioma of the lids and orbit: an analysis of the clinical features and therapeutic result in 101 cases. Ophthalmology. 1979;86:762-92.
69. Kasabach HH, Merritt KK. Capillary hemangioma with extensive purpura: report of a case. Am J Dis Child. 1940;59:1063.
70. Enjolras O, Wassef M, Mazoyer E, Frieden IJ, Rieu PN, Drouet L, et al. Infants with Kasabach-Merrit syndrome do not have "true" hemangiomas. J Pediatr. 1997;130:631-40.
71. Mitchell S, Siegel DH, Shieh JT, Stevenson DA, Grimmer JF, Lewis T, et al. Candidate locus analysis for PHACE & syndrome. Am J Med Genet A. 2012;158A:1363-7.
72. Léauté-Labrèze C, Dumas de la Roque E, Hubiche T, Boralevi F, Thambo JB, Taïeb A. Propranolol for severe hemangiomas of infancy. N Engl J Med. 2008;358:2649-51.
73. Leon-Villapalos, Wolfe K, Kangesu L. GLUT-1: an extra diagnostic tool to differentiate between hemangiomas and vascular malformations. Br J Plast Surg. 2005;58:348-52.
74. Wang Y, Zhang X, Yang Y, Zhang J, Yang Y, Lu Y. Efficacy and safety of 2% topical propranolol cream for the treatment of proliferating infantile strawberry hemangiomas. Indian J Pediatr. 2017;84:425-9.

75. Bayart CB, Tamburro JE, Vidimos AT, Wang L, Golden AB. Atenolol versus propranolol for treatment of infantile hemangiomas during the proliferative phase: a retrospective noninferiority study. Pediatr Dermatol. 2017;34:413-21.
76. Tasani M, Glover M, Martinez AE, Shaw L. Atenolol treatment for infantile hemangioma. Br J Dermatol. 2017;176:1400-2.
77. Greene AK, Couto RA. Oral prednisolone for infantile hemangioma: efficacy and safety using a standardized treatment protocol. Plast Reconstr Surg. 2011;128: 743-52.
78. Filoni A, Ambrogio F, de Marco A, Pacifico A, Bonamonte D. Topical beta-blockers in dermatologic therapy. Dermatol Ther. 2021;34:15016.
79. Greinwald JH Jr. Burke DK, Bonthius DJ, Bauman NM, Smith RJ. An update on the treatment of hemangiomas in children with interferon alfa-2a. Arch Otolaryngol Head Neck Surg. 1999;125:21-7.
80. Payarols JP, Masferrer JP, Bellvert CG. Treatment of life-threatening infantile hemangiomas with vincristine. N Engl J Med. 1995;333:69.
81. Xu WL, Niu AG, Li SL, Li ZD. Pingyangmycin emulsion inducing apoptosis in infantile proliferating capillary hemangiomas. Zhonghua Zheng Xing Wai Ke Za Zhi. 2006;22:362-4.
82. Qiu Y, Ma G, Yang J, Hu X, Chen H, Jin Y, et al. Imiquimod 5% cream versus timolol 0.5% ophthalmic solution for treating superficial proliferating infantile hemangiomas: a retrospective study. Clin Exp Dermatol. 2013;38:845-50.
83. Martinez MI, Sanchez-Carpintero I, North PE, Mihm MC Jr. Infantile hemangioma: clinical resolution with 5% imiquimod cream. Arch Dermatol. 2002;138:881-4.
84. Barry RB, Hughes BR, Cook LJ. Involution of infantile haemangiomas after imiquimod 5% cream. Clin Exp Dermatol. 2008;33:446-9.
85. Ho NT, Lansang P, Pope E. Topical imiquimod in the treatment of infantile hemangiomas: a retrospective study. J Am Acad Dermatol. 2007;56:63-8.
86. Li VW, Li WW, Talcott KE, Zhai AW. Imiquimod as an antiangiogenic agent. J Drugs Dermatol. 2005;4:708-17.
87. Majewski S, Marczak M, Mlynarczyk B, Benninghoff B, Jablonska S. Imiquimod is a strong inhibitor of tumor cell-induced angiogenesis. Int J Dermatol. 2005;44:14-9.
88. Chinnadurai S, Sathe NA, Surawicz T. Laser treatment of infantile hemangioma: a systematic review. Lasers Surg Med. 2016;48:221-33.
89. Batta K, Goodyear HM, Moss C, Williams HC, Hiller L, Waters R. Randomised controlled study of early pulsed dye laser treatment of uncomplicated childhood haemangiomas: results of a 1-year analysis. Lancet. 2002;360:521-7.
90. Witman PM, Wagner AM, Scherer K, Waner M, Frieden IJ. Complications following pulsed dye laser treatment of superficial hemangiomas. Lasers Surg Med. 2006;38:116-23.
91. Blankenship CM. Alster TS. Fractional photo thermolysis of residual hemangioma. Dermatol Surg. 2008;34:1112-4.
92. Aldave AJ, Shields CL, Shields JA. Surgical excision of selected amblyogenic periorbital capillary hemangiomas. Ophthalmic Surg Lasers. 1999;30:754-7.
93. Kennedy RE. Arterial embolization of orbital hemangiomas. Trans Am Ophthalmol Soc. 1978;76:266-77.

17 CHAPTER

Imaging and Artificial Intelligence in Strabismus

Abinaya Valliappan, Sumita Agarkar

ABSTRACT

Strabismus, characterized by misalignment of the eyes, presents a complex array of clinical manifestations, often necessitating precise diagnostic evaluation for optimal management. Advanced imaging modalities have emerged as indispensable tools in this regard, providing detailed anatomical insights and aiding in surgical planning. Magnetic resonance imaging (MRI), with its superior soft-tissue resolution, offers detailed anatomical visualization, particularly useful in evaluating orbital and neurological abnormalities. Computed tomography (CT) complements MRI, providing rapid assessment in trauma cases and delineating bony structures with precision. Anterior segment optical coherence tomography (AS-OCT) has emerged as a valuable tool for assessing extraocular muscle morphology and insertion sites, aiding in surgical planning. Moreover, the chapter also discusses the role of artificial intelligence (AI) in strabismus.

Keywords: Strabismus, imaging modalities, magnetic resonance imaging, computed tomography, optical coherence tomography, ultrasound biomicroscopy, ultrasonography, artificial intelligence

INTRODUCTION

Strabismus, commonly known as *squint* or *crossed eyes*, encompasses a spectrum of ocular misalignment disorders affecting individuals worldwide. While clinical examination remains paramount in diagnosing strabismus, advanced imaging techniques have revolutionized our ability to understand its underlying pathophysiology and guide treatment strategies. This chapter compiles the role of these imaging modalities in the evaluation of strabismus, highlighting their applications and future directions.

Imaging modalities in strabismus include:

- Magnetic resonance imaging (MRI)
- Computed tomography (CT)
- Anterior segment optical coherence tomography (AS-OCT)
- Ultrasound biomicroscopy
- Ultrasonography

MAGNETIC RESONANCE IMAGING

Magnetic resonance imaging is one of the most common imaging modalities advised in varied presentations of strabismus due to its high soft-tissue resolution.[1] MRI is useful in diagnosis, surgical planning, and ruling out other nonocular/orbital abnormalities in a wide range of strabismus patients **(Table 17.1)**.

Indications of imaging[16] include:

- Sudden-onset strabismus
- Sudden-onset diplopia with strabismus
- Signs of raised intracranial tension (headache, nausea, vomiting, and tinnitus)
- Acute limitation of extraocular movements
- Strabismus with variable ptosis
- Strabismus with proptosis
- Strabismus with visual field loss, pupil abnormalities, and disc edema/atrophy
- Congenital strabismus pointing toward cranial nerve abnormalities
- Coexisting infective, vasculopathic, and neurological disorders
- Syndromic presentations with strabismus
- History of antenatal and/or perinatal hypoxic insults
- Known/suspected systemic pathologies such as thyroid disorder/autoimmune conditions
- Developmental delay or regression of milestones

MRI is helpful to get an overview of:

- Neurological abnormalities
- Orbital abnormalities—structural and mass lesions
- Ocular pathologies—muscle morphology or globe-related
- Vascular causes
- Cranial neuropathies and paralytic strabismus
- Post-traumatic—extraocular muscle (EOM) tear, globe architecture assessment, etc.

Magnetic Resonance Imaging Techniques and Inference

- On the T1 pulse sequence, the globe, connective tissue, and the EOMs appear dark, and orbital fat appears bright. T2 fast spin-echo sequences are thus preferred for more rapid image acquisition and soft-tissue resolution within the orbit without the need of intravenous contrast.[17]
- High-resolution surface coil MRI with 2-mm-thick quasi-coronal slices that bisect the long axis of the globe provide useful information on the EOM paths and their innervation.[17]
- Axial images for the horizontal recti and sagittal images for vertical recti are useful.

TABLE 17.1: MRI findings in various conditions associated with strabismus.

Category	*Pathology*	*Findings*
Orbital disorders	Strabismus fixus	Adherence between the globe and the extraocular muscles and Tenon's capsule in the intraconal compartment, with thin, cord-like EOMs[2]
	Myopic strabismus fixus/ heavy eye syndrome	Inferior and medial displacement of the LR and SR, respectively, with severe superotemporal prolapse of the myopic globe **(Fig. 1)**[3]
	Sagging eye syndrome	Age-related degeneration of the LR–SR band and surrounding connective tissues[4]
	Dysthyroid orbitopathy	Disease activity assessment: • MR parameters—T2 signal intensity ratio, T1 signal intensity ratio following gadolinium administration, and apparent diffusion coefficient—correlate positively with the clinical activity score • In T1-weighted images, isointense EOM in inactive TED, with contrast enhancement • In T2-weighted images, hyperintense EOM occurs during active TED and hypointense during inactive TED **(Fig. 2)**[5]
	Congenital fibrosis of EOM and related myopathies	• Atrophy of any EOM • Third nerve aplasia/hypoplasia may be associated[6] • Associated neurological abnormalities in a few cases
	Brown syndrome	Enhancement of the SO tendon–trochlea complex in acquired cases[7]
	Orbital cellulitis	*T2 FLAIR:* High signal characteristics and surrounding soft-tissue swelling:[8] • Diffuse, edematous infiltration of the orbital connective tissue • Ill-defined margins of the extraocular muscles and exophthalmos
	Pulley-related disorders	• On MRI, the EOM with its tendon forms a global layer inserting on the eyeball and an orbital layer, which gets inserted on a connective tissue ring, forming the EOM pulley[9] • The pulley acts as the functional origin of EOM • Coronal plane provides normal locations of EOM pulleys. Malpositioning of pulleys can be appreciated on MRI • Malpositioning of one or more rectus EOM pulleys causes strabismus

Contd...

Contd...

Category	*Pathology*	*Findings*
	Tumors	Mass lesion corresponding to the location and extent of the lesion:[10] • *Hyperintense T1 lesions:* Lipomas, dermoids, melanomas, and mucoceles • *Hypointense T2 lesions:* Lymphomas, round cell tumors, meningiomas, granulomatous diseases such as tuberculosis, Tolosa–Hunt syndrome, sarcoidosis, and calcification in meningiomas
	Congenital aplasia of EOM/ bony abnormalities	• Cord-like EOM missing ocular attachment • EOM volume reduction • Partial absence of a global layer of EOMs suggests embryological insult • Associated craniosynostosis[11]
	Post-traumatic/iatrogenic muscle tear/slipped muscle/ lost muscle/flap tear	• MRI orbit with fat suppression provides a better view of muscles[12] • *Coronal cuts:* To study the relationship between the EOM and the orbital fracture site • *Sagittal and axial cuts:* To locate the EOM position **(Fig. 3)**
Neurological	Cranial nerve palsies	Hypoplasia of cranial nerves is associated with hypoplasia of the supplied EOM and hypertrophy of its antagonist[13]
	Duane retraction syndrome	CN VI aplasia/hypoplasia[14]
	Dysinnervation/ misinnervation syndromes	• *Congenital CN III palsy*: Variable presentation with aplasia/hypoplasia/normal CN III[15] • *Congenital CN IV palsy*: No definite abnormality is seen in 27% of cases, although aplasia with a variable degree of superior oblique hypoplasia is seen in 73% of cases • *Möbius syndrome*: Mostly aplasia in CN VI and VII • *Congenital fibrosis of EOMs*: CN III hypoplasia and the corresponding extraocular muscle hypoplasia
	Intracranial tumors/vascular pathology/encephalomalacia	• MRI is accurate in delineating the anatomic location and vascular component in the space-occupying lesions **(Fig. 4)** • *Encephalomalacia:* Shows loss of brain tissue and is typically isointense to cerebrospinal fluid on all sequences • It is often associated with adjacent gliosis, which is FLAIR hyperintense
	Periventricular leukomalacia	Ischemic lesions in the occipital periventricular region of the visual cortex[14]

(CN: cranial nerve; EOM: extraocular muscle; FLAIR: fluid-attenuated inversion recovery; LR: lateral rectus; MRI: magnetic resonance imaging; SO: superior oblique; SR: superior rectus; TED: thyroid eye disease)

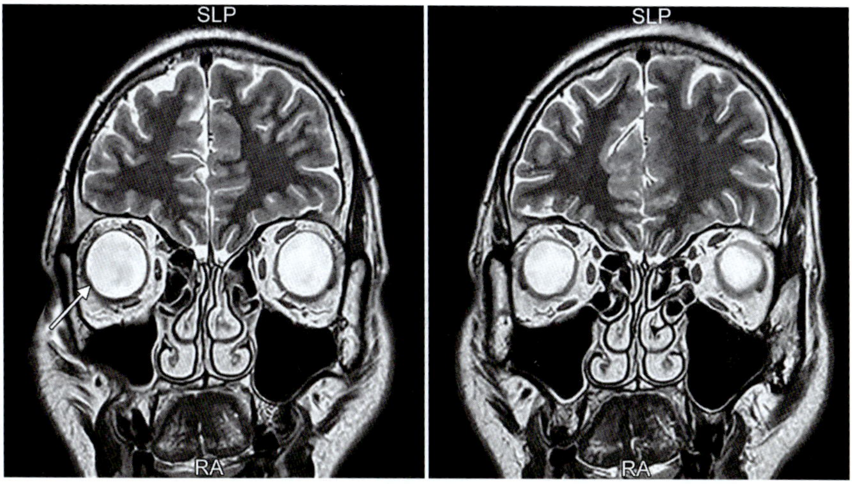

Fig. 17.1: MRI scan of a case of heavy eye syndrome depicting nasalization of the superior and inferior recti with mild inferior displacement of the lateral rectus.

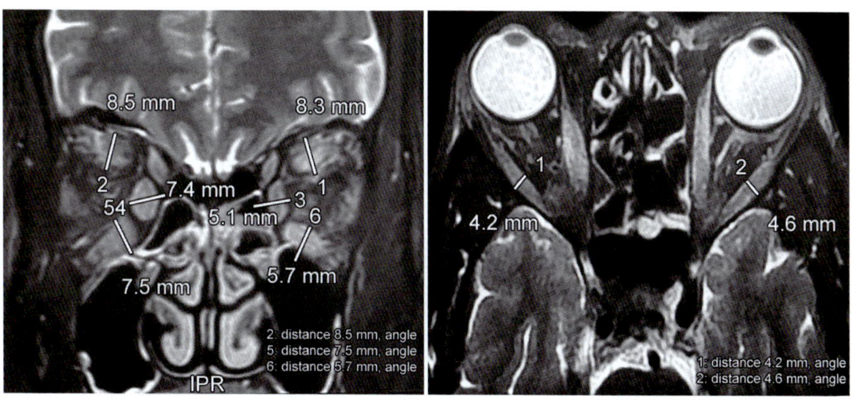

Fig. 17.2: MRI scan of a case of thyroid eye disease—coronal and axial cuts showing selectively enlarged EOMs sparing the muscle tendons with measurements of the width of the muscle. (EOMs: extraocular muscles)

- An 8–10 mm field of view centered on each orbit is acquired to provide orbital and optic nerve details.
- Steady-state coherent fast gradient-echo sequences [three-dimensional (3D)-balanced turbo fluid echo] and fast spin-echo sequences (T2 3D volume isotropic turbo spin-echo acquisition) are commonly used for cranial nerve imaging, as they are well contrasted with background cerebrospinal fluid signal intensity.[18]
- Fast imaging employing steady-state acquisition (FIESTA) and constructive interference steady state (CISS) are also employed in visualization of cranial nerves, especially in the skull base region.[14,16,18]

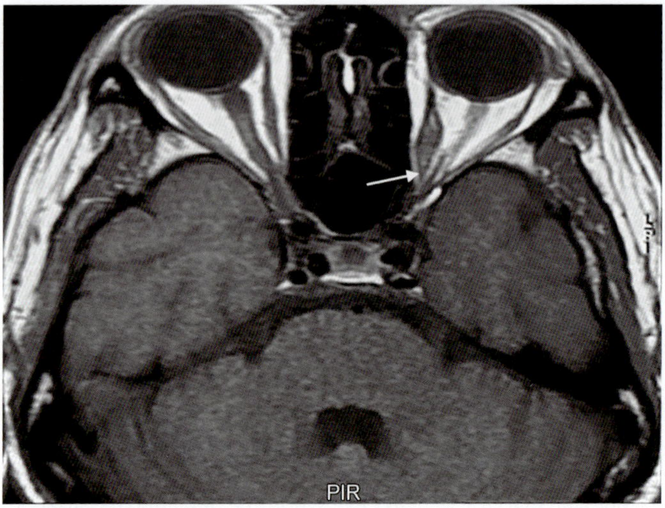

Fig. 17.3: Midorbit level axial MRI cuts showing posteriorly displaced left medial rectus muscle behind the equator suggestive of a lost muscle.

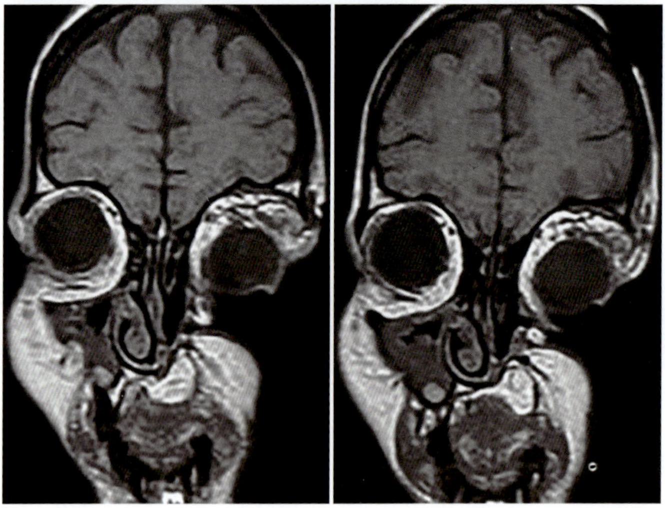

Fig. 17.4: Postradiation and maxillectomy MRI changes with inferior globe dystopia and thinning of surrounding EOMs of the left eye. (EOMs: extraocular muscles)

- Dynamic MRI for assessment of dynamic changes in EOM contractility by changing fixation targets while acquisition of images and digital analysis are useful. Several techniques of dynamic MRI are available, for example, dynamic-multipositional MRI (dmMRI).[19-21] The coronal and axial images are used for assessing horizontal recti movements with additional data on the longitudinal cross-sectional area, which is increased in a contracted muscle.

- In cases of strabismus with proptosis, MRI fat-suppressed postcontrast sequences will be beneficial to characterize any intraorbital lesion distinctively.[10]
- Strabismus with neuro-ophthalmological or neurological disorders requires extensive neuroimaging to identify potential causes, which include:
  - T2 fluid-attenuated inversion recovery (FLAIR) sequence is useful in demyelinating diseases such as multiple sclerosis, where water in edematous and pathologic tissue appears bright.[18]
  - T1 postcontrast (gadolinium) studies with fat suppression sequence of the orbits for better intraorbital visualization, such as in cases of optic nerve sheath meningioma and optic neuritis[22]
  - Diffusion-weighted imaging (DWI) and apparent diffusion coefficient (ADC) in acute ischemic strokes (since changes can be made out even before structural CT and conventional MRI show abnormalities)[23,24]
  - MRI with fat suppression with MRA (angiography)/MRV (venography) is useful in cases of aneurysms/idiopathic intracranial hypertension/venous sinus stenosis or thrombosis.[10]

Advantages

- Nil radiation exposure
- Higher soft-tissue definition

Disadvantages

- *Time-consuming:* Difficult to maintain a steady gaze for scan acquisition
- *Artifacts:* Poor cooperation, especially in children

Contraindications

- Ocular, orbital, or intracranial metallic foreign body
- Intracranial magnetic aneurysm clips
- Cochlear implants
- Metallic orbital floor implants
- Cardiac pacemaker
- Claustrophobic patient[25]

Imaging-based Newer Concepts in Strabismus

- The concept of compartmental innervation of EOM, extraocular muscle pulley position and structural alterations in pattern strabismus are widely described based on MRI studies.[10,26,27]
- Dynamic MRI studies were a useful aid in the diagnosis of a unique entity—synergistic innervational downshoot, which is a type of dysinnervation syndrome.[28]

- The compartmentalization of EOM into orbital and global layer fibers is described with imaging techniques.[29]
- Brain cluster activation evaluation using functional MRI (fMRI) and diffusion tensor imaging (DTI) in patients with strabismic amblyopia revealed reduced stimulation of the occipital calcarine area when seeing with the amblyopic eye, which shows improvement of hemodynamics with vision therapy and patching.[30]

COMPUTED TOMOGRAPHY

Computed tomography of orbits (with or without contrast) is useful in the following conditions associated with strabismus:

- *Thyroid eye disease*: Fusiform enlargement of the muscle bellies with relative tendon sparing—"Coca-cola sign." Barrett's index for quantitative measurement of EOM thickness and apical crowding is derived from CT images. (The vertical index is the division of the sum of vertical muscle diameters by the height of the orbit. The horizontal index is calculated similarly. The greater of the two ratios is Barret's index. An index >67% is predictive of optic neuropathy.)
- CT exophthalmometry for proptosis.[5]
- *Orbital trauma:* To assess fractures of the orbital wall, with or without entrapment of the surrounding muscle and soft tissues **(Figs. 17.5A and B)**[31]
- Craniosynostosis and associated pattern strabismus[32]
- Bony structural abnormalities—congenital and acquired (e.g., orbitofrontal dysplasia, sphenoid wing dysplasia)[16,33]
- Orbital mass lesion causing restrictive strabismus
- *Brown syndrome:* CT scan shows thickening at the trochlear superior oblique tendon region and localized enhancement suggestive of inflammatory changes.[34]

Advantages

- Preferred for trauma cases where the possibility of a foreign body poses a hindrance for an MRI scan
- Faster than MRI, sedation requirement is lesser

Disadvantage

Radiation risk.[25]

ANTERIOR SEGMENT OPTICAL COHERENCE TOMOGRAPHY

A recent imaging tool widely applied for strabismus is the AS-OCT of the extraocular muscles.[35,36] It works on a principle of low coherence interferometry that provides high-resolution multiple cross-sectional images of desired internal structures of biological tissues. The swept source AS-OCT (SS-AS-OCT) has been widely used for this purpose.[37]

Utility in Strabismus

Currently, AS-OCT is used in strabismological practice to look at the insertion of the extraocular muscle from the angle of the eye (measured via an inbuilt caliper). It can additionally comment upon overlying conjunctival scarring, ocular coat status, and muscle morphology to a certain extent.[38] Hence, AS-OCT becomes useful in cases of:

- Preoperative planning of re-surgery cases to note where the recessed muscle is located, especially in cases where primary surgery details are not available[33,39,40]
- In cases of trauma and complex strabismus to locate an EOM at its expected anatomical site
- Suspected cases of slipped/lost muscle to aid in surgical exploration
- Muscle hypertrophy/hypoplasia[37]

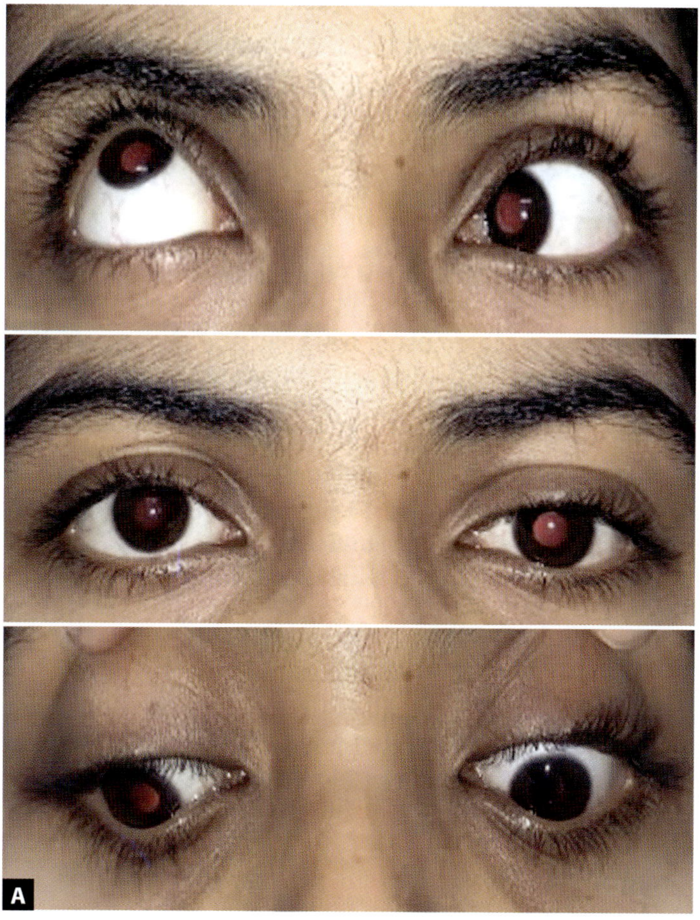

Fig. 17.5A

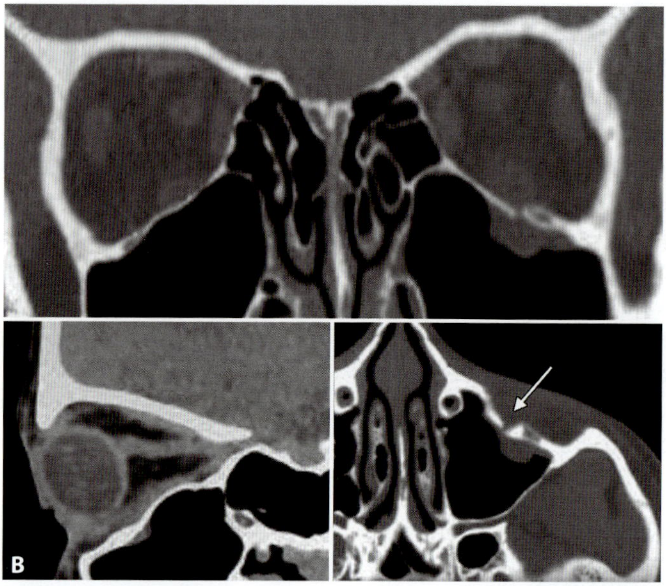

Fig. 17.5B

Figs. 17.5A and B: External photographs showing left hypotropia with limitation of elevation in upgaze with corresponding CT images revealing left orbital floor fracture with inferior rectus muscle entrapment.

Technique

After feeding patient information into the machine, preoperative cataract mode is chosen for the EOM visualization. The patient is positioned comfortably on the machine using the head and chin rest, followed by capturing of the scan at the desired area. The patient is asked to abduct his eyes for scanning the medial rectus muscle and adduct for lateral rectus muscle identification. The eye is positioned opposite to the direction of the muscle imaged. Both horizontal and vertical raster scans are performed to note down the length- and width-wise calibrations of the EOM. The literature says that the calibrations are not significantly affected at various angles of rotation of the eyes, inferring the reliability of measurements to a certain extent even with poor cooperation.[37,41]

Identification and Calibration

- The hyporeflective cleft at a midlevel depth from the anterior surface is detected in the scan when the eye is rotated, which indicates the muscle–sclera junction, vis-à-vis, the insertion site of the EOM.[39]
- An in-built caliper is used to measure the distance from this cleft to the angle.
- The insertion of the EOM from the limbus is obtained by adding 1 mm to the cleft-angle distance, as the limbus is anteriorly placed with respect to the angle.

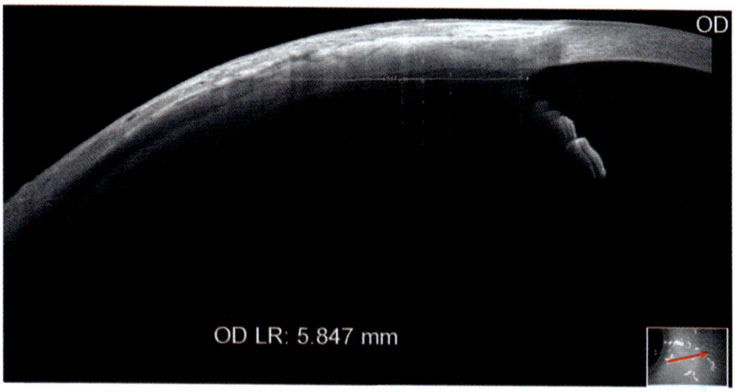

Fig. 17.6: AS-OCT image of the lateral rectus muscle where the distance between the angle and the hyporeflective cleft (muscle–sclera junction) is measured using an in-built caliper. (AS-OCT: anterior segment optical coherence tomography; OD: outer diameter; LR: lateral rectus)

- An average of three measurements can be used to increase the reliability of the calibration **(Figs. 17.6)**.

The identification gets difficult in post-traumatic and previously operated patients. In cases of previous EOM recession, the stump site might appear as an outward bump with surrounding ocular coat thinning, which can be misinterpreted as a mass lesion or insertion site, and a previously resected muscle will have an overall bulky appearance. The AS-OCT of the contralateral unaffected eye is helpful for comparison in such cases.[38]

Advantages

- Fast, reliable, and noncontact method
- No anesthesia required
- Outpatient procedure
- Screening tools are especially useful in re-surgeries and prior EOM exploration procedures. These give a better idea regarding localization of the EOM preoperatively.
- Instant results
- Easy measuring tool
- Supplements the MRI/CT scan by providing more details on the global part of the EOM
- No radiation exposure, safe

Disadvantages

- Easy accessibility
- Definite learning curve
- Difficult in small children with poor cooperation, particularly to position the eye at the desired angle for scan acquisition

- Smaller field of visualization
- Intersubject variability
- Orbital part of the EOM cannot be commented upon

ULTRASOUND BIOMICROSCOPY

Ultrasound biomicroscopy (UBM) is indicated in strabismus practice for measuring muscle insertion sites, especially in previously operated cases. There is a limited role of UBM in recent strabismus practice after the advent of AS-OCT applications for similar indications.

Technique

Under topical anesthesia, a 50-MHz UBM probe is placed over the eye with/without the cup, with the patient reclined. The transducer is held tangentially over the muscle, and the muscle is scanned with the moving probe over the limbus perpendicularly. The direction of the eye should be opposite to that of the desired muscle. The muscle belly appears as a hyporeflective area away from the limbus, and the distance can be measured using built-in calipers.

Ultrasound biomicroscopy findings such as ciliary body edema, choroidal effusion, and secondary shallowing of the anterior chamber in cases of anterior segment ischemia poststrabismus surgery can be used alongside anterior segment fluorescein angiography for diagnostic and prognostic purposes.[42]

The accuracy of prediction of EOM insertion of UBM and AS-OCT ranges from 40.2 to 80% and 60 to 69.5%, respectively.[36,39,41]

ULTRASONOGRAPHY

Ultrasonography is not a preferred modality in delineating EOM in current practice. However, an ocular/orbital ultrasound B scan is helpful in cases of identifying local ocular lesions such as lymphangioma, cysticercosis, and choroidal tumors, which can cause mechanical restriction of EOM[43] and noting globe architecture and related pathologies in traumatic cases.

ROLE OF ARTIFICIAL INTELLIGENCE IN STRABISMUS

As the field of artificial intelligence (AI) is showing promising entry into health care, it is necessary to incorporate datasets, integrate with, and improvise AI in the field of strabismus for aiding early screening and detection and taking one step ahead toward the avoidance of severe impairment. Deep learning models for the detection of strabismus and amblyopia with the help of images, visual acuity, and sensory parameters are upcoming. A classification of version movements based on ocular images through an AI mobile application is under research.

Other AI-based applications for detecting, diagnosing, and framing a basic surgical plan for comitant horizontal strabismus cases are also available in the literature. The future of AI in strabismus looks promising and will help in early detection and referral, especially in regions deprived of targeted pediatric ophthalmology and strabismus practitioners.[44,45]

CONCLUSION

Advanced imaging techniques play a pivotal role in the comprehensive evaluation of strabismus, offering detailed anatomical insights and aiding in treatment planning. From MRI and CT scans to AS-OCT, UBM, and ultrasonography, each modality contributes uniquely to the understanding of strabismus pathophysiology and guides clinical decision-making. Furthermore, the integration of AI promises to revolutionize strabismus management by facilitating early detection and optimizing treatment strategies. As technology continues to evolve, clinicians must harness these advancements to provide optimal care to patients with strabismus, ensuring improved outcomes and quality of life.

REFERENCES

1. Patel JR, Gunton KB. The role of imaging in strabismus. Curr Opin Ophthalmol. 2017;28(5):465-69.
2. Yamada M, Taniguchi S, Muroi T, Satofuka S, Nishina S. Rectus eye muscle paths after surgical correction of convergent strabismus fixus. Am J Ophthalmol. 2002;134(4):630-2.
3. Maiolo C, Fresina M, Campos EC. Role of magnetic resonance imaging in heavy eye syndrome. Eye. 2017;31(8):1163-7.
4. Tan RJD, Demer JL. Heavy eye syndrome versus sagging eye syndrome in high myopia. J AAPOS. 2015;19(6):500-6.
5. Shah SS, Patel BC. Thyroid Eye Disease. In: StatPearls [Internet]. Treasure Island (FL): StatPearls Publishing; 2024 [online]. Available from http://www.ncbi.nlm.nih.gov/books/NBK582134/ [Last accessed September, 2024].
6. Merino P, Gómez de Liaño P, Fukumitsu H, Franco G, Ruiz Y. Congenital fibrosis of the extraocular muscles: magnetic resonance imaging findings and surgical treatment. Strabismus. 2013;21(3):183-9.
7. Lang M, Faraji N, Coffey M, Badve C. MRI of acquired Brown syndrome: a report of two cases. Radiol Case Rep. 2017;13(1):92-5.
8. Jyani R, Ranade D, Joshi P. Spectrum of orbital cellulitis on magnetic resonance imaging. Cureus. 12(8):9663.
9. Demer JL. The orbital pulley system: a revolution in concepts of orbital anatomy. Ann N Y Acad Sci. 2002;956(1):17-32.
10. Kim JD, Hashemi N, Gelman R, Lee AG. Neuroimaging in ophthalmology. Saudi J Ophthalmol. 2012;26(4):401-7.
11. Whitman MC, Jurgens JA, Hunter DG, Engle EC. Congenital fibrosis of the extraocular muscles overview. April 27, 2004 [Updated 2021 Aug 12]. In: Adam MP, Ardinger HH, Pagon RA (Eds). GeneReviews® [Internet]. Seattle (WA): University of Washington, Seattle; 1993-2022.

12. Molinari AD. (2018). Strabismus following extraocular muscle trauma. [online]. Available from https://www.aao.org/education/disease-review/strabismus-following-extraocular-muscle-trauma. [Last accessed September, 2024].
13. Romano N, Federici M, Castaldi A. Imaging of cranial nerves: a pictorial overview. Insights Imaging. 2019;10(1):33.
14. Yoon L, Kim HY, Kwak MJ, Park KH, Bae MH, Lee Y, et al. Utility of magnetic resonance imaging (MRI) in children with strabismus. J Child Neurol. 2019;34(10):574-81.
15. Kim JH, Hwang JM. Imaging of cranial nerves III, IV, VI in congenital cranial dysinnervation disorders. Korean J Ophthalmol. 2017;31(3):183-93.
16. Kim E, Kim JH, Hwang JM, Choi BS, Jung C. MR Imaging of congenital or developmental neuropathic strabismus: common and uncommon findings. Am J Neuroradiol. 2012;33(11):2056-61.
17. Kau HC, Tsai CC, Ortube MC, Demer JL. High-resolution magnetic resonance imaging of the extraocular muscles and nerves demonstrates various etiologies of third nerve palsy. Am J Ophthalmol. 2007;143(2):280-7.
18. Tsuchiya K, Aoki C, Hachiya J. Evaluation of MR cisternography of the cerebellopontine angle using a balanced fast-field-echo sequence: preliminary findings. Eur Radiol. 2004;14(2):239-42.
19. Loba P, Broniarczyk-Loba A, Pajak M, Majos A, Stefanczyk L, Orczykowska M. Morphometric parameters of extraocular rectus muscles evaluated by dynamic-multipositional magnetic resonance. Eur J Ophthalmol. 2015;25(5):373-8.
20. Teodorescu L, Ionescu V. Dynamic nuclear magnetic resonance in strabismus. Oftalmologia. 2010;54(2):123-8.
21. Demer JL, Clark RA. Magnetic resonance imaging of differential compartmental function of horizontal rectus extraocular muscles during conjugate and converged ocular adduction. J Neurophysiol. 2014;112(4):845-55.
22. Guier CP, Stokkermans TJ. Optic Neuritis. In: StatPearls [Internet]. Treasure Island (FL): StatPearls Publishing; 2024 [cited 11 May, 2024]. Available from http://www.ncbi.nlm.nih.gov/books/NBK557853/ [Last accessed September, 2024].
23. Gregory DG, Pelak VS, Bennett JL. Diffusion-weighted magnetic resonance imaging and the evaluation of cortical blindness in preeclampsia. Surv Ophthalmol. 2003;48(6):647-50.
24. Romano A, Bozzao A, Bonamini M, Fasoli F, Ferrante M, Floris R, et al. Diffusion-weighted MR Imaging: clinical applications in neuroradiology. Radiol Med (Torino). 2003;106(5-6):521-48.
25. Nayak BK, Desai S, Maheshwari S. Interpretation of magnetic resonance imaging of orbit: simplified for ophthalmologists (Part I). J Clin Ophthalmol Res. 2013;1(1):29.
26. Sharma P, Gaur N, Phuljhele S, Saxena R. What's new for us in strabismus? Indian J Ophthalmol. 2017;65(3):184-90.
27. Oh SY, Clark RA, Velez F, Rosenbaum AL, Demer JL. Incomitant strabismus associated with instability of rectus pulleys. Invest Ophthalmol Vis Sci. 2002; 43(7):2169-78.
28. Sharma P, Chaurasia S, Rasal A, Angmo D. Synergistic innervational downshoot: a distinct vertical dysinnervation pattern and its unique management. Can J Ophthalmol. 2017;52(1):31-8.

29. Demer JL. Compartmentalization of extraocular muscle function. Eye. 2015;29(2):157-62.
30. Gupta S, Kumaran SS, Saxena R, Gudwani S, Menon V, Sharma P. BOLD fMRI and DTI in strabismic amblyopes following occlusion therapy. Int Ophthalmol. 2016;36(4):557-68.
31. Kubal WS. Imaging of orbital trauma. Radiogr Rev Publ Radiol Soc N Am Inc. 2008;28(6):1729-39.
32. Kim HJ, Roh HG, Lee IW. Craniosynostosis: updates in radiologic diagnosis. J Korean Neurosurg Soc. 2016;59(3):219-26.
33. Kaur S, Vyas S, Singh AK, Sukjiha J. Utility of Anterior Segment Optical Coherence Tomography in Muscle Aplasia. J Pediatr Ophthalmol Strabismus. 2022;59(2):e20–e22.
34. Hermann JS. Acquired Brown's syndrome of inflammatory origin: response to locally injected steroids. Arch Ophthalmol. 1978;96(7):1228-32.
35. Pihlblad MS, Reynolds JD. Anterior segment optical coherence tomography of previously operated extraocular muscles. Am Orthopt J. 2017;67(1):61-6.
36. Rossetto JD, Cavuoto KM, Allemann N, McKeown CA, Capó H. Accuracy of optical coherence tomography measurements of rectus muscle insertions in adult patients undergoing strabismus surgery. Am J Ophthalmol. 2017;176: 236-43.
37. Pujari A, Patil V, Chauhan N, Thangavel R, Phuljhele S, Saxena R. Defining the clinical role of swept-source anterior segment optical coherence tomography in eyes undergoing strabismus surgery. Clin Ophthalmol. 2022;16:1449-65.
38. Pujari A, Maddu SV, Batwani VK, Khokhar S, Jha P, Sharma N. Study 3: Anterior segment optical coherence tomography-guided surgical approach in slipped medial rectus muscle. Indian J Ophthalmol. 2023;71(8):3059-63.
39. Ngo CS, Smith D, Kraft SP. The accuracy of anterior segment optical coherence tomography (AS-OCT) in localizing extraocular rectus muscles insertions. J AAPOS. 2015;19(3):233-6.
40. Pujari A, Agarwal D, Sharma N. Clinical role of swept source optical coherence tomography in anterior segment diseases: a review. Semin Ophthalmol. 2021;1:36.
41. Kaur S, Sukhija J, Korla S, Sachdeva K, Chaurasia S, Raj S. Comparison of the swept-source anterior segment optical coherence tomography and wide-field ultrasound biomicroscopy for imaging previously operated horizontal extraocular muscles. J AAPOS. 2021;25(4):212.
42. Neudorfer M, Mezad-Koursh D, Cohen S, Barzelay A, Stolovtich C. Ultrasound biomicroscopy (UBM) findings in severe anterior ischemic syndrome secondary to transposition surgery. Invest Ophthalmol Vis Sci. 2020;61(7):1872.
43. Ayres B, Kahana A. Ultrasound of orbit tumors and tumorlike lesions. In: Ben Simon G, Greenberg G, Landau Prat D (Eds). Atlas of Orbital Imaging. Cham: Springer International Publishing; 2022. pp. 127-47. [online] Available from https://doi.org/10.1007/978-3-030-62426-2_113. [Last accessed September, 2024].
44. Mao K, Yang Y, Guo C, Zhu Y, Chen C, Chen J, et al. An artificial intelligence platform for the diagnosis and surgical planning of strabismus using corneal light-reflection photos. Ann Transl Med. 2021;9(5):374.
45. de Figueiredo LA, Dias JVP, Polati M, Carricondo PC, Debert I. Strabismus and artificial intelligence app: optimizing diagnostic and accuracy. Transl Vis Sci Technol. 2021;10(7):22.

18 CHAPTER

ChatGPT in Ophthalmology: Application and Future

Divyansh K Mishra, Mahesh P Shanmugam

ABSTRACT

ChatGPT, a large language model (LLM), has emerged as a potential tool in ophthalmology. This chapter explores its applications across clinical practice, education, and research. While ChatGPT demonstrates promise in tasks such as summarizing medical information, generating explanations, and assisting with administrative tasks, limitations remain. Accuracy, potential for bias, and ethical considerations regarding data privacy need to be addressed. The future of ChatGPT in ophthalmology hinges on ongoing development and responsible implementation, ensuring it complements, not replaces, the expertise of ophthalmologists.

Keywords: ChatGPT, large language model (LLM), ophthalmology, future of ChatGPT in ophthalmology

INTRODUCTION: THE EVOLVING LANDSCAPE OF OPHTHALMOLOGY

The field of ophthalmology is constantly evolving, with new technologies and diagnostic tools emerging at an ever-increasing pace. One recent development with significant potential impact is the rise of large language models (LLMs) such as ChatGPT **(Table 18.1)**. These artificial intelligence (AI)-powered chatbots can process vast amounts of information and generate human-like text, raising intriguing possibilities for their application in eye care.[1]

Traditionally, patients seeking second opinions bring in physical examination reports. Today, some arrive with AI-generated interpretations of their fundus images. However, access to these AI tools is often restricted to specific service providers. The future, however, may hold a different reality—a future where patients come armed with diagnoses generated by tools such as ChatGPT, readily available to the public at their fingertips.

This chapter explores the potential of ChatGPT in ophthalmology, examining its strengths and limitations. We will consider scenarios such as the one presented here: a patient who underwent vitreoretinal surgery for a specific condition and now expresses concern due to a conflicting diagnosis

TABLE 18.1: Various large language models (LLMs) available in 2024.[2]

LLM name	*Developer*	*Popular apps*	*Access*
GPT	Open AI	Microsoft products, Duolingo, Stripe, Zapier, Dropbox, and ChatGPT	API
Gemini	Google	Gemini chatbot and some Google Apps features	API
Gemma	Google	(Undisclosed)	Open
Llama 3	Meta	Meta apps features and Meta AI chatbot	Open
Vicuna	LMSYS Org	Chatbot Arena	Open
Claude 3	Anthropic	Slack, Notion, and Zoom	API
Stable Beluga	Stability AI	(Undisclosed)	Open
StableLM 2	Stability AI	(Undisclosed)	Open
Coral	Cohere	HyperWrite, Jasper, and Notion, LongShot	API
Falcon	Technology Innovation Institute	(Undisclosed)	Open
DBRX	Databricks and Mosaic	(Undisclosed)	Open
Mixtral 8x7B and 8x22B	Mistral AI	(Undisclosed)	Open
XGen-7B	Salesforce	(Undisclosed)	Open
Grok	xAI	Grok Chatbot	Chatbot

generated by ChatGPT. Through this example, we will delve into the critical role of ophthalmologists in interpreting information, providing accurate diagnoses, and effectively managing patient anxiety fueled by unvetted AI outputs.

WHAT IS ChatGPT?

ChatGPT is an LLM chatbot developed by Open AI (San Francisco, USA) that uses AI to generate text.[3] It can process information from text and even images and respond in a way that simulates human conversation. It can also create new content, such as poems or code, in a human-like style.

Here is how it works:

- *Generative pretrained transformer (GPT) architecture:* This is the core technology behind ChatGPT. It allows the model to analyze the entire context of a prompt or conversation to generate relevant text.
- *Training on massive datasets:* ChatGPT was trained on a huge amount of text data, including books, articles, and Internet content. This allows it to understand and respond to a wide range of prompts and questions.

- *Fine-tuning:* After the initial training, ChatGPT can be further adjusted for specific tasks through a process called *fine-tuning*. This allows it to perform specialized actions, such as writing different kinds of creative content.

ChatGPT's versatility has made it a popular tool in many fields, including business, entertainment, education, science, law, and healthcare.[4]

ChatGPT'S EVOLUTION

Since its initial release in 2018, ChatGPT has gone through several upgrades. The first version, GPT-1, was introduced in 2018. Subsequent versions, GPT-2 (2019) and GPT-3 (2020), increased in complexity with more training parameters (1.5 billion and 175 billion, respectively). The latest iterations, ChatGPT-3.5 (released in November 2022) and ChatGPT-4 (released in March 2023), have not had their specific technical details disclosed yet.[5]

ChatGPT IN OPHTHALMOLOGY—APPLICATION

Despite the lack of recent information about its internal architecture, ChatGPT's popularity in ophthalmology is undeniable. Its ease of use and accessibility have sparked significant interest within the field, highlighting the ongoing exploration and its few potential applications **(Table 18.2)**.

There is no doubt that ChatGPT is a significant advancement in AI and LLMs. However, questions remain about its suitability for making automated medical decisions.[14,15]

Ongoing improvements to the model's accuracy, reliability, and transparency are crucial. As these aspects are addressed, ChatGPT may reach a level of maturity that inspires trust from various stakeholders in the healthcare field. This could include patients, medical professionals, healthcare systems, researchers, educators, regulatory bodies, and government officials.

Widespread adoption of a trustworthy ChatGPT could usher in a new era for medicine, marking a significant transformation in how we approach healthcare.

Limitations[16]

- *Outdated knowledge:* Trained on data up to November 2022, potentially missing recent medical advancements.
- *Unverified sources:* Relies on Internet sources with unclear credibility, which could lead to inaccurate diagnoses.
- *Data privacy and security:* Uploading patient information, such as facial photographs, raises security concerns.
- *Hallucinations:* Can generate seemingly correct but factually wrong information, risking misdiagnosis.
- *Limited reasoning:* Struggles with complex, multistep questions that are crucial for accurate diagnosis.

TABLE 18.2: Various applications of ChatGPT and its associated pros and cons.

Role of ChatGPT in ophthalmology				
Field	***Application***	***Pros***	***Cons***	***References***
General ophthalmology	Patient triage assistance	Improved efficiency	Inaccurate results	Dossantos et al. (2023)[6]
	Generating patient education materials	Offers educational resources	May contain generic text	Singh et al. (2023)[7]
Retina	Assisting with diagnosis of retinal vascular diseases (English prompts)	Good diagnostic performance (80.05% F1-score)	Lower accuracy than ophthalmologists (89.35 vs. 80.05%)	Liu et al. (2023)[8]
	Providing information on surgical treatment of retinal diseases	High appropriateness in responses (84.6–92.0% for different conditions)	Not a reliable source of information (inappropriate responses 5.1–8.3%)	Momenaei et al. (2023)[9]
Glaucoma	Assisting in glaucoma based on textual descriptions	Achieved an accuracy of 72.7%	Relies on textual descriptions and may miss aspects of a real case	Delsoz et al. (2023)[10] (Investigating use for glaucoma diagnosis)
Cornea	Diagnosing corneal diseases based on textual descriptions	Achieved an accuracy of 85% (ChatGPT-4.0)	Relies on textual descriptions and may miss aspects of a real case	Delsoz et al. (2023)[11] (Investigating use for corneal disease diagnosis)
Neuro-ophthalmology	Assisting in diagnosing neuro-ophthalmic diseases based on textual descriptions	Achieved an accuracy of 82% (ChatGPT-4.0)	Lower inter-rater agreement compared to human experts	Madadi et al. (2023)[12]
Pediatric Ophthalmology and strabismus	Source of information on the topic	Moderate accuracy rate (59.1%)	Information may not be accurate; it requires careful evaluation by a human expert	Verejan (2023)[13] (evaluating knowledge in pediatric ophthalmology)

- *Inability to interpret images:* Neuro-ophthalmology heavily relies on imaging, which ChatGPT cannot analyze (ChatGPT 4 can do—limited access).

ChatGPT IN OPHTHALMOLOGY—FUTURE

Healthcare Professionals and Systems[7,17,18]

- *Improved clinical care:* Virtual assistants can analyze vast amounts of information to support doctors in making diagnoses and planning treatment.
- *Administrative efficiency:* They can handle administrative tasks such as scheduling appointments and managing records, freeing up medical professionals' time for patient care.

Research[19-21]

Research facilitation: Virtual assistants can help researchers with tasks such as generating ideas, finding relevant literature, writing papers, and streamlining data analysis and recruitment.

Training and Education[22-24]

Enhanced learning: Virtual assistants can provide additional explanations for complex medical concepts and translate materials for multilingual learners (patients and allied healthcare professionals). They may also personalize learning experiences.

Patients[25-28]

- *Self-care support:* Virtual assistants can guide patients through self-diagnosis tools and provide educational materials on various health topics. However, anxiety and depression can arise from self-diagnosis, impacting the patient's overall well-being and potentially hindering the effectiveness of the care they receive (studies show a negative outlook can worsen health outcomes).
- *Mental health support:* They can act as virtual therapists, offering resources and tools for managing mental health.
- *Accessibility:* Multilingual support and conversion options (text-to-audio and text-to-image/video) can improve accessibility for patients with language barriers or disabilities.

CONCLUSION

ChatGPT and LLMs are capable of processing vast amounts of text data, presenting intriguing possibilities for ophthalmology. As these LLMs continuously learn and refine themselves, their ability to analyze medical data and assist in diagnoses is expected to improve significantly. It can be harnessed for large-scale population screening for eye diseases such as diabetic retinopathy and retinopathy of prematurity. By taking over routine screening tasks, ChatGPT can free up ophthalmologists' valuable time. Despite its potential, critical challenges remain. ChatGPT's accuracy, particularly in complex medical domains, needs further refinement. Ethical considerations regarding data privacy and potential biases within the model also require careful attention.

Ultimately, ChatGPT's role in ophthalmology lies in supplementing, not replacing, the expertise of healthcare professionals. Responsible implementation, coupled with ongoing development, holds the key to unlock its true potential in improving patient care.

REFERENCES

1. Stokel-Walker C, Van Noorden R. What ChatGPT and generative AI mean for science. Nature. 2023;614(7947):214-6.
2. OpenAI. GPT-4 Technical Report. arXiv. 2023:2303.08774.
3. Seetharaman R. Revolutionizing medical education: can ChatGPT boost subjective learning and expression? J Med Syst. 2023;47:(1)61
4. Yosifova A. (2023). The evolution of chat GPT: History and future. 365data science. [online] Available from https://365datascience.com/trending/the-evolution-of-chatgpt-history-and-future/ [Last accessed September, 2024]
5. Guinness H. The best large language model (LLMs) in 2024. [online] Updated 2 May, 24]. Available from https://zapier.com/blog/best-llm/. [Last accessed September, 2024
6. Dossantos J, An J, Javan R. Eyes on AI: ChatGPT's transformative potential impact on ophthalmology. Cureus. 2023;15(6):40765.
7. Singh S, Djalilian A, Ali MJ. ChatGPT and ophthalmology: exploring its potential with discharge summaries and operative notes. Semin Ophthalmol. 2023;38(5):503-7.
8. Liu X, Wu J, Shao A, Shen W, Ye P, Wang Y, et al. Uncovering language disparity of ChatGPT on retinal vascular disease classification: cross-sectional study. J Med Internet Res. 2024;26:51926.
9. Momenaei B, Wakabayashi T, Shahlaee A, Dirani A, Pandit S, Wang K, et al. Appropriateness and readability of ChatGPT-4-generated responses for surgical treatment of retinal diseases. Ophthalmol Retina. 2023;7(10):862-8.
10. Delsoz M, Raja H, Madadi Y, Tang AA, Wirostko BM, Kahook MY, et al. The use of ChatGPT to assist in diagnosing glaucoma based on clinical case reports. Ophthalmol Ther. 2023;12(6):3121-32.
11. Delsoz M, Madadi Y, Munir WM, Tamm B, Mehravaran S, Soleimani M, et al. Performance of ChatGPT in diagnosis of corneal eye diseases. medRxiv [preprint]. 2023 doi: 10.1101/2023.08.25.23294635.
12. Madadi Y, Delsoz M, Lao PA, Fong JW, Hollingsworth TJ, Kahook MY, et al. ChatGPT assisting diagnosis of neuro-ophthalmology diseases based on case reports. medRxiv. Preprint. 2023 doi: 10.1101/2023.09.13.23295508.

13. Verejan V. Contrast sensitivity and aspects of binocular vision alteration in school-aged children after head injury. Rom J Ophthalmol. 2023;67(4):394-7.
14. Gilson A, Safranek CW, Huang T, Socrates V, Chi L, Taylor RA, et al. How does ChatGPT Perform on the United States medical licensing examination? The implications of large language models for medical education and knowledge assessment. JMIR Med Educ. 2023;9:e45312.
15. Thirunavukarasu AJ, Hassan R, Mahmood S, Sanghera R, Barzangi K, El Mukashfi M, et al. Trialling a large language model (ChatGPT) in general practice with the applied knowledge test: observational study demonstrating opportunities and limitations in primary care. JMIR Med Educ. 2023;9:e46599.
16. Azamfirei R, Kudchadkar SR, Fackler J. Large language models and the perils of their hallucinations. Crit Care. 2023;27(1):120.
17. Singh S, Djalilian A, Ali MJ. ChatGPT and ophthalmology: exploring its potential with discharge summaries and operative notes. Semin Ophthalmol. 2023; 38(5):503-07.
18. Hirosawa T, Harada Y, Yokose M, Sakamoto T, Kawamura R, Shimizu T. Diagnostic accuracy of differential-diagnosis lists generated by generative pretrained transformer 3 chatbot for clinical vignettes with common chief complaints: a pilot study. Int J Environ Res Public Health. 2023;20:3378.
19. Lim MC, Boland MV, McCannel CA, Saini A, Chiang MF, Epley KD, et al. Adoption of electronic health records and perceptions of financial and clinical outcomes among ophthalmologists in the United States. JAMA Ophthalmol. 2018;136(2):164-70.
20. Hutson M. Could AI help you to write your next paper? Nature. 2022;611:192–3.
21. Else H. Abstracts written by ChatGPT fool scientists. Nature. 2023;613:423.
22. Tools such as ChatGPT threaten transparent science; here are our ground rules for their use. Nature. 2023;613:612.
23. Kung TH, Cheatham M, Medenilla A, Sillos C, De Leon L, Elepaño C, et al. Performance of ChatGPT on USMLE: potential for AI-assisted medical education using large language models. PLOS Digit Health. 2023;2:e0000198.
24. Wei J, Wang X, Schuurmans D, Bosma M, Ichter B, Xia F, et al. Chain-of-Thought Prompting Elicits Reasoning in Large Language Models. NeurIPS 2022 Conference. 2022
25. Yang X, Chen A, PourNejatian N, Shin HC, Smith KE, Parisien C, et al. GatorTron: A Large Clinical Language Model to Unlock Patient Information from Unstructured Electronic Health Records. arXiv. 2022:2203.03540.
26. Antaki F, Touma S, Milad D, El-Khoury J, Duval R. Evaluating the Performance of ChatGPT in ophthalmology: an analysis of its successes and shortcomings. Ophthalmol Sci. 2023;3(4):100324.
27. Will ChatGPT transform healthcare? Nat Med. 2023;29:505–6.
28. Sharma A, Lin IW, Miner AS, Atkins DC, Althoff T. Human–AI collaboration enables more empathic conversations in text-based peer-to-peer mental health support. Nat Mach Intell. 2023;5:46–57.

Index

Page numbers followed by *f* refer to figure, *fc* refer to flowchart, and *t* refer to table

D

E

F

G

H

I

N

R